Natural Products and Their Modifications as Agents Used in the Fight against Pathogens

Natural Products and Their Modifications as Agents Used in the Fight against Pathogens

Guest Editor

Anna Duda-Madej

MDPI

Basel • Beijing • Wuhan • Barcelona • Belgrade • Novi Sad • Cluj • Manchester

Guest Editor
Anna Duda-Madej
Department of Microbiology
Wroclaw Medical University
Wrocław
Poland

Editorial Office
MDPI AG
Grosspeteranlage 5
4052 Basel, Switzerland

This is a reprint of the Special Issue, published open access by the journal *Pharmaceuticals* (ISSN 1424-8247), freely accessible at: https://www.mdpi.com/journal/pharmaceuticals/special_issues/L2YS543358.

For citation purposes, cite each article independently as indicated on the article page online and as indicated below:

Lastname, A.A.; Lastname, B.B. Article Title. *Journal Name* **Year**, *Volume Number*, Page Range.

ISBN 978-3-7258-6083-8 (Hbk)
ISBN 978-3-7258-6084-5 (PDF)
https://doi.org/10.3390/books978-3-7258-6084-5

Contents

About the Editor

Anna Duda-Madej

Anna Duda-Madej, Ph.D., is a medical scientist at the Department of Microbiology, Faculty of Medicine, Wroclaw Medical University. Her scientific interests focus on the antimicrobial, anti-inflammatory, and anticancer properties of natural compounds and their chemically modified derivatives. She investigates the interactions between these compounds and the gastrointestinal environment, both under physiological and pathological conditions. Her current research involves in vitro intestinal models used to examine the influence of natural substances on the virulence factors and pathogenic potential of gut-associated bacteria. Additionally, her studies explore the potential of these compounds in overcoming bacterial multidrug resistance, with the aim of identifying novel therapeutic strategies against resistant pathogens.

pharmaceuticals

MDPI

Article

Bioactivities and Chemotaxonomy of Four *Heracleum* Species: A Comparative Study Across Plant Parts

Tugce Ince Kose [1], Gamze Benli Yardimci [2], Damla Kirci [3], Derya Cicek Polat [4], Betul Demirci [5], Mujde Eryilmaz [6,*] and Ceyda Sibel Kilic [4]

1 Department of Pharmaceutical Botany, Graduate School of Health Sciences, Ankara University, 06560 Ankara, Türkiye; tikose@ankara.edu.tr
2 Department of Pharmaceutical Microbiology, Faculty of Pharmacy, Afyonkarahisar Health Sciences University, 03200 Afyonkarahisar, Türkiye; gamze.benli@afsu.edu.tr
3 Department of Pharmacognosy, Faculty of Pharmacy, Izmir Katip Çelebi University, 35620 Izmir, Türkiye; damla.kirci@ikc.edu.tr
4 Department of Pharmaceutical Botany, Faculty of Pharmacy, Ankara University, 06560 Ankara, Türkiye; polatd@ankara.edu.tr (D.C.P.); erdurak@pharmacy.ankara.edu.tr (C.S.K.)
5 Department of Pharmacognosy, Faculty of Pharmacy, Anadolu University, 26210 Eskişehir, Türkiye; bdemirca@anadolu.edu.tr
6 Department of Pharmaceutical Microbiology, Faculty of Pharmacy, Acibadem Mehmet Ali Aydınlar University, 34638 Istanbul, Türkiye
* Correspondence: mujde.eryilmaz@acibadem.edu.tr

Abstract

Background/Objectives: This study investigates the phytochemical profile, essential oil composition, and bioactivities—including antioxidant, antimicrobial, antibio-film, and anti-quorum sensing (QS) activities—of four *Heracleum* L. species (*H. crenatifolium* Boiss, *H. paphlagonicum* Czeczott, *H. sphondylium* subsp. *montanum* Schleich. ex Gaudin, and *H. pastinacifolium* subsp. *incanum* (Boiss. & A.Huet) P.H.Davis). **Methods:** Total phenolic and flavonoid contents were quantified using the Folin–Ciocalteu and aluminum chloride colorimetric methods, respectively. Essential oils were extracted by hydrodistillation and analyzed via Gas Chromatography–Flame Ionization Detector (GC–FID) and Gas Chromatography–Mass Spectrometry (GC–MS), while Principal Component Analysis (PCA) and Hierarchical Cluster Analysis (HCA) evaluated chemical variability among the species. Antioxidant activities were assessed using DPPH and ABTS free radical scavenging assays. Antimicrobial activity was assessed using the broth microdilution method to determine Minimum Inhibitory Concentration (MIC) values, while antibiofilm activity was evaluated using an in vitro microplate-based biofilm model against *Pseudomonas aeruginosa* PAO1. Anti-QS activity was analyzed using a disc diffusion assay with *Chromobacterium violaceum* ATCC 12472 as the reporter strain. **Results:** It was observed that the amounts of total phenolic compounds and total flavonoids were higher in root extracts than in aerial parts extracts for the four species in this study (*H. sphondylium* subsp. *montanum* excluding phenolic content). In the analysis of essential oil, it was determined that the major component in the roots was mostly myristicin, and in the fruits it was mostly octyl acetate. Phenolic and flavonoid contents were positively correlated with antioxidant activity. Methanol and *n*-hexane extracts of *H. pastinacifolium* (aerial parts) and *n*-hexane extracts of *H. paphlagonicum* (root) exhibited notable antimicrobial activity, primarily against Gram-positive bacteria, but none of the extracts showed activity against *Klebsiella pneumoniae* ATCC 13383 or *P. aeruginosa* ATCC 27853. Among methanol extracts, *H. pastinacifolium* (aerial parts) exhibited the highest antibiofilm activity (73.2%), while *H. paphlagonicum* (aerial parts) showed the highest activity among *n*-hexane extracts (75.5%). All *n*-hexane extracts exhibited anti-QS activity, whereas the methanol extracts showed no activity.

Conclusions: These findings underscore the chemical diversity and bioactive potential of *Heracleum* species, contributing to the chemotaxonomic understanding of the genus and supporting their potential applications in medicine and industry. To our knowledge, this is the first study that reveals the antibiofilm and anti-QS properties of these *Heracleum* species.

Keywords: *Heracleum*; antibiofilm; antimicrobial; antioxidant; anti-quorum sensing; essential oils; phytochemical

1. Introduction

The *Apiaceae* (previously known as the *Umbelliferae*) family, known as the Parsley-Celery family, is one of the largest families in the plant kingdom, comprising 300 to 455 genera and approximately 3000 to 3700 species worldwide [1–3]. Members of this family are characterized by their distinctive pungent or aromatic odor, attributed to the presence of essential oils or oleoresins [4]. Among *Apiaceae*, the genus *Heracleum* L. is notable for its diversity and widespread distribution, with approximately 125 taxa primarily found in the Asian continent. In Türkiye, 23 *Heracleum* taxa grow naturally, nine of which are endemics, giving the genus an impressive 41% endemism rate in the country [5–8].

The *Heracleum* genus is known for its traditional and modern uses [9]. In Türkiye, species of *Heracleum* are commonly referred to by various names, including Tavşancıl Otu, Kuruöğrek, Telehaş, Suh, Devesil, Öküz Havucu, and Herkül Otu [10,11]. These plants, often called "hogweed" in Europe, are among the tallest herbaceous plants, sometimes reaching heights of 4 to 5 m, and have been described with adjectives such as "large", "tall", or "giant" [12].

Species of *Heracleum* have been extensively used in traditional Asian medicine for their therapeutic properties. They have been used for a variety of different purposes such as antipyretic, analgesic, diaphoretic, antiseptic, carminative, and digestive, and also in rheumatic transmission, diarrhea, dysentery, lumbago, stomachache, fracture, fracture and fall injuries, as flavoring agents and spices. The fruits of this genus are also used as antiseptic, carminative, digestive, and analgesic in Iranian folk medicine [13,14]. Phytochemical investigations of *Heracleum* species have identified diverse secondary metabolites, including furanocoumarins, anthraquinones, stilbenes, flavonoids, hydrocarbons, monoterpenes, sesquiterpenes, coumarins, and steroids [15].

The essential oils of *Heracleum* species are complex mixtures of bioactive compounds, with significant variations in chemical composition depending on the species and plant parts utilized. These oils are predominantly characterized by the presence of terpenoids, phenylpropanoids, and various oxygenated compounds. Among the major constituents identified are octyl acetate, octyl hexanoate, octyl octanoate, β-pinene, myristicin, limonene, and hexyl butanoate, which collectively contribute to the unique aromatic and biological properties of the oils [16]. This diversity in chemical composition not only reflects the chemotaxonomic value of the *Heracleum* genus but also highlights its potential as a natural resource for bioactive compounds.

Reactive oxygen species (ROS), such as superoxide, peroxides, and hydroxyl radicals are known to cause oxidative stress, leading to conditions such as arthritis, atherosclerosis, and neurodegenerative diseases, including Alzheimer's and Parkinson's. Antioxidant compounds, often derived from medicinal plants, play a critical role in neutralizing these oxidizing agents. Secondary metabolites such as phenolic compounds, alkaloids, and tannins are particularly important in this regard [17].

The growing threat of antibiotic resistance has prompted urgent efforts to discover alternative antibacterial compounds. Resistant bacterial strains have become a global health crisis, causing significant morbidity and mortality [18,19]. Quorum sensing (QS), a bacterial communication system that regulates biofilm formation and virulence, has emerged as a promising target for addressing antibiotic resistance. Recent studies have highlighted the potential of anti-QS and antibiofilm molecules, particularly those derived from natural products, as alternatives to traditional antibiotics [20–22].

A review of the literature indicates that species in the genus *Heracleum* exhibit various biological activities. These include antioxidant, antimicrobial, antifungal, antiepileptic, analgesic, antipyretic, antihyperlipidemic, anxiolytic, anti-inflammatory, antiedema, cytotoxic, antidiabetic, anticonvulsant, and anti-Alzheimer activities. Several species within the *Heracleum* genus have demonstrated notable antimicrobial properties, attributed primarily to their essential oil compositions. For instance, the essential oil extracted from the flowering aerial parts of *H. moellendorffii* comprises 50 compounds, accounting for 92.67% of the oil's composition, and exhibits significant antioxidant and antibacterial activities. Similarly, the essential oil of *Heracleum sphondylium* subsp. *ternatum*, rich in compounds such as 1-octanol (50.3%), octyl butyrate (24.6%), and octyl acetate (7.3%), has been evaluated for its antimicrobial activity using microdilution broth and agar diffusion methods, with 1-octanol identified as the bioactive constituent. These findings underscore the potential of *Heracleum* species as sources of bioactive compounds with antimicrobial efficacy. Additionally, *Heracleum* species have been utilized as odor enhancers and insecticides, showcasing their diverse potential in both medicinal and industrial contexts [13,23–32]. This study investigates the chemical compositions and biological activities of four *Heracleum* species growing in Türkiye, including the endemic *H. crenatifolium* Boiss, *H. paphlagonicum* Czeczott, and *H. sphondylium* subsp. *montanum* Schleich. ex Gaudin, as well as *H. pastinacifolium* subsp. *incanum* Boiss. & A.Huet species. This research aims to carry out the following: (i) Determine the total phenolic and flavonoid contents of methanol extracts; (ii) Analyze the essential oil composition of fruits, aerial parts, and roots of the selected *Heracleum* species; (iii) Evaluate the relationship between total phenolic compound and total flavonoid content with antioxidant activity of methanol extract; (iv) Investigate the antimicrobial, antibiofilm, and anti-QS activities of methanol and *n*-hexane extracts.

2. Results and Discussion

2.1. Determination of Total Phenolic and Total Flavonoid Content

The total phenolic and total flavonoid contents of eight methanol extracts (10 mg/mL), including the aerial parts and roots of *H. crenatifolium*, *H. paphlagonicum*, *H. sphondylium* subsp. *montanum*, and *H. pastinacifolium* subsp. *incanum* were determined (Table S1). Additionally, the yield of each extract was calculated and given in Table S1. See Supplementary Materials (Table S1).

The total phenolic content of methanol extracts prepared from the aerial parts and roots of *H. crenatifolium*, *H. paphlagonicum*, *H. sphondylium* subsp. *montanum*, and *H. pastinacifolium* subsp. *incanum* was determined using Folin–Ciocalteu reagent (FCR). Among the root extracts, *H. pastinacifolium* subsp. *incanum* exhibited the highest total phenolic content (335.744 mg GAEs/g extract). Similarly, among the aerial parts extracts, the highest phenolic content was observed in the *H. pastinacifolium* subsp. *incanum* (37.720 mg GAEs/g extract). In general, it was found that root extracts contained higher amounts of phenolic compounds than aerial parts extracts.

Total flavonoid amounts in methanol extracts prepared from the aerial parts and roots of *H. crenatifolium*, *H. paphlagonicum*, *H. sphondylium* subsp. *montanum*, and *H. pastinacifolium* subsp. *incanum* were determined using the aluminum chloride colorimetric method.

Among the root extracts, the extract containing the highest total of flavonoids was *H. crenatifolium* (154.773 mg QE/g extract). Among the aerial parts extracts, the extract containing the highest amount of flavonoids was *H. pastinacifolium* subsp. *incanum* (70.696 mg QE/g extract). In general, it was observed that the amount of flavonoids was higher in root extracts than in aerial parts extracts.

In literature reviews, it was observed that there might be differences between the total phenol and total flavonoid amounts of the species, and it was thought that the reason for this change may be factors such as the collection locality of the plant, content differences in the subspecies of the plant, collection time, and the status of the plant within the vegetation cycle [33,34].

2.2. *Essential Oils of Heracleum Genus*

The chemical composition of essential oils extracted from three parts (fruits, aerial parts, and roots) of four *Heracleum* species (*H. crenatifolium*, *H. paphlagonicum*, *H. sphondylium* subsp. *montanum* and *H. pastinacifolium* subsp. *incanum*) were analyzed in this study. Across the analyzed plant parts, substantial variations in the main compounds and their yields were identified, emphasizing the nature of the essential oil profiles (Table S2). See Supplementary Materials (Table S2). These findings contribute to the understanding of the phytochemical diversity within the genus *Heracleum*, known for its medicinal and aromatic properties.

Substantial interspecies and interparts variability were observed, particularly in terms of the major compounds and their yields. Additionally, the oil yields varied significantly, reflecting differences in essential oil productivity among the species and plant parts and also demonstrating the uneven distribution of secondary metabolites within and across the *Heracleum* species. The highest yield was recorded in the fruits of *H. sphondylium* subsp. *montanum* (4.39%), while the aerial parts of the same species showed a notably low yield (0.19%). Similarly, the roots of *H. crenatifolium* had a modest yield of 0.42%. This pattern of high oil productivity in fruits compared to other parts is consistent across the studied species, indicating that fruits are the primary sites for essential oil biosynthesis and accumulation. The essential oil profile of *H. crenatifolium* exhibited notable diversity across the fruits, aerial parts, and roots.

2.2.1. Essential Oils Derived from Fruits

In *H. crenatifolium*, the main compound in the fruits' essential oil was octyl acetate, which accounted for 95.4% of the total composition. The aerial parts were characterized by the presence of myristicin (10.6%), while the roots exhibited a distinctive profile, with myristicin being the major component (88.0%). Trace amounts of other monoterpenes such as α-pinene and β-pinene were also detected, highlighting the chemical compositions of this species.

In *H. paphlagonicum*, the fruits' essential oil was found to contain octyl acetate (39.4%), with significant contributions from myristicin (15.1%) and hexyl butyrate (12.9%). The aerial parts showed a high presence of myristicin (42.9%), which was also the main compound in the roots' essential oil, constituting 83.7% of the total composition. These results underscore the prevalence of myristicin in the non-fruit parts of this species, suggesting its potential as a key phytochemical marker.

The fruits' essential oil of *H. sphondylium* subsp. *montanum* demonstrated a rich profile, dominated by octyl acetate (73.7%) and myristicin (8.9%). In contrast, the aerial parts exhibited a balanced distribution, with octyl acetate (56.1%) and hexyl butyrate (4.1%) as the main compounds. The roots' essential oil was highly rich in myristicin (62.6%), further corroborating the trend of myristicin dominance in root oils across species. Additionally, the presence of limonene and octanol in minor amounts adds to the chemical diversity of this subspecies.

The chemical composition of *H. pastinacifolium* subsp. *incanum* showed significant variation across plant parts. The fruit oil was predominantly composed of hexyl butyrate (37.0%), followed by octyl acetate (15.6%). The aerial parts displayed a more complex profile, with myristicin (75.2%) as the major compound, alongside trace levels of methyl chavicol and octyl butyrate. In the root oil, myristicin accounted for 62.6%, consistent with the root-specific patterns observed in other species.

A comparative evaluation of the essential oils from all four species reveals significant interspecies and tissue-specific variations. Octyl acetate and myristicin emerged as the main compounds, with octyl acetate dominating fruit oils and myristicin being the main compound in roots. The fruits of *H. crenatifolium* showed the highest presence of octyl acetate, while *H. pastinacifolium* subsp. *incanum* displayed a more diverse profile with contributions from hexyl butyrate.

In aerial parts, myristicin consistently emerged as the main compound, reflecting a shared chemotype among the species. The roots showed a remarkable trend of myristicin enrichment, underscoring its potential functional significance. Despite these similarities, the presence of minor compounds such as limonene, hexanol, and methyl chavicol adds to the distinctive chemical fingerprints of each species. These results highlight the chemical compositions and adaptive strategies of the *Heracleum* genus.

A clear trend emerges from the comparative analysis of the essential oil yields and chemical compositions across the four *Heracleum* species (according to Tables S2–S5). See Supplementary Materials (Tables S2–S5): (i) Fruits consistently yielded the highest amounts of essential oils, with octyl acetate as the main compound, particularly in *H. crenatifolium* and *H. sphondylium* subsp. *montanum*. (ii) Aerial parts showed the lowest yields across all species, with myristicin prevailing as the main compound. The limited diversity and low productivity may indicate a supplementary defensive role for the aerial parts. (iii) Roots demonstrated moderate yields with main consistent of myristicin in all species. This underscores the evolutionary importance of myristicin as a root-specific secondary metabolite, potentially serving as a chemical barrier against biotic stress. Despite these overarching similarities, the relative presences of minor compounds such as limonene, hexyl butyrate, and methyl chavicol varied among species and plants' parts, contributing to their unique chemical signatures. These interspecies and inter-tissue differences underline the significant chemical plasticity within the *Heracleum* genus and its adaptive responses to ecological pressures.

The results of our study on the fruits of *Heracleum* species, along with the findings from the literature, are presented in Table S3. See Supplementary Materials (Table S3). In our study, the essential oil obtained from the fruits of *H. crenatifolium* was determined to contain 95.4% octyl acetate. Similarly, the fruits of *H. sphondylium* subsp. *montanum* were found to contain 73.7% octyl acetate. In other fruit-focused studies in the literature, octyl acetate has been identified as the main component, with percentages generally ranging between 30 and 70%. For instance, essential oil from the fruits of *H. orphanidis* Boiss. in North Macedonia was reported to contain 84.5% octyl acetate, while in Iran, the octyl acetate content of *H. persicum* Desf. ex Fisch., C.A.Mey. & Avé-Lall fruits varied between 12.3% and 40.8% [35–38]. The high proportions of this compound in *Heracleum* fruits from Türkiye highlight their chemical richness and potential industrial applications.

Additionally, in our study, the fruits of *H. pastinacifolium* subsp. *incanum* were found to contain 37.0% hexyl butyrate and 20.6% octyl butanoate. This species shows notable diversity in its chemical profile compared to other *Heracleum* fruit studies reported in the literature. For example, essential oils from *H. persicum* fruits in Iran have been reported to contain hexyl butyrate in proportions ranging from 13.8% to 56.5%, alongside octyl acetate ranging between 12.3% and 40.8% [35–37]. The high levels of these components in our findings underscore the unique potential of *Heracleum* fruits from Türkiye, due to local environmental conditions and genetic factors [39].

In conclusion, the fruit-focused nature of our study provides a significant advantage when comparing it to other *Heracleum* essential oil studies in the literature. The high proportions of octyl acetate and hexyl butyrate found in our study suggest that the fruits are rich in essential oils, and these components derived from fruits could be valuable for biological and industrial applications. This underscores the importance of further focusing on the chemical profiles of essential oils from fruits.

2.2.2. Essential Oils Derived from Aerial Parts

In our study, the essential oil compositions obtained from the aerial parts of *H. crenatifolium*, *H. paphlagonicum*, *H. sphondylium* subsp. *montanum*, and *H. pastinacifolium* subsp. *incanum*, collected from Türkiye, were analyzed. The results of these species are presented in the first four rows of Table S4, and comparisons were made with data obtained from the literature. See Supplementary Materials (Table S4).

The aerial parts of *H. crenatifolium* were found to contain 85.9% octyl acetate and 10.6% myristicin. *H. sphondylium* subsp. *montanum* exhibited 56.1% octyl acetate and 24.2% myristicin. Similarly, the aerial parts of *H. pastinacifolium* subsp. *incanum* contained 62.6% myristicin, which is notably higher than the values reported for the aerial parts of *H. moellendorffii* Hance. [26]. Compared to these, *H. paphlagonicum* demonstrated a distinct chemical profile with 42.9% myristicin and 30.8% (*E*)-anethole.

According to the literature, *H. anisactis* Boiss. & Hohen from Iran has been reported to contain up to 93.5% myristicin, while *H. orphanidis* from Macedonia exhibited an octyl acetate content of 83.5%. The high octyl acetate levels observed in *H. crenatifolium* and *H. sphondylium* subsp. *montanum* suggest that this compound is produced in greater quantities under the environmental conditions of Türkiye. Additionally, the 30.8% (*E*)-anethole content in *H. paphlagonicum* exceeds the 25.0% reported for species such as *H. persicum* in the literature [40].

In conclusion, the essential oil compositions of *H. crenatifolium*, *H. paphlagonicum*, *H. sphondylium* subsp. *montanum*, and *H. pastinacifolium* subsp. *incanum* analyzed in this study stand out when compared with other *Heracleum* species in the literature, particularly due to their high levels of octyl acetate, myristicin, and (*E*)-anethole.

2.2.3. Essential Oils Derived from Roots

In this study, the essential oil compositions obtained from the roots of *H. crenatifolium*, *H. paphlagonicum*, *H. sphondylium* subsp. *montanum*, and *H. pastinacifolium* subsp. *incanum*, collected from Türkiye, were analyzed. The results for these species are presented in the first four rows of Table S5, while the remaining data were obtained from the literature. See Supplementary Materials (Table S5).

In our study, the root essential oil of *H. crenatifolium* was found to contain 88.0% myristicin. Similarly, the roots of *H. paphlagonicum* contained 83.7% myristicin, while *H. pastinacifolium* subsp. *incanum* exhibited notable richness with 75.2% myristicin. In the roots of *H. sphondylium* subsp. *montanum*, octyl acetate (57.1%) and myristicin (13.8%) were identified as the main compounds. These results indicate that myristicin is a common and main component in the roots across species, suggesting its potential role in the defensive mechanisms of the roots.

According to other studies in the literature, the root essential oils of *H. transcaucasicum* Manden. and *H. anisactis* from Iran contain 96.8% and 95.1% myristicin, respectively. In contrast, the roots of *H. orphanidis* from Macedonia were reported to contain 80.0% (Z)-falcarinol [41]. The high levels of myristicin observed in *H. crenatifolium* and *H. paphlagonicum* in our study highlight the influence of Türkiye's ecological conditions in promoting the biosynthesis of this compound.

The literature data also reveal that certain species exhibit significant proportions of other compounds in their root essential oil profiles, such as β-pinene (17.7–35.1%), limonene (16.0–22.7%), and (Z)-falcarinol [38,41–44]. However, the major of myristicin in the species analyzed in our study underscores the chemical diversity of *Heracleum* roots and highlights the impact of genetic and environmental factors on root chemistry.

In conclusion, the root essential oil compositions of *H. crenatifolium*, *H. paphlagonicum*, *H. sphondylium* subsp. *montanum*, and *H. pastinacifolium* subsp. *incanum* analyzed in our study demonstrates a unique richness in myristicin compared to other *Heracleum* species reported in the literature. The predominance of this compound in roots suggests significant biological activity and potential relevance to plant defense mechanisms.

2.3. Multivariate Analysis of Heracleum Genus

PCA and HCA were used to characterize the volatile compounds of *Heracleum* spp. essential oils, with analyses conducted for the fruit, aerial parts, and root sections using Minitab 19 software [45]. The PCA numbers of the fruits' essential oils for statistical analysis are given in Table S3. See Supplementary Materials (Table S3). PCA analysis is illustrated in Figure 1, while HCA analysis is given in Figure 2. PCA was used to show the interrelationships among the species of the *Heracleum* fruits. In addition, the cluster obtained was confirmed by PCA analysis to evaluate the accuracy of this classification. For the essential oils of *Heracleum* fruits, all variables affected, PC1 (14.8%) and PC2 (13.7%), clarified 27.5% of the accumulated variation of the data analyzed.

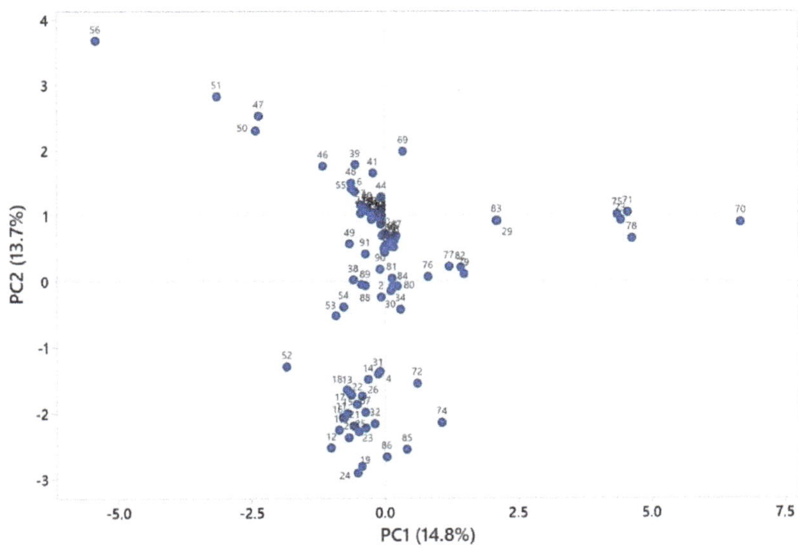

Figure 1. PCA analysis of the major components of the essential oils of fruits.

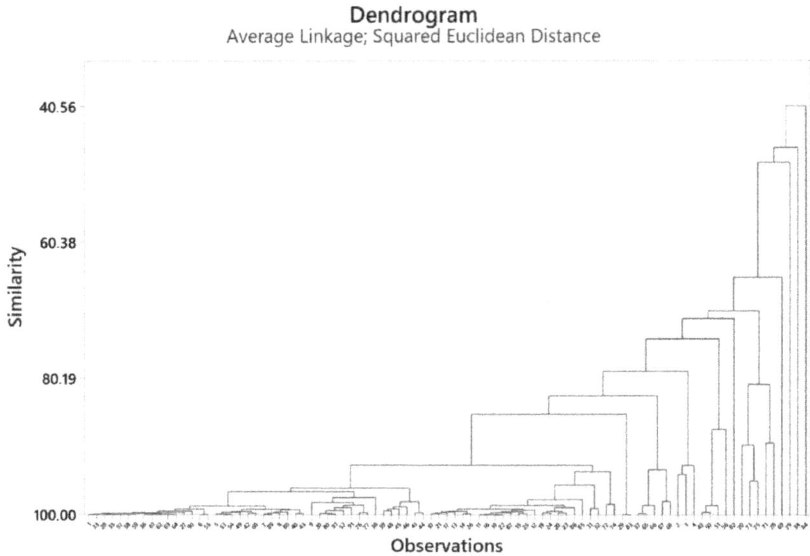

Figure 2. Dendrogram obtained by HCA based on Euclidian distances between groups of the major components of the fruits' essential oils.

The cluster analysis of the fruits' essential oil observations (Figure 2) revealed two main clades, with similarity ranging from 40.56% to 99.99%. The essential oil of *H. crenatifolium* (PCA no: 1) used in this study was clustered with the essential oil of *H. crenatifolium* (Gümüşhane/Türkiye) (PCA no: 33), which suggested that these plants have a closely related origin (99.97%). The similarity between *H. paphlagonicum* (PCA no: 2) and *H. sphondylium* subsp. *montanum* (PCA no: 3) was determined to be 94.12%, while the similarity between *H. pastinacifolium* subsp. *incanum* (PCA no: 4) and PCA 3 was calculated as 92.84%. Among the four essential oils obtained in the study, it was found that the chemical compositions of *H. paphlagonicum* and *H. sphondylium* subsp. *montanum* were more like each other. Additionally, the essential oils were obtained using hydrodistillation (PCA no: 61) and microdistillation (PCA no: 62) methods [46]. The similarity between the oils obtained by these two methods was found to be 99.99%. This result indicates that the change in method does not have a significant effect on the chemical composition of the essential oils.

In conclusion, our study provides a detailed analysis of the essential oils of *H. crenatifolium, H. paphlagonicum, H. sphondylium* subsp. *montanum*, and *H. pastinacifolium* subsp. *incanum*. This analysis is presented alongside a comprehensive review of other *Heracleum* species, with a particular focus on evaluating their chemical variability using PCA and HCA. By incorporating both chemical and statistical data, our findings contribute valuable insights into the chemotaxonomic characteristics of the *Heracleum* genus. Additionally, this study complements previous research by providing a broader perspective on the chemical diversity within the genus.

The results indicate that while certain trends in the essential oil composition can be observed across the analyzed species, variations in specific chemical compounds highlight the complexity and variability inherent within the genus. These findings underscore the importance of using robust statistical tools, such as PCA and HCA, to explore relationships between species and identify chemotaxonomic markers. When viewed in conjunction with earlier studies, this integrated approach offers the potential to clarify phylogenetic relationships and taxonomic classifications within *Heracleum*.

Moreover, our research emphasizes the value of combining essential oil analyses with additional data sources, such as morphological, anatomical, and phytochemical studies. While the essential oil compositions presented in this study provide significant insights, they alone may not be sufficient to fully resolve taxonomic ambiguities within the genus. Future studies should aim to expand this work by examining other plant parts, such as fruits, and exploring secondary metabolites that are commonly found in the *Heracleum* genus. These broader analyses could help refine the understanding of interspecies relationships and support more precise taxonomic adjustments, where needed.

In summary, while this study is not conclusive in redefining the taxonomic hierarchy of the examined species, it provides a critical step toward better understanding the diversity and chemical complexity of the *Heracleum* genus. It also highlights areas where further research is required to fully elucidate the genus's chemotaxonomic framework and phylogenetic relationships. This study thus represents a significant contribution to the growing body of knowledge on *Heracleum* species.

Table S4 shows the PCA numbers of the aerial parts' essential oils used for statistical analysis. See Supplementary Materials (Table S4). Figure 3 presents the results of the PCA analysis, whereas Figure 4 depicts the outcomes of the HCA analysis. PCA was used to show the interrelationships among the species of the *Heracleum* aerial parts. In addition, the cluster obtained was confirmed by PCA analysis to evaluate the accuracy of this classification. For the essential oils of *Heracleum* aerial parts, all variables affected, PC1 (12.6%) and PC2 (10.4%), clarified 23.0% of the accumulated variation of the data analyzed.

The cluster analysis of the aerial parts' essential oil observations (Figure 3) revealed two main clades, with similarity ranging from 34.44% to 99.99%. The essential oil of *H. crenatifolium* (PCA no: 1) used in this study was clustered with the essential oil of *H. orphanidis* (Macedonia) (PCA no: 20), which suggested that these plants have a closely related origin (99.70%) [41].

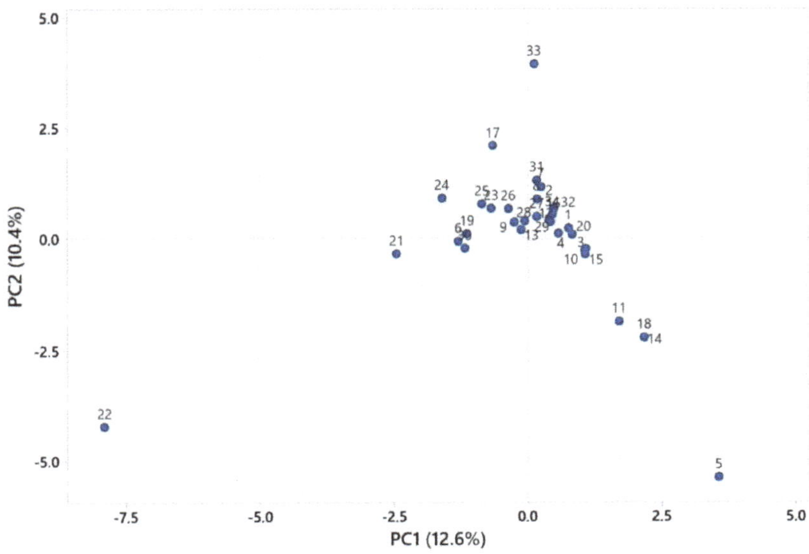

Figure 3. PCA analysis of the major components of the essential oils of aerial parts.

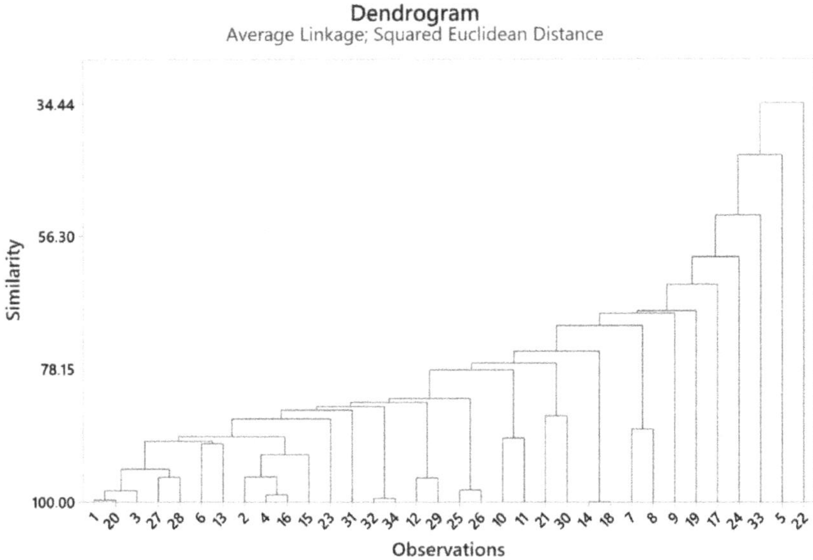

Figure 4. Dendrogram obtained by HCA based on Euclidian distances between groups of the major components of the essential oils of aerial parts.

The similarity between *H. crenatifolium* (PCA no: 1) and *H. sphondylium* subsp. *montanum* (PCA no: 3) was determined to be 98.16%, while the similarity between *H. pastinacifolium* subsp. *incanum* (PCA no: 4) and *H. paphlagonicum* (PCA 2) was calculated as 95.89%. Among the four essential oils obtained in the study, it was found that the chemical compositions of *H. crenatifolium* and *H. sphondylium* subsp. *montanum* were more like each other. The lowest similarity, calculated as 34.44%, was observed between *H. paphlagonicum* from Türkiye (PCA no: 1) and *H. sprengelianum* from India (PCA no: 22). This notable difference can be attributed to several factors, including both geographic and species-related variations. Geographic location plays a critical role in shaping the chemical composition of essential oils due to differences in environmental conditions such as climate, soil type, and altitude. Furthermore, the distinct taxonomic characteristics of the two species contribute significantly to the observed variation. These findings highlight the combined influence of ecological and genetic factors on the chemical profiles of essential oils derived from different *Heracleum* species across diverse regions.

Table S5 shows the PCA numbers of the roots' essential oils used for statistical analysis. See Supplementary Materials (Table S5). Figure 5 presents the results of the PCA analysis, while Figure 6 displays the outcomes of the HCA analyses. PCA was used to show the interrelationships among the species of the *Heracleum* roots. In addition, the cluster obtained was confirmed by PCA analysis to evaluate the accuracy of this classification. For the essential oils of *Heracleum* roots, all variables affected, PC1 (18.8%) and PC2 (17.2%), clarified 36.0% of the accumulated variation of the data analyzed.

The cluster analysis of the roots' essential oil observations (Figure 5) revealed two main clades, with similarity ranging from 35.19% to 99.99%. The essential oil of *H. crenatifolium* (PCA no: 1) used in this study was clustered with the essential oil of *H. paphlagonicum* (PCA no: 2), which suggested that these plants have a closely related origin (99.61%). Also, the essential oil of PCA no: 2 used in this study was clustered with the essential oil of *H. pastinacifolium* subsp. *incanum* (PCA no: 4), which suggested that these plants have a closely related origin (99.94%).

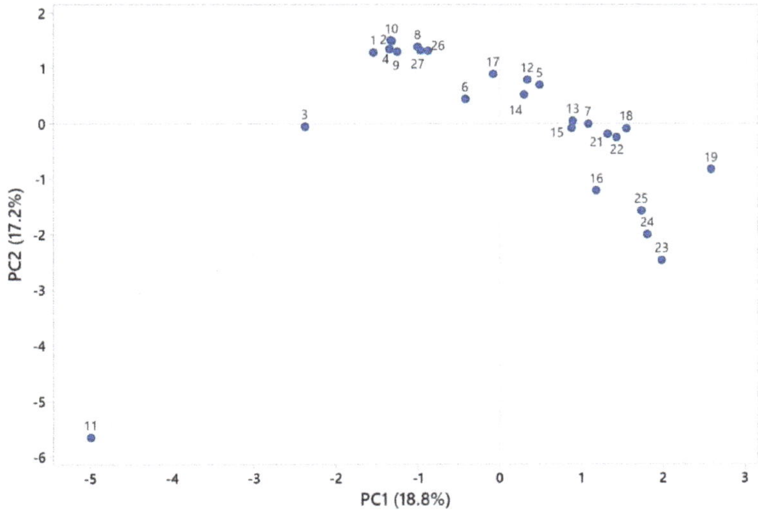

Figure 5. PCA analysis of the major components of the essential oils of roots.

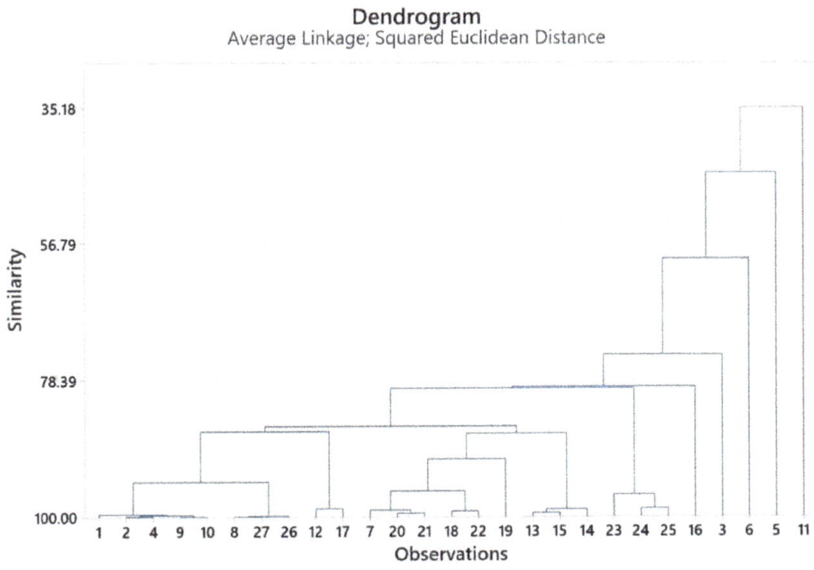

Figure 6. Dendrogram obtained by HCA based on Euclidian distances between groups of the major components of the roots' essential oils.

The similarity rate between *H. crenatifolium* PCA no: 1 and *H. stevenii* (PCA no: 11) was calculated to be 35.19% based on the analyses conducted. This finding indicates a limited shared variance between the analyzed components, thereby suggesting a significant difference in the chemical profiles of the two components. Specifically, PCA no: 11 was identified as belonging to the species *H. stevenii*, which was derived from the essential oil of this species grown in Russia [42]. This information supports broader analyses of regional and species–specific variations in the chemical composition of the essential oil in question, reaffirming the utility of PCA as an effective tool for evaluating such chemical profiles. Furthermore, the similarity rate of 35.19% highlights the potential impact of diverse environmental or genetic factors on the chemical profile.

2.4. Antioxidant Activity

For DPPH free radical scavenging activity, all extracts (8 methanol extracts) were prepared separately at 7 different concentrations (1000–10 μg/mL). IC_{50} values of all, including gallic acid used as standard, were calculated and given in Table 1.

Table 1. Antioxidant activity of methanol extracts.

Plant Extracts		DPPH Radical Scavenging Activity (IC_{50} Value (mg/mL) ± SD [b])	ABTS Free Radical Scavenging Activity (TEAC [a] mg TE/g Extract ± SD [b])
H. crenatifolium	aerial parts	0.216 ± 0.0007	155.622 ± 3.47
	roots	0.765 ± 0.015	143.574 ± 3.47
H. paphlagonicum	aerial parts	0.275 ± 0.001	157.63 ± 3.47
	roots	0.242 ± 0.004	199.799 ± 6.95
H. sphondylium subsp. *montanum*	aerial parts	0.246 ± 0.002	115.461 ± 6.95
	roots	0.416 ± 0.004	282.128 ± 6.95
H. pastinacifolium subsp. *incanum*	aerial parts	1.077 ± 0.007	79.317 ± 3.47
	roots	0.77 ± 0.003	135.542 ± 6.024
Gallic acid		0.001 ± 0.0001	-

[a] TEAC: Trolox equivalent antioxidant capacity, [b] SD: Standard deviation.

For ABTS free radical scavenging activity, all extracts (8 methanol extracts) were prepared at a concentration of 1 mg/mL, and antioxidant activities of all extracts were calculated as mg Trolox equivalent/g extract and given in Table 1.

No antioxidant activity studies have been found on *H. paphlagonicum* and *H. crenatifolium* species, and thus this study was the first to evaluate the aforementioned bioactivity. The DPPH free radical scavenging activity of *H. crenatifolium*, *H. paphlagonicum*, *H. sphondylium* subsp. *montanum*, and *H. pastinacifolium* subsp. *incanum* aerial parts and root methanol extracts was evaluated according to their DPPH bleaching abilities. The most active extract was *H. paphlagonicum* root extract among root extracts; the most active extract among aerial parts extracts was *H. crenatifolium* aerial parts extract.

H. crenatifolium, *H. paphlagonicum*, *H. sphondylium* subsp. *montanum*, and *H. pastinacifolium* subsp. *incanum*, aerial parts and root methanol extracts were evaluated according to the ABTS radical cation scavenging method. The highest trolox equivalent ABTS scavenging effect was in *H. sphondylium* subsp. *montanum* root extract among root extracts; the highest effect was in *H. paphlagonicum* aerial parts extract among aerial parts extracts.

In general, when the DPPH free radical scavenging activity and ABTS free radical scavenging activity results were evaluated, the root extracts of *Heracleum* species showed higher antioxidant activity than aerial parts extracts. It was observed that having a high extract yield had no effect in terms of antioxidant activity. In our study and literature reviews, it was seen that the total phenol and total flavonoid contents of the species were directly proportional to the antioxidant activity, and it was thought that the different antioxidant activities of the species in our study in other literature reviews were due to differences in total phenol and total flavonoid contents [33,34,47].

2.5. Antimicrobial Activity

The MIC values (mg/mL) of the methanol and *n*-hexane extracts of four *Heracleum* species are shown in Table 2. The MIC values of four *Heracleum* species ranged from 0.625 to 10 mg/mL against the tested bacteria and 5 to 10 mg/mL against the tested fungus. Among the tested extracts, the methanol and *n*-hexane extracts of *H. pastinacifolium* subsp. *incanum* (aerial parts) and *n*-hexane extract of *H. paphlagonicum* (root) exhibited the best antimicrobial activity. The extracts demonstrated better antibacterial activity against Gram-positive bacteria. However, none of the extracts showed antibacterial activity against *Klebsiella pneumoniae* ATCC 13383 and *Pseudomonas aeruginosa* ATCC 27853. The observed activities can be considered weak compared to standard antimicrobials (Table 2).

Table 2. MIC values (mg/mL) of the methanol and *n*-hexane extracts of four *Heracleum* species.

Plant Extracts		Gram-Positive Bacteria		Gram-Negative Bacteria			Fungus
		S. aureus	*S. aureus* (MRSA)	*E. coli*	*K. pneumoniae*	*P. aeruginosa*	*C. albicans*
Aerial parts (Methanol)	*H. crenatifolium*	1.25	1.25	-	-	-	-
	H. paphlagonicum	1.25	1.25	-	-	-	-
	H. sphondylium subsp. *montanum*	1.25	1.25	-	-	-	-
	H. pastinacifolium subsp. *incanum*	1.25	0.625	5	-	-	5
Roots (Methanol)	*H. crenatifolium*	2.5	2.5	-	-	-	10
	H. paphlagonicum	1.25	1.25	-	-	-	10
	H. sphondylium subsp. *montanum*	1.25	1.25	10	-	-	5
	H. pastinacifolium subsp. *incanum*	2.5	2.5	-	-	-	5
Aerial parts (*n*-Hexane)	*H. crenatifolium*	-	-	-	-	-	-
	H. paphlagonicum	1.25	1.25	-	-	-	-
	H. sphondylium subsp. *montanum*	1.25	1.25	-	-	-	-
	H. pastinacifolium subsp. *incanum*	0.625	0.625	-	-	-	10
Roots (*n*-Hexane)	*H. paphlagonicum*	0.625	0.625	-	-	-	-
	H. sphondylium subsp. *montanum*	1.25	5	-	-	-	-
Ciprofloxacin		<0.00025	0.0005	<0.00025	<0.00025	<0.00025	NT
Gentamicin		0.0005	<0.00025	0.0005	<0.00025	0.0005	NT
Fluconazole		NT	NT	NT	NT	NT	0.00156
5% DMSO		-	-	-	-	-	-

NT: not tested.

The phytochemical analysis of methanol extracts from *Heracleum* species demonstrated significant variability in total phenolic and flavonoid contents, with root extracts generally exhibiting higher levels than aerial parts.

Among the aerial parts extracts, *H. pastinacifolium* subsp. *incanum* exhibited the highest phenolic content (37.720 mg GAEs/g extract) and was also among the most active extracts against Gram-positive bacteria, including *S. aureus* and MRSA. Phenolic compounds are well documented for their antimicrobial properties, primarily through mechanisms such as bacterial cell wall disruption, inhibition of essential enzymes, and interference with nucleic acid synthesis. The strong activity of *H. pastinacifolium* subsp. *incanum* aerial parts extracts against Gram-positive pathogens may be attributed to their high phenolic content, as these bacteria lack the outer membrane barrier present in Gram-negative bacteria, making them more susceptible to phenolic compounds [48–50].

Similarly, the aerial parts extracts of *H. pastinacifolium* subsp. *incanum*, which exhibited the highest flavonoid content (70.696 mg QE/g extract) among the aerial parts extracts, showed notable antimicrobial activity. Flavonoids have been reported to exert their antimicrobial effects by disrupting bacterial membranes, and inhibiting efflux pumps [51].

The weak or absent activity of the extracts against Gram-negative bacteria aligns with the structural and functional barriers posed by the outer membrane of these bacteria [52]. While phenolic and flavonoid compounds are effective against Gram-positive pathogens, their efficacy against Gram-negative bacteria often requires higher concentrations or synergistic combinations with other bioactive compounds [53].

When comparing the species included in this study with the existing literature, their antimicrobial activities were found to align with previously reported findings [28,29,54]. The phytochemical properties of *Heracleum* species, particularly their high phenolic and flavonoid contents, underpins their antimicrobial properties. The correlation between phytochemical composition and antimicrobial activity reinforces the therapeutic potential of these plants. Future studies should focus on isolating and characterizing individual bioactive compounds to better understand their mechanisms of action and to explore their synergistic potential with existing antimicrobials.

2.6. Antibiofilm Activity

The percentage biofilm inhibition values of the methanol extracts of four *Heracleum* species (10 mg/mL) are presented in Figure 7, while the percentage biofilm inhibition values of the *n*-hexane extracts of four *Heracleum* species (10 mg/mL) are presented in Figure 8. Among the methanol extracts, *H. pastinacifolium* subsp. *incanum* (aerial parts) exhibited the highest antibiofilm activity, whereas *H. paphlagonicum* (aerial parts) showed the highest activity among *n*-hexane extracts, with biofilm inhibition values of 73.2% and 75.5%, respectively. Tables S6 and S7 present the optical density (OD) values and standard deviations (SD) corresponding to the biofilm inhibition percentages displayed in Figures 7 and 8, respectively. See Supplementary Materials (Tables S6 and S7).

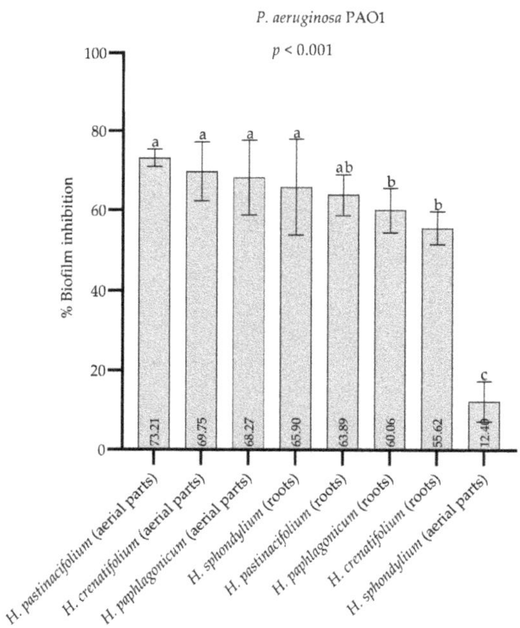

Figure 7. The percentage biofilm inhibition values of the methanol extracts of four *Heracleum* species. Data were represented as mean values with standard deviations. Different letters indicate the statistical difference. One-way ANOVA and Tukey's tests were conducted to compare mean values of % biofilm inhibition between groups.

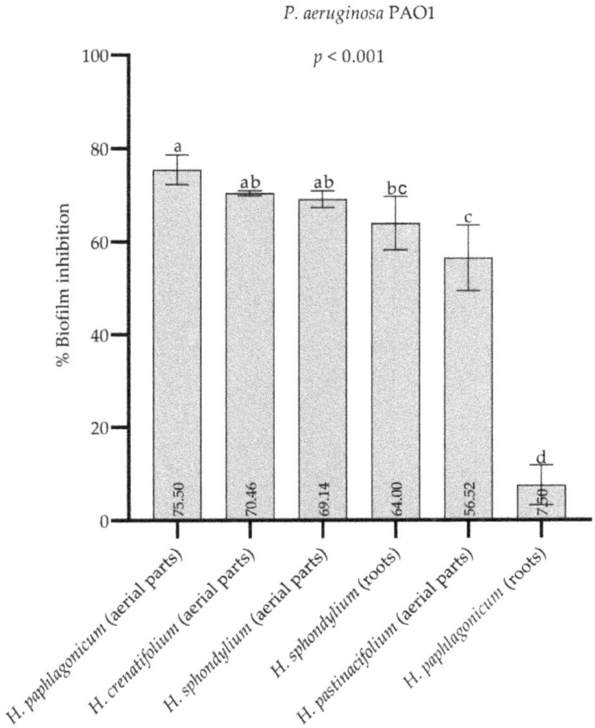

Figure 8. The percentage biofilm inhibition values of the *n*-hexane extracts of four *Heracleum* species. Data were represented as mean values with standard deviations. Different letters indicate the statistical difference. One-way ANOVA and Tukey's tests were conducted to compare mean values of % biofilm inhibition between groups.

The strong antibiofilm activity observed in the methanol extracts of *H. pastinacifolium* subsp. *incanum* (aerial parts) aligns with its high phenolic and flavonoid content. Phenolic compounds are known to interfere with bacterial adhesion and QS pathways, both of which are critical for biofilm formation [55]. Flavonoids, similarly, can disrupt bacterial communication and inhibit enzymes necessary for biofilm matrix development [50,56]. These findings suggest that the phenolic and flavonoid constituents in *H. pastinacifolium* subsp. *incanum* methanol extracts play a significant role in their antibiofilm activity.

Biofilm-associated infections pose a substantial challenge in medical settings, particularly in relation to implanted medical devices, chronic wounds, and respiratory tract infections [57]. The strong antibiofilm activity of *H. pastinacifolium* subsp. *incanum* (aerial parts) methanol extract positions them as potential candidates for further development into antibiofilm agents. To the best of our knowledge, this is the first study investigating the antibiofilm activity of the four *Heracleum* species included in this research (*H. crenatifolium*, *H. paphlagonicum*, *H. sphondylium* subsp. *montanum*, and *H. pastinacifolium* subsp. *incanum*). This study highlights the distinctive bioactive properties of these species, particularly their ability to inhibit biofilm formation—a feature that has not been previously investigated.

2.7. Anti-Quorum Sensing Activity

The anti-QS activity test was carried out based on the MIC values of the extracts of four *Heracleum* species against *C. violaceum* ATCC 12472 (Figures S1 and S2). See Supplementary Materials (Figures S1 and S2). No violacein inhibition zone was observed in methanol extracts, but it was observed in all *n*-hexane extracts. Based on the anti-QS activity results, *n*-hexane extracts exhibited better activity.

3. Materials and Methods

3.1. Plant Material

The *Heracleum* species used in this study—*H. crenatifolium*, *H. paphlagonicum*, *H. sphondylium* subsp. *montanum*, and *H. pastinacifolium* subsp. *incanum*—were collected from the localities given in Table 3 (fruiting period). The plant materials were identified by Tugçe Ince Kose, Prof. Dr. Hayri Duman, and Prof. Dr. Ahmet Duran. Voucher specimens were deposited at the herbarium of Ankara University Faculty of Pharmacy (AEF).

Table 3. Localities and herbarium registry numbers of collected *Heracleum* species.

Plant	Locality	Date of Collection	Herbarium Number
H. crenatifolium	Konya; Hadim 810–820 m 37.0282, 32.6936	15.07.2023	AEF 31001
H. paphlagonicum	Kastamonu; Ilgaz Dağı 1800–1850 m 41.0772, 33.7299	22.07.2023	AEF 30999
H. sphondylium subsp. *montanum*	Ankara; Çamlıdere 1100–1150 m 40.5436, 32.5636	23.07.2023	AEF 31000
H. pastinacifolium subsp. *incanum*	Karabük; Keltepe 1950–2000 m 41.0866, 32.4623	05.08.2023	AEF 30998

3.2. Preparation of Extracts

3.2.1. Methanol Extract

Plant extracts were obtained using the maceration method. A total of 100 g of plant material (roots and aerial parts) was ground using a grinder (Renas Makine ve Otomasyon Teknolojileri RBT-200, İstanbul, Türkiye). The ground material was macerated three times for 8 h with methanol at room temperature using magnetic stirrers (Heidolph MR 3001, Darmstadt, Germany), (VELP ARE, VELP AREC.X, Usmate Velate, Italy). The extracts were filtered using Filtros Anonia, S.A. filter paper (Barcelona, Spain), and the methanol was evaporated under reduced pressure at a maximum temperature of 65 °C using a rotary evaporator (Büchi Rotavapor R-200, Flawil, Switzerland).

3.2.2. *n*-Hexane Extract

n-Hexane extracts were prepared using a Soxhlet apparatus. Approximately 25–30 g of plant material (roots and aerial parts) was placed in the Soxhlet apparatus cartridge, and *n*-hexane (Emplura®, Darmstadt, Germany) was added and flushed once. The extraction process was carried out for 4 h, after which the solvent was removed using a rotary evaporator. Due to insufficient plant material, *n*-hexane extracts could not be prepared from the roots of *H. pastinacifolium* subsp. *incanum* and *H. crenatifolium*.

3.3. Phytochemical Composition

3.3.1. Determination of Total Phenolic Compounds

The total phenolic content of the extracts was determined using the FCR method, following the protocol outlined by Büyüktuncel [58]. Gallic acid, at concentrations ranging from 50 to 500 μg/mL, was used as a standard to construct the calibration curve. Absorbance measurements were taken at 765 nm using a spectrophotometer (Shimadzu UV Spectrophotometer UV-1800, Kyoto, Japan). The total phenolic content was calculated as gallic acid equivalents (GAE) based on the calibration curve and expressed as milligrams of GAE per gram of extract (mg GAE/g extract). Each experiment was performed in triplicate to ensure reproducibility and reliability.

3.3.2. Determination of Total Flavonoids

The total flavonoid content of the extracts was determined using the aluminum chloride colorimetric method, as described by Demir et al. [59] and Keskin et al. [60]. Quercetin, at concentrations ranging from 50 to 800 μg/mL, was used as a standard to construct the calibration curve. Absorbance was measured at 510 nm using a spectrophotometer. Based on the quercetin calibration curve, the total flavonoid content was calculated and expressed as milligrams of quercetin equivalents (mg QE) per gram of extract (mg QE/g extract). All experiments were performed in triplicate to ensure accuracy and reproducibility.

3.4. *Essential Oils*

Essential oils were isolated from the fruits, roots, and aerial parts of the *Heracleum* species and analyzed for their chemical compositions using Gas Chromatography with Flame Ionization Detection (GC–FID) and Gas Chromatography–Mass Spectrometry (GC–MS). To assess the variation in essential oil compositions across different *Heracleum* species, Hierarchical Cluster Analysis (HCA) and Principal Component Analysis (PCA) were performed.

3.4.1. Isolation of the Essential Oils

Air-dried fruits, aerial parts, and roots of the *Heracleum* species (fruiting period) were subjected to hydrodistillation for 3 h using a Clevenger-type apparatus, following the protocol recommended by the [61]. Obtained essential oils were dried over anhydrous sodium sulfate to remove moisture and stored in sealed vials at +4 °C, protected from light, to preserve their quality until further analysis and testing.

3.4.2. GC–MS Analysis

GC–MS analysis was carried out with an Agilent 5975 GC-MSD system (Santa Clara, CA, USA). Innowax FSC column (60 m × 0.25 mm, 0.25 mm film thickness) was used with helium as carrier gas (0.8 mL/min). The GC oven temperature was initially maintained at 60 °C for 10 min, then increased to 220 °C at a rate of 4 °C/min, where it was held constant for 10 min. Subsequently, the temperature was increased to 240 °C at a rate of 1 °C/min. The split ratio was set to 40:1, and the injector temperature was adjusted to 250 °C. Mass spectra were recorded at 70 eV with a mass range of m/z 35 to 450 [62].

3.4.3. GC–FID Analysis

GC analysis was carried out using an Agilent 6890N GC system. The flame ionization detector (FID) temperature was set to 300 °C. To obtain the same elution order on the GC–MS, simultaneous auto-injection was carried out on the same type of column (Innowax FSC column, 60 m × 0.25 mm, 0.25 μm film thickness) under identical operational conditions. The relative percentage amounts of the separated compounds were calculated from FID chromatograms, respectively [62].

3.4.4. Identification of the Volatile Compounds

The identification of essential oil components was performed by comparing their relative retention times with those of authentic reference samples or by comparing their relative retention indices (RRIs) to a series of n-alkanes. Computer matching against commercial (Wiley GC/MS Library, MassFinder Software 4.0), and in-house "Başer Library of Essential Oil Constituents" built up by genuine compounds and components of known oils [62].

3.4.5. Statistical Analysis

Statistical analysis was performed to evaluate the chemical variability among the essential oils. Original variables were defined as essential oil contents that exceeded 3.0%

of the overall essential oil composition in at least one species. After normalization, the data was subjected to HCA and PCA. Minitab 19 was used to conduct the statistical analysis (State College, PA, USA). Using the rescaled distances in the dendrogram and a cut-off point (Euclidean distance) that allows the attainment of consistent clusters, the number of clusters was computed. To determine the similarity among the essential oils regarding the contents of their chemical constituents, the PCA and the HCA were utilized [45].

3.5. Antioxidant Activity

3.5.1. DPPH Free Radical Scavenging Activity

The DPPH free radical scavenging effect of the extracts was evaluated according to their DPPH bleaching ability. The experiment is based on the DPPH redox change reaction [63]. The reaction mixture contained 100 μM of DPPH dissolved in methanol and extracts at different concentrations. The absorbance values of the test substances kept at room temperature for 30 min were measured at 517 nm and the free radical capture percentages were calculated. The experiment was performed in triplicate. Gallic acid was used as a reference. Calibration curves were determined for gallic acid and each sample according to the % inhibition formula given below. IC50 values were determined according to these curves for gallic acid and all samples.

The free radical scavenging effect was calculated according to the % inhibition formula:

$$\% \text{ Inhibition} = [(\text{Acontrol}^* - \text{Asample}^*/\text{Acontrol}^*)] \times 100$$

Acontrol*: Absorbance of control; Asample*: Absorbance of extract

3.5.2. ABTS Free Radical Scavenging Activity

Total antioxidant activity was determined using the standard TEAC (Trolox equivalent antioxidant capacity) method [64]. ABTS used during the experiment is a mixture of 2.45 mM potassium persulfate and 7 mM ABTS aqueous solution. The mixture was left to stand in the dark at room temperature overnight (12 to 16 h) and blue-green colored radical formation was achieved. The obtained ABTS radical cation was diluted with methanol (pH 7.4). The samples were diluted with ABTS solution at a ratio of 1/10. After waiting for 6 min, the absorbance value at 734 nm was measured and the amount of inhibition was calculated.

Trolox (water-soluble α-tocopherol analogue) was used as a standard. Calibration curve was obtained according to 5 different concentrations and absorption values of Trolox. Antioxidant activity of 8 different extracts was calculated according to this calibration curve. The results were given as Trolox equivalent antioxidant capacity (TEAC). The experiment was performed in triplicate.

3.6. Antimicrobial Activity

The antimicrobial activity of the extracts was assessed using the broth microdilution method to determine the MIC values, following the guidelines provided by the Clinical and Laboratory Standards Institute [65,66]. The test organisms included *S. aureus* ATCC 25923, methicillin-resistant *S. aureus* ATCC 43300 (MRSA), *E. coli* ATCC 25922, *P. aeruginosa* ATCC 27853, *K. pneumoniae* ATCC 13883 as bacterial strains, and *C. albicans* ATCC 10231 as the fungal strain. The plant extracts were dissolved in 5% dimethyl sulfoxide (DMSO), and all experiments were conducted in triplicate to ensure reproducibility.

For the antibacterial activity test, serial two-fold dilutions of the extracts, ranging from 10 to 0.78 mg/mL, were prepared in Mueller Hinton Broth (Merck, Darmstadt, Germany). Inoculums were prepared from 24-h subcultures, and the final bacterial suspension concentration was adjusted to 5×10^5 CFU/mL. After incubation at 35 °C for 18–24 h, the

MIC value (µg/mL) was determined as the lowest concentration that completely inhibited visible bacterial growth. Negative controls consisted of inoculated broth with 5% DMSO, while ciprofloxacin and gentamicin were used as standard antibiotics.

For the antifungal activity test, serial two-fold dilutions of the extracts (10 to 0.78 mg/mL) were prepared in RPMI 1640 broth (ICN-Flow, Aurora, OH, USA). The final fungal suspension concentration was adjusted to 0.5 to 2.5 × 10^3 CFU/mL. The microplate was incubated at 35 °C for 48 h. The MIC value (µg/mL) was defined as the lowest concentration that completely inhibited visible fungal growth. Negative controls consisted of 5% DMSO and RPMI 1640 broth, with fluconazole serving as the standard antifungal agent.

3.7. Antibiofilm Activity

The antibiofilm activity of the extracts against *Pseudomonas aeruginosa* PAO1 was evaluated using the crystal violet assay, based on an in vitro microplate-based biofilm model. Before the test, the MIC values of the extracts were determined against *P. aeruginosa* PAO1 [20,21].

For biofilm formation, *P. aeruginosa* PAO1 was cultured in Brain Heart Infusion (BHI) broth at 37 °C for 24 h. Final inoculum suspensions (~10^6 CFU/mL) were prepared in BHI enriched with 2% sucrose. In total, 100 µL of the inoculum suspensions were added to 96-well microtiter plates for all test conditions. The plates were incubated at 37 °C for 72 h to allow the formation of mature biofilms.

After biofilm formation, the medium was aspirated, and non-adherent cells were removed by washing the wells with sterile phosphate-buffered saline (PBS, pH 7.2). Subsequently, 100 µL of plant extracts were added to each well containing the mature *P. aeruginosa* biofilms. The plates were incubated at 37 °C for 24 h. After incubation, the wells were washed with PBS to remove non-adherent cells and dried at room temperature for 1 h. An amount of 100 µL of 0.5% crystal violet solution was added to each well to stain the biofilm cells. After 30 min, the wells were washed three times with PBS, and a 30:70 (*v/v*) acetone-alcohol solution was added to dissolve the bound dye within the biofilm matrix. BHI broth enriched with 2% sucrose was used as the control. The optical density (OD) of the dissolved crystal violet was measured at 620 nm using a microplate reader (Thermo Scientific Multiskan GO Microplate Spectrophotometer, Vantaa, Finland). The percentage biofilm inhibition values were calculated using the following formula:

$$\text{Biofilm Inhibition (\%)} = [(\text{OD (Growth control)} - \text{OD (Sample)})/\text{OD (Growth control)}] \times 100$$

Data were represented as means ± SD. Statistical differences were analyzed using One-way ANOVA and Tukey's test for post-hoc comparisons with GraphPad Prism software (version 8.0, GraphPad, Boston, MA, USA).

3.8. Anti-Quorum Sensing Activity

The anti-quorum sensing (anti-QS) activity of the plant extracts was evaluated using the disc diffusion method with *Chromobacterium violaceum* ATCC 12472 as the reporter strain, following the protocols described by Çiçek Polat et al. [21] and Junejo et al. [22]. Before the test, the MIC values of the extracts against *C. violaceum* ATCC 12472 were determined.

An overnight bacterial culture was prepared, and its density was adjusted to 1.5 × 10^8 CFU/mL. The bacterial suspension was then inoculated onto Luria-Bertani (LB) agar plates. Sterile blank discs (6 mm diameter; Bioanalyse®, Ankara, Turkey) were impregnated with 20 µL of the plant extracts and placed on the agar surface. The plates were incubated at 30 °C for 24 h. Following the incubation at 30 °C for 24 h, the plates were examined for the presence of a violacein inhibition zone. The formation of an inhibition zone around the discs indicated positive anti-QS activity.

4. Conclusions

This study presents a comprehensive investigation into the bioactivities and chemotaxonomic characteristics of four *Heracleum* species (*H. crenatifolium*, *H. paphlagonicum*, *H. sphondylium* subsp. *montanum*, and *H. pastinacifolium* subsp. *incanum*), three of which are endemic to our country, focusing on their phytochemical profiles, essential oil compositions, and some bioactivities across different plant parts.

The root extracts consistently demonstrated higher phenolic and flavonoid contents, correlating with their antioxidant activities. Among the essential oils, while it was demonstrated that octyl acetate dominated the essential oil of the fruits, myristicin was prevalent in the roots, highlighting potential ecological and functional adaptations and defining the distinctive chemical fingerprints of these species. The study also demonstrates the utility of PCA and HCA in elucidating chemotaxonomic relationships and interspecies chemical variability, offering valuable insights for further research in phylogenetics and taxonomy of the *Heracleum* genus.

The observed antimicrobial, antibiofilm, and anti-QS activities further underscore the pharmaceutical potential of these species, particularly against Gram-positive bacteria and biofilm-forming pathogens.

Future studies should expand on these findings by exploring additional plant parts, such as seeds, and investigating seasonal and geographic variations in chemical composition. Integrating morphological, anatomical, and genomic data is crucial for understanding taxonomic relationships within the genus and maximizing the pharmaceutical and industrial potential of *Heracleum* species.

Supplementary Materials: The following supporting information can be downloaded at: https://www.mdpi.com/article/10.3390/ph18040576/s1. Table S1. Total phenolic and flavonoid content and yield of methanol extracts; Table S2. Essential oil compounds of *Heracleum* species; Table S3. Studies on the essential oils of *Heracleum* spp. fruits; Table S4. Studies on the essential oils of *Heracleum* spp. aerial parts; Table S5. Studies on the essential oils of *Heracleum* spp. roots; Table S6. *P. aeruginosa* PAO1 OD values; Table S7. *P. aeruginosa* PAO1 OD values; Figure S1. The anti-QS activity of methanol extracts of four *Heracleum* species; Figure S2. The anti-QS activity of n-hexane extracts of four *Heracleum* species. References [13,26,27,33,35,37,38,40–44,46,67–86] are cited in the supplementary materials.

Author Contributions: Conceptualization, M.E., T.I.K. and C.S.K.; methodology, M.E., T.I.K., G.B.Y., D.C.P., D.K., B.D. and C.S.K.; software, M.E., D.C.P., D.K. and B.D.; validation, M.E., D.C.P., D.K. and B.D.; formal analysis, M.E., T.I.K., G.B.Y., D.C.P., D.K. and B.D.; investigation, M.E., G.B.Y., T.I.K., D.C.P., D.K. and B.D.; resources, M.E., T.I.K., D.C.P., D.K., B.D. and C.S.K.; data curation, M.E., T.I.K., G.B.Y., D.C.P., D.K., B.D. and C.S.K.; writing—original draft preparation, M.E., G.B.Y., T.I.K., D.C.P., D.K., B.D. and C.S.K.; writing—review and editing, M.E., T.I.K. and C.S.K.; visualization, M.E. and D.K.; supervision, M.E. and C.S.K.; project administration, M.E. and C.S.K.; funding acquisition, M.E., D.C.P., D.K., B.D. and C.S.K. All authors have read and agreed to the published version of the manuscript.

Funding: This research received no external funding.

Institutional Review Board Statement: Not applicable.

Informed Consent Statement: Not applicable.

Data Availability Statement: The data that support the findings of this study are available from the corresponding author upon reasonable request. The data are not publicly available due to ethical reasons, as they are part of an ongoing related project and currently under restricted access.

Acknowledgments: We are very grateful to Basar Karaca from Ankara University (Ankara, Türkiye) for his support in our study.

Conflicts of Interest: The authors declare no conflicts of interest.

References

1. Das, G.; Das, S.; Talukdar, A.D.; Venil, C.K.; Bose, S.; Banerjee, S.; Shin, H.-S.; Gutierrez-Grijalva, E.P.; Heredia, J.B.; Patra, J.K. Pharmacology and ethnomedicinal potential of selected plants species from *Apiaceae* (*Umbelliferae*). *Comb. Chem. High. Throughput Screen.* **2023**, *26*, 256–288. [PubMed]
2. Al-Jaboury, K.R. Checklist of the Umbelliferae family in the herbarium of Iraq natural history museum. *GSC Biol. Pharm. Sci.* **2021**, *15*, 177–181.
3. Kaval, U.; Tonçer, Ö. Apiaceae Lindley familyasına dâhil bitkilerin antibakteriyal, antifungal ve antiviral aktiviteleri üzerine bir derleme. *Batman Univ. J. Life Sci.* **2020**, *10*, 163–182.
4. Singh, V.; Jain, D.K. *Taxonomy of Angiosperms*, 6th ed.; Rastogi Publications: Meerut, India, 2007; p. 298.
5. Pimenov, M.G.; Leonov, M.V. The Asian Umbelliferae biodiversity database (ASIUM) with particular reference to South-West Asian taxa. *Turk. J. Bot.* **2004**, *28*, 139–145.
6. Bakış, Y.; Babaç, M.T.; Uslu, E. Updates and improvements of Turkish Plants Data Service (TÜBİVES). In Proceedings of the 6th International Symposium on Health Informatics and Bioinformatics (HIBIT), İzmir, Türkiye, 2–5 May 2011.
7. Güner, A.; Aslan, S.; Ekim, T.; Vural, M.; Babaç, M.T. *Türkiye Bitkileri Listesi (Damarlı Bitkiler)*; Nezahat Gökyiğit Botanik Bahçesi ve Flora Araştırmaları Derneği Yayını: İstanbul, Türkiye, 2012.
8. Gürbüz, P. Flavonoid glycosides from *Heracleum pastinaca* Fenzl. *Turk. J. Pharm. Sci.* **2019**, *16*, 191–195.
9. Butola, J.S.; Samant, S.S.; Vashistha, R.K.; Malik, A.R. Propagation and cultivation techniques for *Heracleum candicans* Wall.: A himalayan medicinal resource in Peril. In *Medicinal Plants and Sustainable Development*; Nova Sciences Publishers, Inc.: New Delhi, India, 2011; pp. 65–76.
10. Yazlık, A. *Heracleum* (Apiaceae) taksonlarının Türkiye'de dağılımı, çevresel ve sosyoekonomik etkileri ve önemi. *KFBD* **2021**, *11*, 544–556.
11. Bizim Bitkiler. Available online: www.bizimbitkiler.org.tr (accessed on 7 December 2024).
12. Güneş Özkan, N.; Yazlık, A.; Jabran, K. Düzce'de doğal olarak yayılış yapan *Heracleum* L. taksonları, habitatları ve bu habitatların floristik kompozisyonu. *Eurasian J. Forest Sci.* **2020**, *8*, 264–284.
13. Habibi, Z.; Eshaghi, R.; Mohammadi, M.; Yousefi, M. Chemical composition and antibacterial activity of essential oil of *Heracleum rechingeri* Manden from Iran. *Nat. Prod. Res.* **2010**, *24*, 1013–1017.
14. Hosseinzadeh, Z.; Ramazani, A.; Razzaghi-Asl, N. Plants of the genus *Heracleum* as a source of coumarin and furanocoumarin. *J. Chem. Rev.* **2019**, *1*, 78–98.
15. Kuljanabhagavad, T.; Sriubolmas, N.; Ruangrungsi, N. Chemical composition and antimicrobial activity of essential oil from *Heracleum siamicum*. *J. Health Res.* **2010**, *24*, 55–60.
16. Bahadori, M.B.; Dinparast, L.; Zengin, G. The genus *Heracleum*: A comprehensive review on its phytochemistry, pharmacology, and ethnobotanical values as a useful herb. *Compr. Rev. Food Sci. Food Saf.* **2016**, *15*, 1018–1039. [PubMed]
17. Mazandarani, M.; Makari, S.; Bajian, G.R.; Moghaddam, P.Z.; Abrodi, M. Evaluation of phytochemical and antioxidant activity in different parts of *Heracleum gorganicum* Rech. F. in Golestan province of Iran. *Iran. J. Plant Physiol.* **2012**, *2*, 381–386.
18. Antimicrobial Resistance Collaborators. Global burden of bacterial antimicrobial resistance in 2019: A systematic analysis. *Lancet* **2022**, *399*, 629–655.
19. World Health Organization. Implementation of the Global Action Plan on Antimicrobial Resistance. 2017. Available online: https://www.who.int/publications/i/item/9789240074668 (accessed on 27 November 2024).
20. Önder, A.; Rızvanoğlu, S.S.; Gündoğdu, E.F.; Demirci, B.; Eryılmaz, M. Chemical composition and antimicrobial, anti-biofilm, and anti-quorum sensing activities of *Mentha longifolia* subsp. *typhoides* essential oil. *Plant Biosyst.* **2024**, *158*, 1085–1092.
21. Çiçek Polat, D.; Gümüşok, S.; Rızvanoğlu, S.S.; Eryılmaz, M. Bioactivities of *Cotinus coggygria* and its HPLC-DAD phenolic profiles. *Plant Biosyst.* **2023**, *157*, 1061–1066.
22. Junejo, B.; Eryilmaz, M.; Rizvanoglu, S.S.; Palabiyik, I.M.; Ghumro, T.; Mallah, A.; Solangi, A.R.; Hyder, S.I.; Maleh, H.K.; Dragoi, E.N. Pharmacological assessment of Co_3O_4, CuO, NiO and ZnO nanoparticles via antibacterial, anti-biofilm and anti-quorum sensing activities. *Water Sci. Technol.* **2023**, *87*, 2840–2851.
23. Koriem, K.M.M.; Asaad, G.F.; Megahed, H.A.; Zahran, H.; Arbid, M.S. Evaluation of the antihyperlipidemic, anti-inflammatory, analgesic, and antipyretic activities of ethanolic extract of *Ammi majus* Seeds in albino rats and mice. *Int. J. Toxicol.* **2012**, *31*, 294–300.
24. Kumar, D.; Bhat, Z.A.; Kumar, V.; Shah, M.Y. Coumarins from *Angelica archangelica* Linn. and their effects on anxiety-like behavior. *Prog. Neuropsychopharmacol. Biol. Psychiatry* **2013**, *40*, 180–186.
25. Lino, C.; Taveira, M.; Viana, G.; Matos, F. Analgesic and antiinflammatory activities of *Justicia pectoralis* Jacq and its main constituents: Coumarin and umbelliferone. *Phytother. Res.* **1997**, *11*, 211–215.

26. Chu, S.S.; Cao, J.; Liu, Q.Z.; Du, S.S.; Deng, Z.W.; Liu, Z.L. Chemical composition and insecticidal activity of *Heracleum moellendorffii* Hance essential oil. *Chemija* **2012**, *23*, 108–112.
27. Chauhan, R.S.; Nautiyal, M.C.; Tava, A.; Cecotti, R. Essential oil composition from leaves of *Heracleum candicans* Wall.: A sustainable method for extraction. *J. Essent. Oil Res.* **2014**, *26*, 130–132.
28. Uysal, A.; Özer, Ö.Y.; Zengin, G.; Stefanucci, A.; Mollica, A.; Picot-Allain, C.M.N.; Mahomoodally, M.F. Multifunctional approaches to provide potential pharmacophores for the pharmacy shelf: *Heracleum sphondylium* L. subsp. *ternatum* (Velen.) Brummitt. *Comput. Biol. and Chem.* **2019**, *78*, 64–73.
29. Ocal, M.; Altunoglu, Y.C.; Angeloni, S.; Mustafa, A.M.; Caprioli, G.; Zengin, G.; Paksoy, M.Y.; Baloglu, M.C. Comparative content, biological and anticancer activities of *Heracleum humile* extracts obtained by ultrasound-assisted extraction method. *Chem. Biodivers.* **2022**, *19*, e202101040.
30. Ghavam, M. *Heracleum persicum* Desf. ex Fisch., C.A. Mey. & Avé-Lall. fruit essential oil: Content, antimicrobial activity and cytotoxicity against ovarian cancer cell line. *BMC Complement. Med. Ther.* **2023**, *23*, 87.
31. Wu, Z.; Zhong, A.; Shen, P.; Zhu, J.; Li, L.; Xia, G.; Zang, H. Chemical constituents, antioxidant and antibacterial activities of essential oil from the flowering aerial parts of *Heracleum moellendorffii* Hance. *Cogent Food Agric.* **2024**, *10*, 2325198.
32. İşcan, G.; Demirci, F.; Kürkçüoğlu, M.; Kıvanç, M.; Can Başer, K. The bioactive essential oil of *Heracleum sphondylium* L. subsp. *ternatum* (Velen.) *Brummitt. Z. Für Naturforschung C* **2003**, *58*, 195–200.
33. Firuzi, O.; Asadollahi, M.; Gholami, M.; Javidnia, K. Composition and biological activities of essential oils from four *Heracleum* species. *Food Chem.* **2010**, *122*, 117–122.
34. Matejic, J.S.; Dzamic, A.M.; Mihajilov-Krstev, T.; Ristic, M.S.; Randelovic, V.N.; Krisovej, Z.D.; Marin, P.D. Chemical composition, antioxidant and antimicrobial properties of essential oil and extracts from *Heracleum sphondylium* L. *J. Essent. Oil Bear. Pl.* **2016**, *19*, 944–953.
35. Hajhashemi, V.; Sajjadi, S.E.; Heshmati, M. Anti-inflammatory and analgesic properties of *Heracleum persicum* essential oil and hydroalcoholic extract in animal models. *J. Ethnopharmacol.* **2009**, *124*, 475–480.
36. Radjabian, T.; Salimi, A.; Rahmani, N.; Shockravi, A.; Mozaffarian, V. Essential oil composition of some wild populations of *Heracleum persicum* Desf. Ex *Fischer* growing in Iran. *J. Essent. Oil Bear. Pl.* **2013**, *16*, 841–849.
37. Radjabian, T.; Salimi, A.; Rahmani, N. Essential-oil composition of the fruits of six *Heracleum* L. species from Iran: Chemotaxonomic significance. *Chem. Biodivers.* **2014**, *11*, 1945–1953.
38. Usjak, L.J.; Drobac, M.M.; Niketić, M.S.; Petrović, S.D. Chemosystematic significance of essential oil constituents and furanocoumarins of underground parts and fruits of nine *Heracleum* L. taxa from Southeastern Europe. *Chem. Biodivers.* **2018**, *15*, e1800412.
39. Jahodová, Š.; Trybush, S.; Pyšek, P.; Wade, M.; Karp, A. Invasive species of *Heracleum* in Europe: An insight into genetic relationships and invasion history. *Divers. Distrib.* **2007**, *13*, 99–114.
40. Tkachenko, K.G. Essential oils from leaves of several *Heracleum* species growing in Leningrad oblast. *Chem. Nat. Compd.* **2010**, *46*, 319–321.
41. Usjak, L.; Petrović, S.; Drobac, M.; Soković, M.; Stanojković, T.; Ćirić, A.; Niketić, M. Chemical composition and bioactivity of the essential oils of *Heracleum pyrenaicum* subsp. *pollinianum* and *Heracleum orphanidis*. *Nat. Prod. Commun.* **2016**, *11*, 1934578X1601100428.
42. Tkachenko, K.G. Composition of the essential oils of *Heracleum stevenii* Manden. *J. Essent. Oil Res.* **1994**, *6*, 535–537.
43. George, V.; Chacko, S.; Sethuraman, M.G. Chemical composition of the essential oil from the rhizomes of *Heracleum candolleanum*. *J. Essent. Oil Res.* **2001**, *13*, 80–81.
44. Karuppusamy, S.; Muthuraja, G. Chemical composition and antioxidant activity of *Heracleum sprengelianum* (Wight and Arnott) essential oils growing wild in peninsular India. *Iran. J. Pharm. Res.* **2011**, *10*, 769.
45. Fan, S.; Chang, J.; Zong, Y.; Hu, G.; Jia, J. GC-MS analysis of the composition of the essential oil from *Dendranthema indicum* var. *aromaticum* using three extraction methods and two columns. *Molecules* **2018**, *23*, 576.
46. Özek, T.; Özek, G.; Baser, K.H.C.; Duran, A. Comparison of the essential oils of three endemic Turkish *Heracleum* species obtained by different isolation techniques. *J. Essent. Oil Res.* **2005**, *17*, 605–610.
47. Fierascu, R.C.; Padure, I.M.; Avramecu, S.M.; Ungureanu, C.; Bunghez, R.I.; Ortan, A.; Dinu-pirvu, C.; Fierascu, I.; Soare, L.C. Preliminary assessment of the antioxidant, antifungal and germination inhibitory potential of *Heracleum sphondylium* L. (APIACEAE). *Farmacia* **2016**, *64*, 3.
48. Cowan, M.M. Plant products as antimicrobial agents. *Clin. Microbiol. Rev.* **1999**, *12*, 564–582. [PubMed]
49. Khameneh, B.; Eskin, N.A.M.; Iranshahy, M.; Fazly Bazzaz, B.S. Phytochemicals: A promising weapon in the Arsenal against antibiotic-resistant bacteria. *Antibiotics* **2021**, *10*, 1044. [CrossRef] [PubMed]
50. Lobiuc, A.; Pavăl, N.-E.; Mangalagiu, I.I.; Gheorghiță, R.; Teliban, G.-C.; Amăriucăi-Mantu, D.; Stoleru, V. Future antimicrobials: Natural and functionalized phenolics. *Molecules* **2023**, *28*, 1114. [CrossRef] [PubMed]

51. Biharee, A.; Sharma, A.; Kumar, A.; Jaitak, V. Antimicrobial flavonoids as a potential substitute for overcoming antimicrobial resistance. *Fitoterapia* **2020**, *146*, 104720.
52. Nikaido, H. Molecular basis of bacterial outer membrane permeability revisited. *Microbiol. Mol. Biol. Rev.* **2003**, *67*, 593–656.
53. Miklasińska-Majdanik, M.; Kępa, M.; Wojtyczka, R.D.; Idzik, D.; Wąsik, T.J. Phenolic compounds diminish antibiotic resistance of *Staphylococcus aureus* clinical strains. *Int. J. Environ. Res. Public Health* **2018**, *15*, 2321. [CrossRef]
54. Buruk, K.; Sokmen, A.; Aydin, F.; Erturk, M. Antimicrobial activity of some endemic plants growing in the Eastern Black Sea Region, Turkey. *Fitoterapia* **2006**, *77*, 388–391.
55. Cushnie, T.P.; Lamb, A.J. Recent advances in understanding the antibacterial properties of flavonoids. *Int. J. Antimicrob. Agents* **2011**, *38*, 99–107.
56. Xie, Y.; Yang, W.; Tang, F.; Chen, X.; Ren, L. Antibacterial activities of flavonoids: Structure-activity relationship and mechanism. *Curr. Med. Chem.* **2015**, *22*, 132–149.
57. Bouhrour, N.; Nibbering, P.H.; Bendali, F. Medical device-associated biofilm infections and multidrug-resistant pathogens. *Pathogens* **2024**, *13*, 393. [CrossRef] [PubMed]
58. Büyüktuncel, E. Main spectrophotometric methods for the determination of total phenolic content and antioxidant capacity. *Marmara Pharm. J.* **2013**, *17*, 93–103.
59. Demir, F.; Aliyazıcıoğlu, Y.; Demir, S. Asidifikasyon işleminin *Laurocerasus officinalis* ekstraktlarının antioksidan özellikleri üzerine etkisinin incelenmesi. *El-Cezeri* **2017**, *4*, 365–373.
60. Keskin, S.; Sirin, Y.; Cakir, H.E.; Kaya, G.; Keskin, M. Phenolic composition and antioxidant properties of *Spiraea nipponica*. *Int. J. Sci. Technol. Res.* **2019**, *5*, 87–92.
61. *European Pharmacopoeia*, 5th ed.; Council of Europe: Strasbourg, France, 2005; Volume 1, p. 217.
62. Demirci, B.; Kırcı, D.; Öztürk, G.; Demirci, F. Effect of extraction time on *Origanum onites* L. infusions and essential oils—biological evaluation, statistical principal component and hierarchial cluster analyses. *Chem. Biodivers.* **2022**, *19*, e202200482.
63. Blois, M.S. Antioxidant determinations by the use of a stable free radical. *Nature* **1958**, *181*, 1199–1200.
64. Re, R.; Pellegrini, N.; Proteggente, A.; Pannala, A.; Yang, M.; Rice-Evans, C. Antioxidant activity applying an improved ABTS radical cation decolorization assay. *Free Radic. Biol. Med.* **1999**, *26*, 1231–1237.
65. *CLSI Standard M07*; Methods for Dilution Antimicrobial Susceptibility Tests for Bacteria That Grow Aerobically, 11th ed. Clinical and Laboratory Standards Institute (CLSI): Wayne, PA, USA, 2018.
66. *CLSI Standard M27*; Reference Method for Broth Dilution Antifungal Susceptibility Testing of Yeasts, 4th ed. Clinical and Laboratory Standards Institute (CLSI): Wayne, PA, USA, 2017.
67. Maggi, F.; Quassinti, L.; Bramucci, M.; Lupidi, G.; Petrelli, D.; Vitali, L.A.; Papa, F.; Vittori, S. Composition and biological activities of hogweed [*Heracleum sphondylium* L. subsp. *ternatum* (Velen.) Brummitt] essential oil and its main components octyl acetate and octyl butyrate. *Nat. Prod. Res.* **2014**, *28*, 1354–1363.
68. Pirbalouti, A.G.; Sedaghat, L.; Hamedi, B.; Tirgir, F. Chemical composition and antioxidant activity of essential oils of three endemic medicinal plants of Iran. *Bangladesh J. Bot.* **2014**, *42*, 327–332.
69. Akcin, A.; Seyis, F.; Akcin, T.A.; Cayci, Y.T.; Coban, A.Y. Chemical composition and antimicrobial activity of the essential oil of endemic *Heracleum platytaenium* Boiss. from Turkey. *J. Essent. Oil Bear. Pl.* **2013**, *16*, 166–171.
70. Özkırım, A.; Keskin, N.; Kürkçüoğlu, M.; Başer, K.H.C. Evaluation of some essential oils as alternative antibiotics against American foulbrood agent *Paenibacillus larvae* on honey bees *Apis mellifera* L. *J. Essent. Oil Res.* **2012**, *24*, 465–470. [CrossRef]
71. Kuljanabhagavad, T.; Sriubolmas, N.; Ruangrungsi, N. Chemical composition, antibacterial and antifungal activities of essential oil from *Heracleum siamicum* Craib. *Pharm. Chem. J.* **2011**, *45*, 178–182.
72. Tosun, F.; Kızılay, Ç.A.; Erol, K.; Kılıç, F.S.; Kürkçüoğlu, M.; Başer, K.H.C. Anticonvulsant activity of furanocoumarins and the essential oil obtained from the fruits of *Heracleum crenatifolium*. *Food Chem.* **2008**, *107*, 990–993. [CrossRef]
73. John, A.J.; Karunakaran, V.P.; George, V.; Sethuraman, M.G. Chemical composition of leaf and fruit oils of *Heracleum candolleanum*. *J. Essent. Oil Res.* **2007**, *19*, 358–359. [CrossRef]
74. Iscan, G.; Ozek, T.; Ozek, G.; Duran, A.; Baser, K.H.C. Essential oils of three species of *Heracleum*. anticandidal activity. *Chem. Nat. Compd.* **2004**, *40*, 544–547. [CrossRef]
75. Baser, K.H.C.; Kürkçüoglu, M.; Adigüzel, N.; Aytaç, Z.; Joulain, D.; Laurent, R. Composition of the essential oil of *Heracleum paphlagonicum* Czeczott. *J. Essent. Oil Res.* **2000**, *12*, 385–386. [CrossRef]
76. Mishyna, M.; Laman, N.; Prokhorov, V.; Maninang, J.S.; Fujii, Y. Identification of octanal as plant growth inhibitory volatile compound released from *Heracleum sosnowskyi* fruit. *Nat. Prod. Commun.* **2015**, *10*, 771–774. [CrossRef]
77. Özdemir, F.G.G.; Tosun, B.; Şanlı, A.; Karadoğan, T. Bazı *Apiaceae* uçucu yağlarının *Meloidogyne incognita* (Kofoid & White, 1919) Chitwood, 1949 (Nematoda: *Meloidogynidae*)'ya karşı nematoksik etkisi. *Ege Üniv Ziraat Fak Derg* **2022**, *59*, 529–539.
78. Hasheminya, S.M.; Dehghannya, J. Chemical composition, antioxidant, antibacterial, and antifungal properties of essential oil from wild *Heracleum rawianum*. *Biocatal. Agric. Biotechnol.* **2021**, *31*, 101913.

79. Yılmaz, A.; Çiftçi, V. Determination of essential oil composition of naturally growing *Heracleum platytaenium* L. plant in Bolu ecological conditions. *ISPEC J. Agric. Sci.* **2021**, *5*, 344–349.
80. Shokri, H.; Sharifzadeh, A.; Tamai, I.A. Anti-Candida zeylanoides activity of some Iranian plants used in traditional medicine. *J. Mycol. Med.* **2012**, *22*, 211–216. [CrossRef] [PubMed]
81. Guleria, S.; Saini, R.; Jaitak, V.; Kaul, V.K.; Lal, B.; Rahi, P.; Gulati, A.; Singh, B. Composition and antimicrobial activity of the essential oil of *Heracleum thomsonii* (Clarke) from the cold desert of the western Himalayas. *Nat. Prod. Res.* **2011**, *25*, 1250–1260. [CrossRef] [PubMed]
82. Li Wei, L.W.; Chen LinLin, C.L.; Wu Chun, W.C.; Xin JiaYing, X.J. Analysis of the essential oil from seed of *Heracleum moellendorffii* Hance cultivated in northeast China. *Asian J. Chem.* **2013**, *25*, 4701–4702. [CrossRef]
83. Miladinović, D.L.; Ilić, B.S.; Mihajilov-Krstev, T.M.; Nikolić, D.M.; Cvetković, O.G.; Marković, M.S.; Miladinović, L.C. Antibacterial activity of the essential oil of *Heracleum sibiricum*. *Nat. Prod. Commun.* **2013**, *8*, 1309–1311. [CrossRef]
84. Torbati, M.; Nazemiyeh, H.; Lotfipour, F.; Asnaashari, S.; Nemati, M.; Fathiazad, F. Composition and antibacterial activity of *Heracleum transcaucasicum* and *Heracleum anisactis* aerial parts essential oil. *Adv. Pharm. Bull.* **2013**, *3*, 415–418.
85. Papageorgiou, V.P.; Ochir, G.; Motl, O.; Argyriadou, N.; Dunkel, H. Composition of the essential oil from *Heracleum dissectum*. *J. Nat. Prod.* **1985**, *48*, 851–853. [CrossRef]
86. Sefidkon, F.; Dabiri, M.; Mohammad, N. Analysis of the oil of *Heracleum persicum* L. (leaves and flowers). *J. Essent. Oil Res.* **2002**, *14*, 295–297. [CrossRef]

pharmaceuticals

MDPI

Article

Antimicrobial and Antiherpetic Properties of Nanoencapsulated *Hypericum perforatum* Extract

Yoana Sotirova [1], Nadezhda Ivanova [1,*], Neli Ermenlieva [2], Neli Vilhelmova-Ilieva [3], Lora Simeonova [3], Miroslav Metodiev [3], Viliana Gugleva [1] and Velichka Andonova [1]

[1] Department of Pharmaceutical Technologies, Faculty of Pharmacy, Medical University of Varna, 9000 Varna, Bulgaria; yoana.sotirova@mu-varna.bg (Y.S.); viliana.gugleva@mu-varna.bg (V.G.); velichka.andonova@mu-varna.bg (V.A.)

[2] Department of Microbiology and Virology, Faculty of Medicine, Medical University of Varna, 9000 Varna, Bulgaria; neli.ermenlieva@mu-varna.bg

[3] Department of Virology, Stephan Angeloff Institute of Microbiology, Bulgarian Academy of Sciences, 26 G. Bonchev Str., 1113 Sofia, Bulgaria; nelivili@gmail.com (N.V.-I.); losimeonova@gmail.com (L.S.); mnmetodiev@microbio.bas.bg (M.M.)

* Correspondence: nadejda.ivanova@mu-varna.bg

Abstract

Background/Objectives: This study aims to gain insights into the antimicrobial and antiherpetic activity of hyperforin-rich *Hypericum perforatum* L. (HP) extract using nanostructured lipid carriers (NLCs) as delivery platforms. **Methods**: Two established NLC specimens, comprising glyceryl behenate and almond oil or borage oil, and their extract-loaded counterparts (HP-NLCs) were utilized. Their minimal bactericidal/fungicidal concentrations (MBC; MFC) were investigated against *Escherichia coli* ATCC 25922, *Staphylococcus aureus* ATCC 25923, *Pseudomonas aeruginosa* ATCC 10145, *Klebsiella pneumoniae* ATCC 10031, and *Candida albicans* ATCC 10231. The anti-herpesvirus (HSV-1) potential was evaluated concerning antiviral and virucidal activity and impact on viral adsorption. **Results**: The borage oil-based extract-loaded nanodispersion (HP-NLC2) exhibited pronounced microbicidal activity against *S. aureus* (MBC 6.3 mg/mL), *K. pneumoniae* (MBC 97.7 μg/mL), and *C. albicans* (MFC < 48.8 μg/mL), unlike the almond oil-containing sample (HP-NLC1), which showed only weak inhibition of the fungal growth. HP-NLC2 was found to be less cytotoxic and to suppress HSV-1 replication slightly more than HP-NLC1, but generally, the effects were weak. Neither the empty lipid nanoparticles nor the HP extract-loaded carriers expressed activity against *E. coli*, *P. aeruginosa*, the HSV-1 extracellular virions, or viral adhesion. **Conclusions**: It could be concluded that both HP-NLC samples revealed only minor antiherpetic potential of the hyperforin-rich extract, but HP-NLC2 demonstrated significant antibacterial and antimycotic activity. Therefore, the latter was featured as a more convenient HP-carrier system for nano-designed dermal pharmaceutical formulations. Such a thorough investigation of hyperforin-determined anti-HSV-1 effects and antibacterial and antimycotic properties, being the first of its kind, contributes to the fundamental knowledge of HP and reveals new perspectives for the utilization, limitations, and therapeutic designation of its non-polar components.

Keywords: antibacterial activity; antifungal activity; antimicrobial activity; antiviral activity; herpesvirus; hyperforin; lipid nanoparticles; nanostructured lipid carriers; phloroglucinols; St. John's wort

 https://doi.org/10.3390/ph18030366

1. Introduction

St. John's wort (*Hypericum perforatum* L.; HP) has a history as a medicinal plant dating back to ancient times. Apart from its well-known application in mental disorders (depression, melancholy, anxiety, and hyperarousal), it has also been used for treating various skin pathologies such as hemorrhages, infections, inflammations, burns, wounds, bruises, etc. [1–3]. The technological evolution in scientific research satisfies the growing interest in the herb; multiple biochemical, pharmacological, pharmacokinetic, and clinical trials have been conducted and have identified its antioxidant, anti-inflammatory, antibacterial, and antiviral properties, as well as the mechanisms underlying them [4–7]. Moreover, after a detailed phytochemical analysis, it has been revealed that several groups of biologically active compounds (BACs) in St. John's wort contribute to these effects, viz., phloroglucinols, naphthodianthrones, phenolic acids and depsides, flavonoids, and xanthones [8,9].

Concerning the antibacterial activity of HP, phloroglucinols and naphthodianthrones stand out as the main microbicidal constituents (Figure 1) [5]. Numerous studies testify to the pronounced effect of the herb against Gram-positive bacteria. Among the most susceptible representatives are reported to be *Staphylococcus aureus* (including methicillin-resistant strains), *Bacillus cereus*, and *Enterococcus faecalis* [10–12]. Most of the research indicates an absence of activity of St. John's wort preparations against Gram-negative bacteria and fungi [13–16]. However, some reports contradict the latter statement by reporting antimicrobial effects against *Escherichia coli*, *Klebsiella pneumoniae*, *Pseudomonas aeruginosa*, and *Candida albicans* [12,17,18].

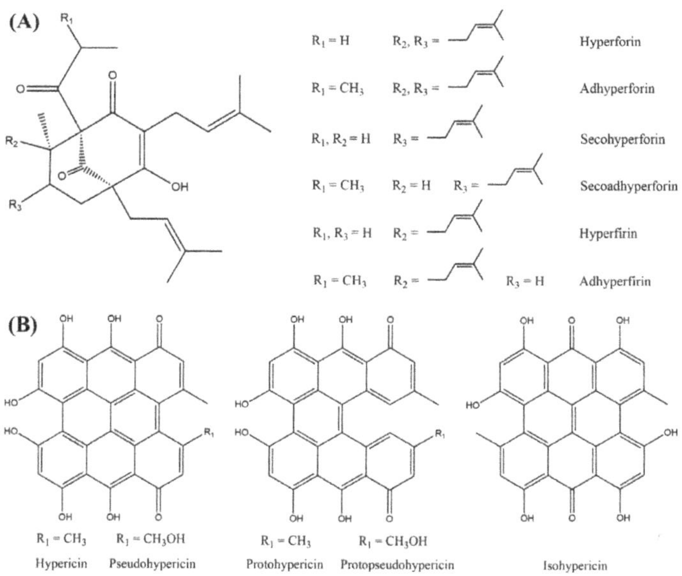

Figure 1. Chemical structures of the main phloroglucinols (**A**) and naphthodianthrones (**B**) present in *Hypericum perforatum* L.

As for the antiviral properties of St. John's wort, the herbal substance is reported to be effective against encapsulated viruses—HIV-1, Influenza Virus Type A, Avian Infectious Bronchitis Virus, SARS-CoV-2, as well as others [7,19–21]. Interestingly, only naphthodianthrones (hypericin, pseudohypericin) have been tested and proven to exhibit anti-herpesvirus activity. Their action is determined to a significant extent by photoactivation upon daylight exposure [22]. However, when activated in the presence of oxygen, naphthodianthrones become powerful generators of singlet oxygen, superoxide anions, and other reactive oxygen species. The latter activate various cytotoxic cascades in cells, the ultimate result of which is cell death. This effect is used in the so-called photodynamic therapy but may turn into a "defect" in other skin pathological conditions [23].

A major hindrance to the topical application of HP phloroglucinols is their inherent chemical instability. In particular, the main phytochemical from that class, hyperforin, is photosensitive and highly reactive to oxygen [24]. A successful approach for preserving such labile BACs is their incorporation into nanoscale drug-delivery systems. Among the first such created were polymer and metal nanoparticles, liposomes, and nanoemulsions [25]. In the early 1990s, the Müller and Gasco teams pioneered the idea of solid lipid nanoparticles (SLNs) [26,27]. SLNs are presented as a safer, non-toxic alternative to other types of nanoparticles. Moreover, they are physically more stable than liposomes and, in addition, their production is more cost-effective [28]. SLNs have a solid lipid core surrounded by a stabilizing surfactant layer. Their key advantages as drug carriers are biocompatibility, biodegradability, lack of toxicity, and the possibility of modified drug release [29]. Their main disadvantages, namely low drug-loading capacity and rapid drug release, are related to their highly organized crystalline lipid matrix [30]. To overcome the aforementioned drawbacks of SLNs, the so-called nanostructured lipid carriers (NLCs) were subsequently introduced [31]. In contrast to SLNs, their stability is increased, and their drug-loading capacity is much higher as well. The NLCs' superiority over SLNs is determined by the liquid lipids included in the cores of the former [30].

Our previous work aimed to obtain a hyperforin-rich St. John's wort extract and incorporate it into a suitable NLC system prior to topical application in wound healing [32,33]. To the best of our knowledge, our study on isolating and "preserving" such an extract by a lipid nanocarrier-based approach is the first of its kind. The herein presented work on the antimicrobial activity of the nanocarriers in question is also sui generis. We have already proven the wound-healing properties of HP-NLCs. Here, we aim to further emphasize their therapeutic importance by investigating their effect against "classic" pathogens causing wound infections—*S. aureus*, *E. coli*, *K. pneumoniae*, *P. aeruginosa*, and *C. albicans*. We also believe that preserving the main phloroglucinol in the extract via nanoencapsulation would allow us to acquire insights into its anti-herpesvirus potential.

2. Results

2.1. "Blank" and HP-Loaded NLCs

All data concerning the HP extraction, NLC formulation, and characterization have already been published elsewhere [32,33]. We summarize herein some of the critical findings that could be related to the current results.

The concentration of hyperforin in the HP extracts was found to be 8.9 μg/mL, i.e., its extraction yield was 44.35%; knowing that, the hyperforin content, and not the total HP extract content, was applied for the calculation of the entrapment efficiency (EE) [32]. The HP extract was incorporated into the NLCs in a concentration of 1.25% (*w*/*w*) as according to the Attenuated Total Reflectance (ATR)-FTIR study, higher amounts led to the formation of extract–nanoparticle co-aggregates [32]. The "blank" nanodispersions (NLC1 and NLC2) were observed as milky-white liquids, while the HP-loaded ones (HP-NLC1 and HP-NLC2) inherited the extract's green shade (Figure 2A). Dynamic Light Scattering (DLS) analysis revealed an initial mean hydrodynamic size of about 150 nm (Figure 2B). The EE (%), derived from the ratio of the theoretically loaded hyperforin to the actual HPLC-detected hyperforin, was in the range of 70.44–74.49% (Figure 2C). Further, Transmission Electron Microscopy (TEM) discovered the particles' irregular shape and well-defined core and shell. In the presence of the plant extract, the bilayer structure of the nanoparticles appeared to be more amorphous, but the encapsulation did not affect their matrix organization or integrity (Figure 2D). Except for HP-NLC1, the nanocarriers retained their average particle diameter below 200 nm during one month of storage at 4 °C (Figure 2B). The almond oil-based extract-loaded nanoplatforms also demonstrated a significant deterioration of homogeneity, expressed as the highest polydispersity index (Figure 2B). Moreover, their ability to encapsulate and preserve HP extract was also lower than that of HP-NLC2. However, in the search of a better choice for the most suitable HP carrier, despite the obvious advantageous physicochemical properties of the borage-based HP-NLC specimen so far, we decided to subject both samples to antimicrobial and antiviral tests.

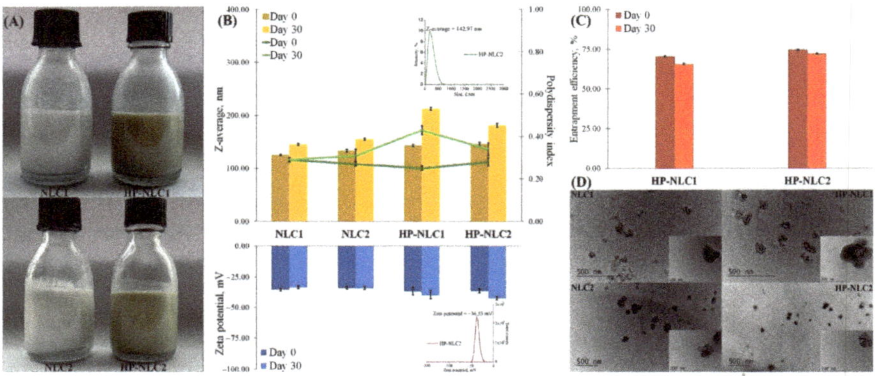

Figure 2. Physicochemical characteristics of "blank" and hyperforin-rich HP extract-loaded lipid nanoparticles. Subfigure (**A**) presents the visual appearance of the obtained lipid nanodispersions. The extract-loaded ones were stored in amber glass vials but were photographed in transparent ones to display their qualitative characteristics. Mean particle size (Z-average), polydispersity index, zeta potential (**B**), and entrapment efficiency (**C**) of the nanoparticles were assessed immediately after their preparation and after 30-day storage at 4 °C. Subfigure (**D**) demonstrates the shape and inner morphology of the nanocarriers. Data from the study of Sotirova et al. [32] were used for constructing the figure.

2.2. Antiviral Activity

Before conducting the antiviral experiments, we established the non-toxic range of the investigated samples to exclude a toxic effect on the cells. NLC1 and NLC2 showed no toxicity even at the highest concentration tested. Nanoparticles carrying the active extract showed cytotoxicity close to that of the reference Acyclovir {[9-(2-hydroxyethoxymethyl)-guanine]; ACV}, but slightly stronger—in the range of 2.5–3 times more toxic. HP-NLC2 demonstrated lower cytotoxicity against Madin–Darbey bovine kidney (MDBK) cells compared with HP-NLC1 (Table 1).

Table 1. Cytotoxicity and antiviral activity of the HP-loaded test samples.

Sample	MDBK Cell Line		HSV-1 (Victoria Strain)	
	CC_{50} Mean ± SD (µg/mL)	MTC (µg/mL)	IC_{50} Mean ± SD (µg/mL)	SI
HP-NLC1	87.5 ± 2.3 **	12.5	25.3 ± 2.2 **	3.5
HP-NLC2	94.7± 3.6 *	12.5	23.7 ± 2.1 **	4.0
ACV	291.0 ± 9.4	nd	0.33 ± 0.03	881.8

CC_{50}—cytotoxic concentrations 50%; SD—standard deviation; MTC—maximum tolerable concentration; IC_{50}—inhibitory concentration 50%; SI—selectivity index, which was calculated from the CC_{50}/IC_{50} ratio; nd—no data; * $p < 0.05$—when comparing the value of each compound with the reference substance ACV; ** $p < 0.001$—when comparing the value of each compound with the reference substance ACV.

The anti-herpesvirus activity of the studied nanocarriers was determined within the defined non-toxic concentration range. The two "blank" specimens did not show any effect on human herpes simplex virus type 1 (HSV-1) replication. The two samples loaded with the extract demonstrated a weak effect on the viral replication of HSV-1 with selectivity index (SI) ≤ 4. However, a stronger effect was established for HP-NLC2 with SI = 4.0 (Table 1).

"Blank" and loaded NLCs were also examined for their impact on extracellular HSV-1 virions. The effect was monitored for different time intervals within 120 min. In all the time intervals studied, none of the samples induced a significant drop in the viral titer (Table 2), indicating that they act only as carriers that do not release the extract outside the cell.

Table 2. Virucidal activity of the test samples against HSV-1 virions (Victoria strain).

Sample	Δlg				
	15 min	**30 min**	**45 min**	**60 min**	**120 min**
NLC1	0.5	0.5	0.5	0.5	0.5
HP-NLC1	1.0	1.0	1.0	1.0	1.0
NLC2	0.5	0.5	0.5	0.5	0.5
HP-NLC2	0.5	0.5	0.75	0.75	0.75
70% ethanol	8.0	8.0	8.0	8.0	7.75

The results obtained so far show that the effect of HP-NLCs occurs only intracellularly, but we decided to check the possibility that they have an effect on the step of virus adsorption by influencing the cell membrane and the binding of cell receptors to the viral structures responsible for the attachment of the virus to the cell. Time intervals of different duration within the viral adsorption (60 min) were investigated. None of the samples showed an effect on this stage at any of the time intervals examined (Table 3). This is more evidence that the studied nanocarriers exert their effect only intracellularly.

Table 3. Influence of the test samples on the stage of adsorption of HSV-1 (Victoria strain) to sensitive MDBK cells.

Sample	Δlg			
	15 min	**30 min**	**45 min**	**60 min**
NLC1	0.25	0.25	0.25	0.5
HP-NLC1	0.25	0.25	0.5	0.5
NLC2	0.0	0.25	0.25	0.5
HP-NLC2	0.25	0.25	0.5	0.75

2.3. *Antimicrobial and Antifungal Activity*

During this study, all test tubes acquired the opaque off-white appearance inherent in the NLC/HP-NLC suspensions; therefore, determination of minimal inhibitory concentrations by visual assessment of microbial growth-related turbidity was not possible. As a next step, minimal bactericidal/fungicidal concentrations (MBC; MFC) were recorded after transfer to blood agar and another incubation. The NLCs themselves (or their components within the composition) were not found to possess any activity against the targeted pathogenic microorganisms (Figure 3). The control antimicrobial agent, chlorhexidine diacetate, showed MBCs of 35.3 μg/mL (*S. aureus*), 141.2 μg/mL (*E. coli*), 564.8 μg/mL (*K. pneumoniae*), 1130.0 μg/mL (*C. albicans*), and 2260.0 μg/mL (*P. aeruginosa*).

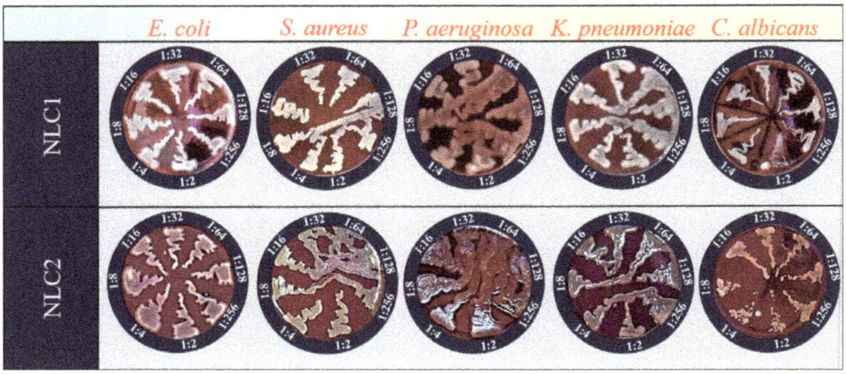

Figure 3. Antibacterial and antifungal activity of the "blank" NLC samples.

HP-NLC2 demonstrated a distinct microbicidal effect against *K. pneumoniae* and *C. albicans*, with MBC/MFC of 97.7 µg/mL (dilution 1:128) and <48.8 µg/mL (dilution 1:256), respectively. A weaker but still present activity of the nanosuspension in question was recorded against *S. aureus*, with an MBC of 6.3 mg/mL (dilution 1:2) (Figure 4). No antimicrobial activity was established in the extract-loaded nanoparticles against the Gram-negative *E. coli* and *P. aeruginosa*.

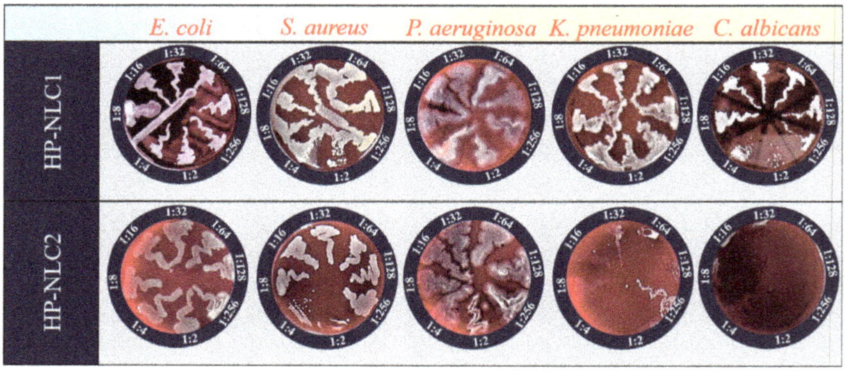

Figure 4. Antibacterial and antifungal activity of the HP-NLC samples.

3. Discussion

The results so obtained testify that the established antimicrobial and anti-herpesvirus action of HP-NLCs is owing to the hyperforin-rich extract and not to the delivery nanoplatforms employed. However, because of the main compound's extreme chemical instability, the formulation of the extract into the nano-sized lipid particles could be regarded as a requirement for the activity to be manifested. This observation only highlights the practical importance of the current study and the obtained results. Moreover, it explains the reason why standard hyperforin-rich extract cannot be used as a reference formulation.

An ideal nanocarrier system should provide physical endurance over time, high loading capacity, chemical inertness, drug stability or stabilization, lack of toxicity, biocompatibility, and expedient drug permeation and release [34]. According to our previous and current results, the formulation HP-NLC2 fulfills all these criteria and also contributes to an explicit potentiation of the antibacterial and antimycotic activities against *K. pneumoniae*, *S. aureus*, and *C. albicans*. A reasonable explanation for this phenomenon might be sought in the presence of borage oil as the liquid lipid in the nanocarriers' composition.

Several scientific reports have confirmed its antimicrobial action, as well as that of its major polyunsaturated fatty acids, i.e., linoleic and γ-linolenic acids [35], including against the herein-investigated pathogens [36–38]. It is likely that the relative content of borage oil within the lipid nanoparticles was below its minimal inhibitory concentrations, and because of this, we did not observe its own antimicrobial effect when applying the "empty" NLC2 sample. We hypothesize that the oil's permeation-enhancing properties [39] may also have reinforced the HP extract's activity by facilitating its intracellular passage through the bacterial walls.

The results of any preferential mechanism of action of the hyperforin-rich extract against Gram-positive or Gram-negative pathogens remain inconclusive. It is evident that along with *C. albicans*, the Gram-negative *K. pneumoniae* stands out as the most susceptible to the extract's action, while the Gram-positive *S. aureus* is affected at much higher doses. Still, the other Gram-negative representatives in this study, *E. coli* and *P. aeruginosa*, demonstrated resistance to the extract's action in the applied doses. Low susceptibility to antimicrobial agents is unique to *P. aeruginosa*. Its rich resistome, multiple efflux systems, and ability to form biofilms contribute to its high resistance [40]. In addition, the lipopolysaccharides and porin proteins in its outer membrane are distinct from those of the Enterobacteriaceae family, which also ensures its much lower permeability to exogenous substances [41].

There are numerous extraction solvents and techniques that could be applied for the production of St. John's wort extracts, and they all result in a highly differentiating qualitative and quantitative content of BACs. Unless the herbal preparations are traditional or standardized, their established effects are hard to relate to any other data from the scientific literature [42]. In this regard, directive 2004/24/EC of the European Parliament and of the Council provides a list of several traditional HP preparations. These include the dry extract obtained with the extraction solvent ethanol 45% (*v*/*v*), which contains hypericin of approximately 0.3–0.7% and hyperforin between 0.3 and 1.6%; the liquid extract obtained with the extraction solvent maize oil in a drug–extractant ratio (DER) of 1:13, with an approximate content of hypericin of 0.0013% and hyperforin of 0.01%; the liquid extract obtained with the extraction solvent other vegetable oils (DER 1:4–20), in which hypericin is at least 0.005%; and finally, the ethanolic 45–50% (*v*/*v*) tinctures (DER 1:5 or 1:10), the ethanolic 50% (*v*/*v*) extract (DER 1:2), the expressed juice from the fresh herb, the comminuted herbal substance for tea infusion, and the powdered substance for solid dosage forms [43]. On the other hand, the European Pharmacopoeia (Ph. Eur.) regards the production of quantified St. John's wort dry extract from the herbal substance by using ethanol (50–80%, *v*/*v*) or methanol (50–80%, *v*/*v*) with a total content of hypericins, expressed as hypericin, in the range of 0.10–0.30%; flavonoids, expressed as rutin, minimum 6.0%; and hyperforin of maximum 6.0% [44]. The herbal substance is defined as a whole or as fragmented, dried flowering tops of HP with a minimal total content of hypericins, expressed as hypericin 0.08%. As the phloroglucinol derivative hyperforin is lipophilic, it is best retrieved by non-polar extractants such as supercritical CO_2, ethyl acetate, petroleum ether, *n*-hexane, dichloromethane, and *n*-heptane [45–47]. Indeed, the highest production yield of hyperforin is achieved with the aid of supercritical CO_2 extraction; therefore, this method is now also commercially established [46,48]. Taking into account all the above, we related the results of this study with reports providing analytic proof of hyperforin content as the main BAC in the extract or at least using solvents capable of extracting the phloroglucinol.

Drozdov et al. reported the lack of antibacterial activity of St. John's wort supercritical extract against bacteria and fungi. Interestingly, the authors isolated the pure hyperforin from the extract and demonstrated its antimicrobial effect against *P. aeruginosa* [49]. Naeem et al. established an equivalent efficacy of *n*-butanol and ethyl acetate St. John's wort extracts against Gram-positive and Gram-negative bacteria (*Bacillus subtilis*, *Sarcina lutea*, *P. aeruginosa*, and *E. coli*) but did not observe any antibacterial activity of *n*-hexane and dichloromethane-retrieved extracts [50]. Schempp et al., on the other side, proved hyperforin to be active only against Gram-positive bacteria, viz., *S. aureus*, *Streptococcus pyogenes*, *Streptococcus agalactiae*, and *Corynebacterium diphteriae* [51]. Similar results were obtained by Avato et al., who found hyperforin and a hyperforin-containing ethyl acetate St. John's wort extract to be effective against different strains of *S. aureus*, as well as against *B. cereus*, *Bacillus subtilis*, and *E. faecalis*, but ineffective against Gram-negative bacteria and fungi [52]. Despite the relative controversy in these results, it should be acknowledged that the investigated extracts were of different chemical compositions and were applied in different doses. Most importantly, none of the above reports used a nano-delivery system for the hyperforin-containing herbal preparations, and neither did they follow the stability of the phloroglucinol. As for the antiherpetic activity of HP, only the naphthodianthrones in the herb, viz. the hypericins, have been reported so far to possess such [22]; thus, we came to conclude that the current study presents a first thorough investigation of the hyperforin-rich HP extract's potency against HSV-1.

4. Materials and Methods

4.1. Materials

All materials used in the study were of pharmaceutical grade. St. John's Wort air-dried ground flowers, leaves, and shoots were supplied by Bilec Company, Troyan, Bulgaria; anhydrous methylene chloride $\geq$ 99.7% and sorbitan monooleate were supplied by Thermo Fisher Scientific, Waltham, MA, USA; double-distilled water was obtained in laboratory conditions (Gesellschaft für Labortechnik GmbH, Burgwedel, Germany); almond oil and borage oil were purchased from Alteya Organics, Stara Zagora, Bulgaria; polyoxyethylene (20) sorbitan monooleate was supplied by Sigma-Aldrich, St. Louis, MO, USA. Glyceryl behenate (Compritol® ATO 888) was a kind gift from Gattefossé, Saint-Priest, France.

4.2. Methods

4.2.1. Preparation of Hyperforin-Rich HP Extract

The extraction procedure for the preparation of hyperforin-rich HP extract was recently established [32]. The extract was obtained by applying a maceration method under conditions that align with the high reactivity of hyperforin. The extraction was carried out in amber glass flasks under an argon atmosphere in the condition of darkness. Anhydrous methylene chloride was employed as an extractant, and the plant material-to-solvent ratio was set to be 30:100 (w/v). The extract obtained after separation of the plant residue, filtration, and removal of the organic solvent was dissolved in anhydrous methanol (to a concentration of 20.0 µg/mL) and subjected to an HPLC-UV analysis. The presence of hyperforin was determined by the retention time reported using a hyperforin standard, and its concentration in the isolated extract was determined by the absolute calibration method [32].

4.2.2. Preparation of "Blank" and HP-Loaded NLCs

The optimal carriers for the thus-obtained extract were identified based on a thorough physicochemical characterization of twenty potential specimens by DLS, Laser Doppler Electrophoresis, EE determination, ATR-FTIR Spectroscopy, X-ray Diffraction Analysis, and TEM. The samples currently labeled as NLC1 and NLC2 were recognized to be a "best fit" to the particles' designation [32]. Herein, a total of four specimens (two "blank", viz., NLC1 and NLC2, and the corresponding hyperforin-rich St. John's wort extract-loaded samples, i.e., HP-NLC1 and HP-NLC2) were obtained as previously described [32]. They all comprised a 10% (*w*/*w*) lipid phase with a glyceryl behenate-to-almond oil (NLC1 and HP-NLC1) or glyceryl behenate-to-borage oil (NLC2 and HP-NLC2) ratio of 7:3. The employed surfactant mixture (5% *w*/*w*) for their preparation was in a polyoxyethylene (20) sorbitan monooleate-to-sorbitan monooleate ratio of 3:2. "Blank" nanodispersions were developed as follows: the aqueous phase (double-distilled water and polyoxyethylene (20) sorbitan monooleate) was heated to 80 $\pm$ 2 °C and added dropwise to the lipid phase (a mixture of glyceryl behenate, almond or borage oil, and sorbitan monooleate), which was pre-heated to the same temperature, under continuous stirring at a speed of 750 rpm for 3 min. The resulting macroemulsion was homogenized for 3 min at 10,000 rpm and then ultrasonified for 15 min at 25 °C. Hyperforin-rich St. John's wort extract-loaded samples were prepared by incorporating the extract (1.25% *w*/*w*) into the lipid phase before the emulsification under dark conditions.

4.2.3. Microbial Strains

Reference strains of *Escherichia coli* ATCC 25922, *Staphylococcus aureus* ATCC 25923, *Pseudomonas aeruginosa* ATCC 10145, *Klebsiella pneumoniae* ATCC 10031, and *Candida albicans* ATCC 10231 were provided as MicroSwabs® from Ridacom, Bulgaria. The microbial strains were activated according to manufacturer's instructions, initially plating them on blood agar (HiMedia, supplied by Ridacom, Bulgaria). Prior to preparing the bacterial inoculum, each bacterial strain was cultured for 24 h in Brain Heart Infusion broth (HiMedia, supplied by Ridacom, Bulgaria) and subsequently plated again on agar medium. Single colonies were transferred to sodium chloride solution to obtain a suspension with turbidity corresponding to 0.5 McFarland standard (Grant Bio DEN-1, Grant Instruments, Cambridge, UK).

4.2.4. Cells

MDBK cells were provided by the National Bank for Industrial Microorganisms and Cell Cultures in Sofia, Bulgaria. They were grown in DMEM medium (Gibco, Grand Island, NY, USA) supplemented with 10% FCS (Gibco BRL, Paisley, Scotland, UK), 10 mM HEPES buffer (AppliChem GmbH, Darmstadt, Germany), and antibiotics (100 IU/mL penicillin, 100 µg/mL streptomycin) (Sigma-Aldrich Chemie GmbH, Taufkirchen, Germany) at 37 °C and 5% CO_2 atmosphere (Radobio Scientific Co., Ltd., Shanghai, China).

4.2.5. Virus

Victoria strain of HSV-1 was obtained from the National Center for Infectious and Parasitic Diseases (Sofia, Bulgaria) and was propagated in a confluent monolayer of MDBK cells in DMEM (Gibco BRL, Paisley, Scotland, UK) with 0.5% fetal calf serum (Gibco BRL, Scotland, UK) and antibiotic mix added. After incubation at 37 °C and 5% CO_2, viral stock was collected, aliquoted, and stored at −80 °C. The infectious titer was determined to be $10^{8.5}$ $CCID_{50}$/mL.

4.2.6. Reference Substance

ACV was kindly provided by the Deutsches Kresforschung Zentrum, Heidelberg, with a stock concentration of 3.0 mg/mL solution in DMSO, which was diluted in DMEM maintenance medium to the required concentration.

4.2.7. Cytotoxicity Assay

Confluent MDBK cell monolayers grown in 96-well plates (Costar®, Corning Inc., Kennebunk, ME, USA) were treated with 0.1 mL/well of the test samples ("blank" and loaded with HP-rich extract NLCs), diluted 10-fold in DMEM maintenance medium, and then were placed at 37 °C and 5% CO_2 for 48 h. After microscopic evaluation, the test sample was removed and its influence on the cell monolayer viability was determined by Neutral Red (Sigma-Aldrich Chemie GmbH, Germany) Uptake Assay, as described previously, and read spectrophotometrically [53]. The 50% cytotoxic concentration (CC_{50}) was estimated for the HP-loaded specimens as the extract's dose that reduced cell survival by 50% compared with untreated cells. Each sample was tested in triplicate, with four wells per test sample. Maximum tolerable concentration (MTC) of the hyperforin-rich HP extract in each NLC specimen was the highest concentration (lowest dilution) at which the cell monolayer was not affected and the treated cells' appearance was similar to the cells in the non-treated control.

4.2.8. Determination of Infectious Viral Titers

After MDBK cells reached confluence in 96-well plates, they were infected with 0.1 mL of virus suspension at 10-fold falling dilutions. Following 1 h, the unadsorbed virus was discarded and 0.1 mL/well DMEM medium was added to the cells. The plates were incubated at 37 °C and 5% CO_2 in CO_2 incubator (Radobio Scientific Co., Ltd., Shanghai, China) for 48 h. Infectious viral titer was determined by microscopic observation of the cell monolayer and cytopathic effect (CPE) determination. Visually determined CPE was confirmed by Neutral Red Uptake Assay as described in the previous section. Viral titers are expressed as lg IU (infectious units) ($CCID_{50}$)/mL.

4.2.9. Antiviral Activity Assay

Confluent MDBK cells in 96-well plates were inoculated with 100-cell culture infectious dose of 50% ($CCID_{50}$) in 0.1 mL. After 60 min of viral adsorption to host cells, the unadsorbed virus was removed and the test sample was added following 10-fold dilution step. Cells were incubated for 48 h at 37 °C and 5% CO_2. The CPE was determined by the Neutral Red Uptake Assay, and the percentage of CPE inhibition for each concentration of the test sample was calculated by an established calculation protocol [53]. The concentration at which 50% of the cytopathic effect was inhibited compared with the mock-control was defined as the inhibitory concentration 50% (IC_{50}). From the obtained IC_{50} and toxicity CC_{50} values determined so far, the SI for the HP extract in each loaded NLC sample was determined using the CC_{50}/IC_{50} ratio.

4.2.10. Virucidal Activity (Effect on Extracellular Virions)

Samples containing virus (10^5 $CCID_{50}$) and test sample at its MTC were mixed in a 1:1 ratio and then stored at 20 °C for 15, 30, 60, 90, and 120 min intervals. The residual infectious virus content in each sample was then determined by titration [54], and the reduction in viral titer in samples containing the test products compared with the untreated viral control was assessed by determining the difference in viral titers Δlg (delta log).

4.2.11. Effect on Viral Adsorption

Monolayers of MDBK cell culture in 24-well plates were pre-cooled to 4 °C and inoculated simultaneously with 10^4 $CCID_{50}$ of HSV-1 and MTC of the test sample. This was followed by incubation at 4 °C for the time of virus adsorption. At various time intervals (15, 30, 45, and 60 min), cells were washed with PBS to remove both test components and unattached virus, and then covered with maintenance medium and incubated at 37 °C for 24 h. Triple freezing and thawing of the obtained samples was followed by an estimation of the infectious virus titer of each sample by an end-point dilution method. Δlg was calculated on the basis of differences in viral titers compared with the viral control (untreated with the products). Each sample was prepared in quadruplicate.

4.2.12. Antibacterial and Antifungal Activity

The antibacterial and antifungal activities of the NLC samples, "blank" and loaded with HP-rich extract, were tested against *E. coli*, *S. aureus*, *P. aeruginosa*, *K. pneumoniae*, and *C. albicans*. The starting extract concentration in the extract-loaded samples (HP-NLC1 and HP-NLC2) was 12.5 mg/mL. A serial 2-fold dilution of the samples was carried out in 1.0 mL Mueller–Hinton broth-containing sterile tubes up to 1:256 dilution of the stock solutions. The vials were then inoculated with 0.1 mL standardized to 0.5 McFarland turbidity equivalent microbial suspension corresponding to cell count density of approximately 1.5×10^8 CFU/mL. Samples for positive control were set by combining 0.1 mL of each microbial suspension with 1.0 mL Mueller–Hinton broth; non-inoculated mixtures of the test samples with Mueller–Hinton broth in a 1:1 ratio were left as negative controls. The antimicrobial susceptibility of all strains was assessed by using chlorhexidine diacetate as a control inhibitor. All experiments were repeated in triplicate. The test vials contaminated with bacterial strains were incubated for 24 h at 37 °C, and the ones contaminated with *C. albicans* for 48 h at 35 °C. The MBC and MFC were determined by transferring all test suspensions in a single-bacterial-loop-volume onto blood agar. The so-obtained specimens were incubated once again under the same conditions as described above. The lowest concentration at which bacterial/fungal growth appeared to be inhibited at ≥99.9% was reported as MBC/MFC.

4.2.13. Statistical Analysis

The values of CC_{50} were calculated using non-linear regression analysis (GraphPad 4 Software, San Diego, CA, USA). The values were presented as means ± SD from three independent experiments. The difference significance between the cytotoxicity values of the samples and the reference substance ACV, as well as between the effects of the test products on the viral replication, was performed by Student's *t*-test, where *p*-values of < 0.05 were considered significant.

5. Conclusions

In our study, we investigated the anti-herpesvirus and antimicrobial properties of NLC-incorporated St. John's wort extract rich in hyperforin. We reported slight activity against HSV-1, which covered viral replication but did not affect either extracellular virions or viral adsorption. By comparing the effects of the loaded and the "blank" NLCs, we also proved the latter is owing to the extract. The antimicrobial properties of the HP-NLCs were also assessed as being present due to the extract itself. A more pronounced activity was exhibited by HP-NLC2. The latter was highly effective against *K. pneumoniae* and *C. albicans*, while its activity against *S. aureus* was manifested at much higher extract concentrations. Assuming all obtained results, we can conclude that HP-NLC2 serves as a more efficient nanocarrier of the hyperforin-rich St. John's wort extract.

Author Contributions: Conceptualization, Y.S. and N.I.; methodology, Y.S., N.I., N.E., L.S., N.V.-I. and M.M.; software, L.S. and N.V.-I.; validation, N.E., L.S., N.V.-I., V.G. and V.A.; formal analysis, Y.S. and N.I.; investigation, Y.S., N.I., N.E., L.S., N.V.-I. and M.M.; resources, Y.S., N.E., L.S. and N.V.-I.; data curation, Y.S., N.I., N.E., L.S. and N.V.-I.; writing—original draft preparation, Y.S., N.I., L.S. and N.V.-I.; writing—review and editing, V.G. and V.A.; visualization, Y.S., N.E. and N.I.; supervision, N.I. and V.A.; project administration, N.I.; funding acquisition, N.I., V.G. and V.A. All authors have read and agreed to the published version of the manuscript.

Funding: This study was funded by Fund "Nauka" at the Medical University of Varna, Bulgaria, grant number Project No. 23011.

Institutional Review Board Statement: Not applicable.

Informed Consent Statement: Not applicable.

Data Availability Statement: The data presented in this study are available on request from the corresponding author.

Acknowledgments: The graphical abstract of this article was created in BioRender. ivanova, n. (2025) https://BioRender.com/v07w921 (accessed 10 February 2025). The authors would like to thank Ilina Amer of Sofia University St. Kl. Ochridski for the linguistic revision and editing of the text.

Conflicts of Interest: The authors declare no conflicts of interest. The funders had no role in the design of the study; in the collection, analyses, or interpretation of data; in the writing of the manuscript; or in the decision to publish the results.

References

1. Galeotti, N. *Hypericum perforatum* (St John's wort) beyond depression: A therapeutic perspective for pain conditions. *J. Ethnopharmacol.* **2017**, *200*, 136–146. [CrossRef] [PubMed]
2. Ersoy, E.; Özkan, E.E. *Hypericum perforatum* (St John's Wort) for Depression Treatment from Past to Present-What Do We Know? *J. Lit. Pharm. Sci. J.* **2020**, *9*, 137–148. [CrossRef]
3. Zhang, R.; Ji, Y.; Zhang, X.; Kennelly, E.J.; Long, C. Ethnopharmacology of Hypericum species in China: A comprehensive review on ethnobotany, phytochemistry and pharmacology. *J. Ethnopharmacol.* **2020**, *254*, 112686. [CrossRef]
4. Estrada, M.; Chávez-Nomberto, R.E.; Tsuneto, A.P.; Crestani, A.S.; Awad, C.; Takahiro Chone, C.; Kimura, D.; Quiroz Robladillo, D.; de Azevedo Lopes, E.; Ibrahim Abdullah, H.; et al. Anti-inflammatory Effects of Topical *Hypericum perforatum*: A Systematic Review. *Princ. Pract. Clin. Res. J.* **2023**, *9*, 47–52. [CrossRef]
5. Wölfle, U.; Seelinger, G.; Schempp, C.M. Topical application of St. John's wort (*Hypericum perforatum*). *Planta Med.* **2014**, *80*, 109–120. [PubMed]
6. Saddiqe, Z.; Naeem, I.; Maimoona, A. A review of the antibacterial activity of *Hypericum perforatum* L. *J. Ethnopharmacol.* **2010**, *131*, 511–521. [CrossRef] [PubMed]
7. Birt, D.F.; Widrlechner, M.P.; Hammer, K.D.; Hillwig, M.L.; Wei, J.; Kraus, G.A.; Murphy, P.A.; McCoy, J.; Wurtele, E.S.; Neighbors, J.D.; et al. Hypericum in infection: Identification of anti-viral and anti-inflammatory constituents. *Pharm. Biol.* **2009**, *47*, 774–782. [CrossRef]
8. Klemow, K.M.; Bartlow, A.; Crawford, J.; Kocher, N.; Shah, J.; Ritsik, M. Medical Attributes of St. John's Wort (*Hypericum perforatum*). In *Herbal Medicine: Biomolecular and Clinical Aspects*, 2nd ed.; Benzie, I.F.F., Wachtel-Galor, S., Eds.; CRC Press: Boca Raton, FL, USA, 2011; pp. 211–237, ISBN 978-042-913-094-6.
9. Alahmad, A.; Alghoraibi, I.; Zein, R.; Kraft, S.; Dräger, G.; Walter, J.G.; Scheper, T. Identification of Major Constituents of *Hypericum perforatum* L. Extracts in Syria by Development of a Rapid, Simple, and Reproducible HPLC-ESI-Q-TOF MS Analysis and Their Antioxidant Activities. *ACS Omega* **2022**, *7*, 13475–13493. [CrossRef]
10. Maltas Cagil, E.; Uysal, A.; Yildiztugay, E.; Aladağ, M.; Yildiz, S.; Kucukoduk, M. Investigation of antioxidant and antibacterial activities of some Hypericum species. *Fresenius Environ. Bull.* **2013**, *22*, 862–869.
11. Kisa, O.; Oksuz, L.; Servi, H.; Aysal, A.I. Antibacterial activity of *Hypericum perforatum* L. (St. John's wort) extracts against Gram-positive bacteria and characterisation of its secondary metabolites. *Nat. Prod. Res.* **2023**, *39*, 1019–1026. [CrossRef]
12. Sherif, M.M.; Elshikh, H.H.; Abdel-Aziz, M.M.; Elaasser, M.M.; Yosri, M. In Vitro Antibacterial and Phytochemical Screening of *Hypericum perforatum* Extract as Potential Antimicrobial Agents against Multi-Drug-Resistant (MDR) Strains of Clinical Origin. *BioMed Res. Int.* **2023**, *2023*, 6934398. [CrossRef] [PubMed]
13. Hodžić, S.; Osmanović, S.; Huseinović, S.; Grbić, S. In vitro inhibitory effect of *Hypericum perforatum* L. ethanol extract on microbial growth. *Acta Agric. Serb.* **2010**, *15*, 95–101.
14. Nazlı, O.; Baygar, T.; Demirci Dönmez, Ç.E.; Dere, Ö.; Uysal, A.İ.; Aksözek, A.; Işık, C.; Aktürk, S. Antimicrobial and antibiofilm activity of polyurethane/*Hypericum perforatum* extract (PHPE) composite. *Bioorg. Chem.* **2019**, *82*, 224–228. [CrossRef]
15. Kakouri, E.; Daferera, D.; Trigas, P.; Charalambous, D.; Pantelidou, M.; Tarantilis, P.A.; Kanakis, C.D. Comparative Study of the Antibacterial Activity, Total Phenolic and Total Flavonoid Content of Nine Hypericum Species Grown in Greece. *Appl. Sci.* **2023**, *13*, 3305. [CrossRef]
16. Afqir, H.; Belmalha, S.; Farihi, A.; Elbouzidi, A.; Bouhrim, M.; Elrherabi, A.; Boutagayout, A.; Oubihi, A.; Ouhssine, M. Comparative Analysis of Phenolic and Flavonoid Content, Antioxidant, Antibacterial Activities, and Functional Groups of Chemicals from *Hypericum perforatum* L. and Papaver Rhoeas L. Flower Extracts. *Ecol. Eng. Environ. Technol.* **2024**, *25*, 88–101. [CrossRef]
17. Radulović, N.; Stankov-Jovanović, V.; Stojanović, G.; Šmelcerović, A.; Spiteller, M.; Asakawa, Y. Screening of in vitro antimicrobial and antioxidant activity of nine Hypericum species from the Balkans. *Food Chem.* **2007**, *103*, 15–21. [CrossRef]

18. Zamani Faradonbeh, M.; Barzegar, H.; Hojjati, M.; Alizadeh Behbahani, B.; Taki, M. Active packaging coating based on Ocimum basilicum seed mucilage and *Hypericum perforatum* extract: Preparation, characterization, application and modeling the preservation of ostrich meat. *Appl. Food Res.* **2024**, *4*, 100524. [CrossRef]
19. Pu, X.; Liang, J.; Wang, X.; Xu, T.; Hua, L.; Shang, R.; Liu, Y.; Xing, Y. Anti-influenza A virus effect of *Hypericum perforatum* L. Extract. *Virol. Sin.* **2009**, *24*, 19–27. [CrossRef]
20. Chen, H.; Muhammad, I.; Zhang, Y.; Ren, Y.; Zhang, R.; Huang, X.; Diao, L.; Liu, H.; Li, X.; Sun, X.; et al. Antiviral Activity Against Infectious Bronchitis Virus and Bioactive Components of *Hypericum perforatum* L. *Front. Pharmacol.* **2019**, *10*, 1272. [CrossRef]
21. Bajrai, L.H.; El-Kafrawy, S.A.; Hassan, A.M.; Tolah, A.M.; Alnahas, R.S.; Sohrab, S.S.; Rehan, M.; Azhar, E.I. In vitro screening of anti-viral and virucidal effects against SARS-CoV-2 by *Hypericum perforatum* and Echinacea. *Sci. Rep.* **2022**, *12*, 21723. [CrossRef]
22. Cao, K.; Zhang, Y.; Yao, Q.; Peng, Y.; Pan, Q.; Jiao, Q.; Ren, K.; Sun, F.; Zhang, Q.; Guo, R.; et al. Hypericin blocks the function of HSV-1 alkaline nuclease and suppresses viral replication. *J. Ethnopharmacol.* **2022**, *296*, 115524. [CrossRef]
23. Korzeniowska, K.; Malesza, K.; Pawlaczyk, M. The phototoxic properties of *Hypericum perforatum*—Case report and review of the literature. *Farm. Współczesna* **2019**, *12*, 107–112.
24. Li, X.X.; Yan, Y.; Zhang, J.; Ding, K.; Xia, C.Y.; Pan, X.G.; Shi, Y.J.; Xu, J.K.; He, J.; Zhang, W.K. Hyperforin: A natural lead compound with multiple pharmacological activities. *Phytochemistry* **2023**, *206*, 113526. [CrossRef]
25. Liu, Q.; Zou, J.; Chen, Z.; He, W.; Wu, W. Current research trends of nanomedicines. *Acta Pharm. Sin. B.* **2023**, *13*, 4391–4416. [CrossRef]
26. Gasco, M.R. Method for Producing Solid Lipid Microspheres Having a Narrow Size Distribution. US Patent US5250236A, 5 October 1993.
27. Lucks, S.; Müller, R. Medication Vehicles Made of Solid Lipid Particles (Solid Lipid Nanospheres—SLN). European Patent EP0605497A1, 20 March 1996.
28. Scioli Montoto, S.; Muraca, G.; Ruiz, M.E. Solid Lipid Nanoparticles for Drug Delivery: Pharmacological and Biopharmaceutical Aspects. *Front. Mol. Biosci.* **2020**, *7*, 587997. [CrossRef]
29. Sivadasan, D.; Ramakrishnan, K.; Mahendran, J.; Ranganathan, H.; Karuppaiah, A.; Rahman, H. Solid Lipid Nanoparticles: Applications and Prospects in Cancer Treatment. *Int. J. Mol. Sci.* **2023**, *24*, 6199. [CrossRef]
30. Khan, S.; Sharma, A.; Jain, V. An Overview of Nanostructured Lipid Carriers and its Application in Drug Delivery through Different Routes. *Adv. Pharm. Bull.* **2023**, *13*, 446–460. [CrossRef]
31. Müller, R.H.; Jenning, V.; Mäder, K.; Lippacher, A. Lipid Particles on the Basis of Mixtures of Liquid and Solid Lipids and Method for Producing Same. WIPO (PCT). WO2000067728A2, 16 November 2000.
32. Sotirova, Y.; Gugleva, V.; Stoeva, S.; Kolev, I.; Nikolova, R.; Marudova, M.; Nikolova, K.; Kiselova-Kaneva, Y.; Hristova, M.; Andonova, V. Bigel Formulations of Nanoencapsulated St. John's Wort Extract—An Approach for Enhanced Wound Healing. *Gels* **2023**, *9*, 360. [CrossRef]
33. Sotirova, Y.; Stoeva, S.; Nikolova, R.; Andonova, V. Nanostructured lipid carriers as a promising dermal delivery platform for St. John's Wort extract: Preliminary studies. *J. IMAB* **2023**, *29*, 4911–4919. [CrossRef]
34. Tomeh, A. Design and Development of Novel Nanocarriers for Targeted Drug Delivery. Available online: https://etheses.whiterose.ac.uk/29256/1/Mhd%20Anas%20Tomeh_PhD%20Thesis%20Final%20Edition.pdf (accessed on 10 December 2024).
35. Casas-Cardoso, L.; Mantell, C.; Obregón, S.; Cejudo-Bastante, C.; Alonso-Moraga, Á.; de la Ossa, E.J.M.; de Haro-Bailón, A. Health-Promoting Properties of Borage Seed Oil Fractionated by Supercritical Carbon Dioxide Extraction. *Foods* **2021**, *10*, 2471. [CrossRef]
36. Yaghmour, R.; Garajah, M.; Kayali, I.; Al-Rimawi, F. Antioxidant, Antimicrobial and Formulation of Borage (*Borago officinalis*) Seeds Oil and Leaves Extracts as Microemulsion. *J. Pharm. Res. Int.* **2021**, *33*, 136–148. [CrossRef]
37. Hobby, C.R.; Herndon, J.L.; Morrow, C.A.; Peters, R.E.; Symes, S.J.K.; Giles, D.K. Exogenous fatty acids alter phospholipid composition, membrane permeability, capacity for biofilm formation, and antimicrobial peptide susceptibility in Klebsiella pneumoniae. *MicrobiologyOpen* **2019**, *8*, e00635. [CrossRef]
38. Wang, S.; Wang, P.; Liu, J.; Yang, C.; Wang, Q.; Su, M.; Wei, M.; Gu, L. Antibiofilm Activity of Essential Fatty Acids Against *Candida albicans* from Vulvovaginal Candidiasis and Bloodstream Infections. *Infect. Drug Resist.* **2022**, *15*, 4181–4193. [CrossRef] [PubMed]
39. Tisserand, R.; Young, R. Chapter 4: Kinetics and Dosing. In *Essential Oil Safety*, 2nd ed.; Churchill Livingstone: London, UK, 2013; pp. 39–67, ISBN 978-070-205-434-1.
40. Lorusso, A.B.; Carrara, J.A.; Barroso, C.D.N.; Tuon, F.F.; Faoro, H. Role of Efflux Pumps on Antimicrobial Resistance in Pseudomonas aeruginosa. *Int. J. Mol. Sci.* **2022**, *23*, 15779. [CrossRef]
41. Pottinger, P.; Reller, L.B.; Ryan, K.J.; Weissman, S. Pseudomonas and Other Opportunistic Gram-negative Bacilli. In *Sherris Medical Microbiology*, 7th ed.; Ryan, K.J., Ed.; McGraw-Hill Education: New York, NY, USA, 2018; pp. 653–664; ISBN 978-125-985-980-9.
42. Hadzhieva, B.; Dimitrov, M.; Petkova, V. Pharmaceutical regulation of herbal medicinal products in the countries of the European Union, the USA, Canada and Japan. *Acta Med. Bulg.* **2023**, *50*, 71–74. [CrossRef]

43. European Union Herbal Monograph on *Hypericum perforatum* L., Herba. Available online: https://www.ema.europa.eu/en/documents/herbal-monograph/final-european-union-herbal-monograph-hypericum-perforatum-l-herba-revision-1_en.pdf (accessed on 12 December 2024).
44. European Directorate for the Quality of Medicines & HealthCare of the Council of Europe (EDQM). *European Pharmacopoeia*; Council of Europe: Strasbourg, France, 2019; pp. 1391–1394.
45. Orth, H.C.J.; Rentel, C.; Schmidt, P.C. Isolation, Purity Analysis and Stability of Hyperforin as a Standard Material from *Hypericum perforatum* L. *J. Pharm. Pharmacol.* **1999**, *51*, 193–200. [CrossRef]
46. Cossuta, D.; Vatai, T.; Báthori, M.; Hohmann, J.; Keve, T.; Simándi, B. Extraction of Hyperforin and Hypericin from St. John's Wort (*Hypericum perforatum* L.) with Different Solvents. *J. Food Process Eng.* **2011**, *35*, 222–235. [CrossRef]
47. Gaid, M.; Haas, P.; Beuerle, T.; Scholl, S.; Beerhues, L. Hyperforin production in *Hypericum perforatum* root cultures. *J. Biotechnol.* **2016**, *222*, 47–55. [CrossRef]
48. Römpp, H.; Seger, C.; Kaiser, C.S.; Haslinger, E.; Schmidt, P.C. Enrichment of hyperforin from St. John's Wort (*Hypericum perforatum*) by pilot-scale supercritical carbon dioxide extraction. *Eur. J. Pharm. Sci.* **2004**, *21*, 443–451. [CrossRef]
49. Drozdov, A.L.; Beleneva, I.A.; Lepeshkin, F.D.; Krutikova, A.A.; Ustinovich, K.B.; Pokrovskii, O.I.; Parenago, O.O. The effect of St. John's wort supercritical extract and hyperforin solution on biological subjects. *Russ. J. Phys. Chem. B.* **2014**, *7*, 854–862. [CrossRef]
50. Naeem, I.; Saddiqe, Z.; Patel, A.; Hellio, C. Analysis of Flavonoid and Antimicrobial Activity of Extracts of *Hypericum perforatum*. *Asian J. Chem.* **2010**, *22*, 3596–3600.
51. Schempp, C.M.; Pelz, K.; Wittmer, A.; Schöpf, E.; Simon, J.C. Antibacterial activity of hyperforin from St John's wort, against multiresistant Staphylococcus aureus and gram-positive bacteria. *Lancet* **1999**, *353*, 2129. [CrossRef] [PubMed]
52. Avato, P.; Raffo, F.; Guglielmi, G.; Vitali, C.; Rosato, A. Extracts from St John's Wort and their antimicrobial activity. *Phytother. Res.* **2004**, *18*, 230–232. [CrossRef] [PubMed]
53. Ivanova, N.; Ermenlieva, N.; Simeonova, L.; Kolev, I.; Slavov, I.; Karashanova, D.; Andonova, V. Chlorhexidine–Silver Nanoparticle Conjugation Leading to Antimicrobial Synergism but Enhanced Cytotoxicity. *Pharmaceutics* **2023**, *15*, 2298. [CrossRef]
54. Reed, L.J.; Muench, H. A simple method of estimating fifty percent endpoints. *Am. J. Hyg.* **1938**, *27*, 493–497.

pharmaceuticals

Article

In Vitro Evaluation of Rosemary Essential Oil: GC-MS Profiling, Antibacterial Synergy, and Biofilm Inhibition

Daniel E. K. Kabotso [1], David Neglo [1], Sarah E. Gaba [2], Emmanuel K. Danyo [3], Alberta D. Dayie [4], Anastasia A. Asantewaa [5], Fleischer C. N. Kotey [5] and Nicholas T. K. D. Dayie [5,*]

1 Department of Basic Sciences, School of Basic and Biomedical Sciences, University of Health and Allied Sciences, PMB 31, Ho 00233, Ghana; ekabotso@uhas.edu.gh (D.E.K.K.); dneglo@uhas.edu.gh (D.N.)
2 Department of Biomedical Sciences, School of Basic and Biomedical Sciences, University of Health and Allied Sciences, PMB 31, Ho 00233, Ghana; esinamgaba@gmail.com
3 Department of Technologies for Organic Synthesis, Institute of Chemical Technology, Ural Federal University, Mira Street 28, 620002 Ekaterinburg, Russia; e.kdanyo@gmail.com
4 Department of Chemistry, University of Cape Coast, Cape Coast 00233, Ghana; alberta.dayie@ucc.edu.gh
5 Department of Medical Microbiology, University of Ghana Medical School, Korle Bu, Accra 00233, P.O. Box KB 4236, Ghana; fcnkotey@flerholiferesearch.com (F.C.N.K.)
* Correspondence: ntkddayie@ug.edu.gh; Tel.: +233-208449415

Abstract: Background: Antimicrobial resistance (AMR) has become precarious, warranting investments in antimicrobial discovery. **Aim:** To investigate the antibacterial activity of rosemary essential oil (REO), alone and in combination with selected conventional antibiotics. **Methods:** REO was subjected to antimicrobial susceptibility testing (including minimum bactericidal concentration (MBC) and minimum inhibitory concentration (MIC) determination) and investigation of anti-pre-biofilm and antibiofilm activities. **Results:** The phytochemical composition of the REO was eucalyptol (42.68%), bornanone (33.20%), endo-borneol (9.37%), α-terpeneol (7.95%), linalool (2.10%), bornyl acetate (1.81%), caryophyllene (1.09%), 4-terpeneol (0.94%), and anethole (0.87%). The antibacterial inhibition zones generally increased with increasing REO concentration (i.e., 10, 20, 50, 100, and 200 mg/mL). The MIC and MBC ranges of REO for all bacteria were 3.13–6.25 mg/mL and 3.12–12.5 mg/mL, respectively. The MICs (in μg/mL) of ciprofloxacin, chloramphenicol, streptomycin, tetracycline, and ampicillin, respectively, were *Escherichia coli* (0.98, 3.92, 1.96, 7.81, and 250), *Klebsiella pneumoniae* (1.25, 7.81, 125, 7.81, and 1000), MRSA (62.5, 7.81, 3.91, 7.81, and 250), *Streptococcus mutans* and *Bacillus subtilis* (125, 15.68, 250, 31.25, and 1000), *Pseudomonas aeruginosa* (125, 31.25, 500, 31.25, and 1000), and *Salmonella* Typhi (0.98, 15.68, 125, 1.96, and 1000). The MBC-MIC ratios of REO against all bacteria were in the range 1–2, indicating bactericidal effects. Mainly synergy (FICI = 0.16–0.37) was observed between REO and the conventional antibiotics. The IC50 values (in μg/mL) of REO against the bacteria, pre-biofilm vs. biofilm formation, were *E. coli* (1342.00 vs. 4.00), *K. pneumoniae* (106.00 vs. 3.00), MRSA (134.00 vs. 6.00), *S. mutans* (7259.00 vs. 7.00), *B. subtilis* (120.00 vs. 7.00), *P. aeruginosa* (4989.00 vs. 7.00), and *S.* Typhi (10.00 vs. 2.00). **Conclusions:** Rosemary essential oil had significant bactericidal effects on the bacteria tested, and its MIC and MBC values were low. Overall, it was synergistic with known conventional antibiotics and, thus, has encouraging prospects in combination therapy involving conventional antibiotics, even in the treatment of infections with multidrug-resistant bacteria, including biofilm-forming ones.

Keywords: *Rosmarinus officinalis*; essential oil; antibacterial activity; *Escherichia coli*; *Klebsiella pneumoniae*; MRSA; *Streptococcus mutans*; *Bacillus subtilis*; *Pseudomonas aeruginosa*; *Salmonella* Typhi

1. Introduction

Antimicrobial resistance (AMR), which had its onset shortly after the discovery of the first antibiotic, penicillin, has become more precarious in the 21st century, creating a seemingly perpetual global public health crisis [1]. To illustrate, it accounted for about

5 million deaths in 2019 alone and can result in an annual death toll of double this figure by 2050 [1–3]. While antimicrobial stewardship efforts have consequentially been intensified to curtail the anthropogenic drivers of AMR, they are not enough to obliterate the AMR menace. It is imperative to concurrently complement these efforts with investments in sustainable discovery of newer antimicrobials, such as from plant sources [4,5].

One plant that has a huge potential for exploitation in antimicrobial chemotherapy is *Rosmarinus officinalis* L., which is commonly referred to as rosemary [6–8]. Historically, its leaves and essential oils have been used in the preservation and spicing of food as well as in alternative medicine [9]. Furthermore, phytochemical analyses of its essential oils have demonstrated the presence of such bioactive agents as 3-carene, pinenes, camphene, camphor, and 1,8-cineole, which account for its antimicrobial activity [10–12]. There have also been sporadic reports on its antimicrobial effects, such as against bacteria like *Listeria monocytogenes, Klebsiella pneumoniae, Pseudomonas aeruginosa, Staphylococcus aureus,* and *Salmonella* Typhimurium [7,8,10,13].

One key blind spot of investigations on the antibacterial activity of rosemary essential oil (REO) is the general absence of data on the exploration of its synergistic effects when combined with conventional antibiotics. In addition, these studies hardly originate from sub-Saharan Africa, where the bulk of the AMR problem is felt [1]. Meanwhile, AMR patterns of bacterial strains are geographically dynamic, as is the distribution of the various bioactive compounds within the essential oils. To help clarify the "blind spot" and provide further insights, this study investigated the antimicrobial activity of REO, alone and in combination with selected conventional antibiotics, using REO extracted from rosemary plants in Ghana, one of the AMR hotspots in sub-Saharan Africa.

2. Results

2.1. Gas Chromatographic–Mass Spectrometric-Based Phytochemical Analysis of REO

The phytochemicals present in REO, based on gas chromatography, were diverse, and their relative proportions decreased across eucalyptol (42.68%), bornanone (33.20), endo-borneol (9.37%), α-terpeneol (7.95%), linalool (2.10%), bornyl acetate (1.81%), caryophyllene (1.09%), 4-terpeneol (0.94%), and anethole (0.87%). Further details of the gas chromatographic analysis are presented in Table 1.

Table 1. Major phytochemical constituents of the REO.

S/N	RT	Structure of Compound	Area %	MW/CID *	Molecular Formula	Common Name	IUPAC Nomenclature
1	8.037	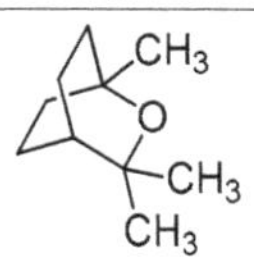	42.681	154 2758 *	$C_{10}H_{18}O$	Eucalyptol	(1S,4S)-1,3,3-trimethyl-2-oxabicyclo [2.2.2]octane
2	9.724	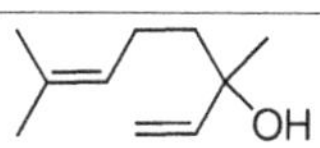	2.101	154 6549 *	$C_{10}H_{18}O$	Linalool	3,7-dimethylocta-1,6-dien-3-ol
3	9.944	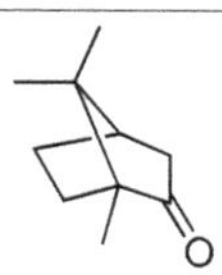	33.198	152 2537 *	$C_{10}H_{16}O$	(+)-2-Bornanone, camphor	(1S)-1,7,7-Trimethylbicyclo [2.2.1]heptan-2-one
4	10.641	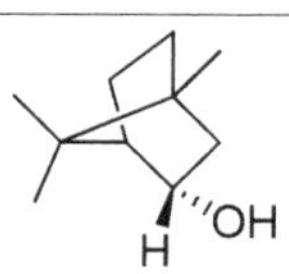	9.372	154 439,569 *	$C_{10}H_{18}O$	Endobornoel, camphol	(1S-endo)-1,7,7-Trimethylbicyclo [2.2.1]heptan-2-ol

Table 1. *Cont.*

S/N	RT	Structure of Compound	Area %	MW/CID *	Molecular Formula	Common Name	IUPAC Nomenclature
5	10.714	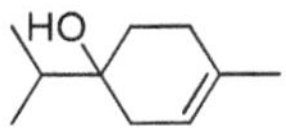	0.938	154 11,230 *	$C_{10}H_{18}O$	4-Terpineol, terpinen-4-ol	(R)-4-methyl-1-(1-methylethyl)-3-cyclohexen-1-ol
6	10.916	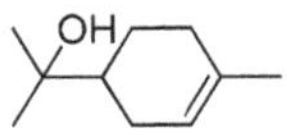	7.947	154 1700 *	$C_{10}H_{18}O$	α-Terpineol	2-(4-Methylcyclohex-3-en-1-yl)propan-2-ol
7	11.887	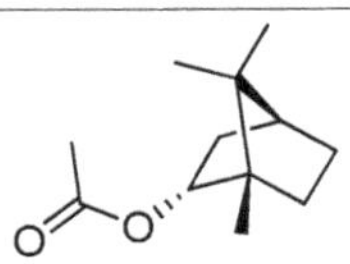	1.808	196 93,009 *	$C_{12}H_{20}O_2$	Bornyl acetate	(1S,2R,4S)-1,7,7-trimethylbicyclo [2.2.1]heptan-2-yl acetate
8	12.052	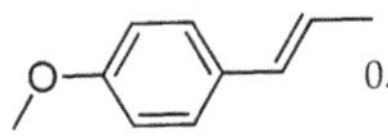	0.868	148 637,563 *	$C_{10}H_{12}O$	Anethole	(E)-1-methoxy-4-(prop-1-en-1-yl)benzene
9	13.758	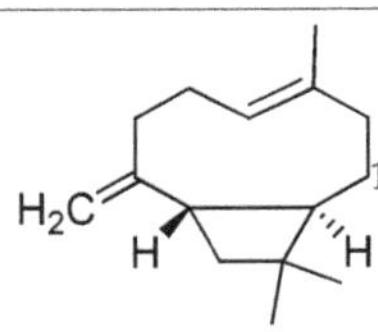	1.086	204 5,281,522 *	$C_{15}H_{24}$	Caryophyllene	(1R,4Z,9S)-4,11,11-trimethyl-8-methylenebicyclo [7.2.0]undec-4-ene

* = PubChem ID.

2.2. Susceptibility of Selected Bacterial Pathogens to Varying Concentrations of REO

Generally, there was a trend of increasing size of the inhibition zone with an increasing concentration of REO for the bacteria tested, even for MRSA. In the case of *K. pneumoniae*, of the five concentrations of REO examined (10 mg/mL, 20 mg/mL, 50 mg/mL, 100 mg/mL, and 200 mg/mL), only the highest tested REO concentration—200 mg/mL—demonstrated an inhibitory effect. Regarding *S. mutans*, the inhibitory effects were observed starting with the 50 mg/mL REO concentration, whereas in the other bacteria tested—*E. coli*, MRSA, *B. subtilis*, *P. aeruginosa*, and *S.* Typhi—inhibitory effects were observed even at the lowest REO concentration tested (10 mg/mL). Details of the susceptibility of various bacterial pathogens to varying concentrations of REO are presented in Table 2 and Figure S1.

Table 2. Zones of inhibition (in millimeters) of different bacterial strains to rosemary essential oil.

Bacterial Strains	Concentration of Rosemary Essential Oil (mg/mL)					Control	
	200	100	50	20	10	Positive	Negative
E. coli	17.50 ± 1.32	16.67 ± 1.53	8.00 ± 1.00	9.00 ± 2.00	7.67 ± 1.53	25.50 ± 0.87	–
K. pneumoniae	18.50 ± 1.32	0.00 ± 0.00	0.00 ± 0.00	0.00 ± 0.00	0.00 ± 0.00	11.67 ± 0.58	–
MRSA	16.33 ± 1.15	14.67 ± 0.58	11.33 ± 1.15	11.00 ± 0.00	9.67 ± 0.58	30.33 ± 1.15	–
S. mutans	11.67 ± 0.58	10.00 ± 0.00	9.67 ± 1.15	0.00 ± 0.00	0.00 ± 0.00	22.67 ± 1.15	–
B. subtilis	14.67 ± 0.58	13.00 ± 1.15	13.33 ± 1.15	10.67 ± 1.15	9.33 ± 1.15	24.67 ± 1.15	–
P. aeruginosa	13.00 ± 0.00	12.67 ± 0.58	11.33 ± 1.15	10.67 ± 0.58	10.00 ± 0.00	21.67 ± 0.58	–
S. Typhi	25.67 ± 2.52	16.83 ± 2.02	12.33 ± 0.58	7.67 ± 1.15	5.50 ± 0.50	39.33 ± 0.58	–

Positive control = 30 µg chloramphenicol; Negative control = 20% DMSO in 0.5% Tween 80

2.3. Minimum Inhibitory and Bactericidal Concentrations of REO Against the Bacterial Pathogens

Table 3 details out the minimum inhibitory concentration (MIC) and the minimum bactericidal concentration (MBC) of REO and a range of conventional antibiotics against various strains of bacteria. *B. subtilis*, *P. aeruginosa*, and *S.* Typhi had the lowest MIC values for REO (3.13 mg/mL), while *B. subtilis* and *P. aeruginosa* had the least MBC values (3.12 mg/mL). Overall, the MIC values ranged from 3.13 mg/mL to 6.25 mg/mL, and the MBC values ranged from 3.12 mg/mL to 12.5 mg/mL. The ratio (R) between the MBC and the MIC, which informs on whether the effect is bactericidal (R $\leq$ 4) or bacteriostatic (R > 4) recorded against each of the bacterial pathogens, shows that REO was bactericidal against all the bacteria tested.

Table 3. Minimum inhibitory effect of rosemary essential oil and antibiotics on different bacterial strains.

Bacterial Strains	Concentration of REO			CIP	CHL	STR	TET	AMP
	MIC (mg/mL)	MBC (mg/mL)	R	MIC (µg/mL)	MIC (µg/mL)	MIC (µg/mL)	MIC (µg/mL)	MIC (µg/mL)
E. coli	6.25	6.25	1	0.98	3.92	1.96	7.81	250
K. pneumoniae	6.25	6.25	1	1.25	7.81	125	7.81	1000
MRSA	6.25	12.5	2	62.5	7.81	3.91	7.81	250
S. mutans	6.25	12.5	2	125	15.68	250	31.25	1000
B. subtilis	3.13	3.13	1	125	15.68	250	31.25	1000
P. aeruginosa	3.13	3.12	1	125	31.25	500	31.25	1000
S. Typhi	3.13	6.25	2	0.98	15.68	125	1.96	1000

REO = Rosemary essential oil, MIC = minimum inhibitory concentration, MBC = minimum bactericidal concentration, R = ratio of MBC to MIC, R $\leq$ 4 = bactericidal, R > 4 = bacteriostatic, CIP = ciprofloxacin, CHL = chloramphenicol, STR = streptomycin, TET = tetracycline, AMP = ampicillin; details of the interpretative criteria can be found in the EUCAST guidelines.

2.4. *Synergistic Effects of Various REO–Conventional Antibiotic Combinations Against a Range of Bacterial Pathogens*

The synergistic effect of REO, when combined with various antibiotics, is presented in Table 4. The fractional inhibitory concentration index (FICI), which is used to interpret the effect (values 0.5 representing synergism, >0.5 and 1 representing partial synergism, =1 representing an additive effect, >1 and 4 representing indifference or no difference, and >4 representing antagonism), showed that for most of the bacteria, the combination of REO with various antibiotics had synergistic or partially synergistic effects.

Table 4. Synergistic effect of rosemary essential oil on antibiotics against different bacterial strains.

Bacterial Strain	FICI		FICI		FICI		FICI		FICI	
	CIP + REO	INT	CHL + REO	INT	STR + REO	INT	TET + REO	INT	AMP + REO	INT
E. coli	1.00	I	1.03	I	16.07	A	40.19	A	0.25	S
K. pneumoniae	0.79	PS	1.06	I	0.37	S	4.13	A	0.16	S
MRSA	0.31	S	2.12	I	8.12	A	0.62	PS	0.25	S
S. mutans	0.37	S	2.12	I	0.25	S	1.12	I	0.16	S
B. subtilis	0.19	S	2.12	I	0.25	S	1.13	I	0.16	S
P. aeruginosa	0.19	S	0.56	PS	0.19	S	1.13	I	0.16	S
S. Typhi	1.03	I	1.06	I	0.37	S	8.10	A	0.16	S

FICI = Fractional inhibitory concentration index, FICI $\leq$ 0.5 = synergism (S), FICI > 0.5 and < 1 = partial synergism (PS), FICI = 1 = additive (AD), FICI > 1 and $\leq$ 4 = indifference or no difference (I), FICI > 4 = antagonism (A), INT = interpretation.

2.5. REO Inhibition of Pre-Biofilms and Biofilms of Various Bacterial Pathogens

Table 5 presents the IC50 values for REO's inhibition of pre-biofilms and biofilms of various bacteria. There were lower IC50 values for biofilm formation, indicating that REO is more effective in inhibiting biofilm formation than it is in inhibiting pre-biofilm formation for all the tested bacterial pathogens.

Table 5. IC50 values for inhibition of pre-biofilm and biofilm formation of different bacterial strains by rosemary essential oil.

Bacterial Strains	IC50 (μg/mL)	
	Pre-Biofilm	Biofilm
E. coli	1342.00	4.00
K. pneumoniae	106.00	3.00
MRSA	134.00	6.00
S. mutans	7259.00	7.00
B. subtilis	120.00	7.00
P. aeruginosa	4989.00	7.00
S. Typhi	10.00	2.00

Moreover, Figures 1 and 2 depict the changes in percentage inhibition with increasing REO concentration for pre-biofilms and biofilms, respectively.

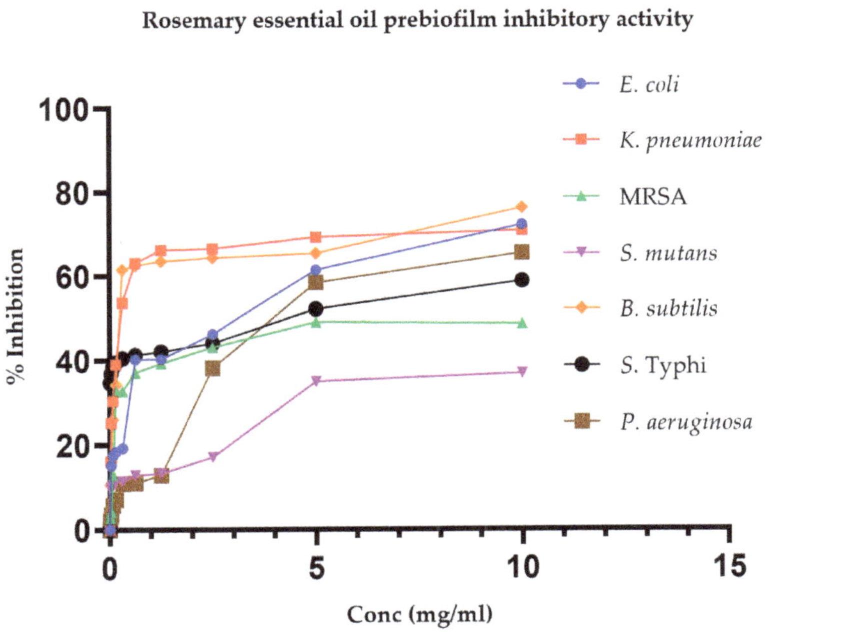

Figure 1. Inhibition of pre-biofilm formation potential of different bacterial strains by rosemary essential oil.

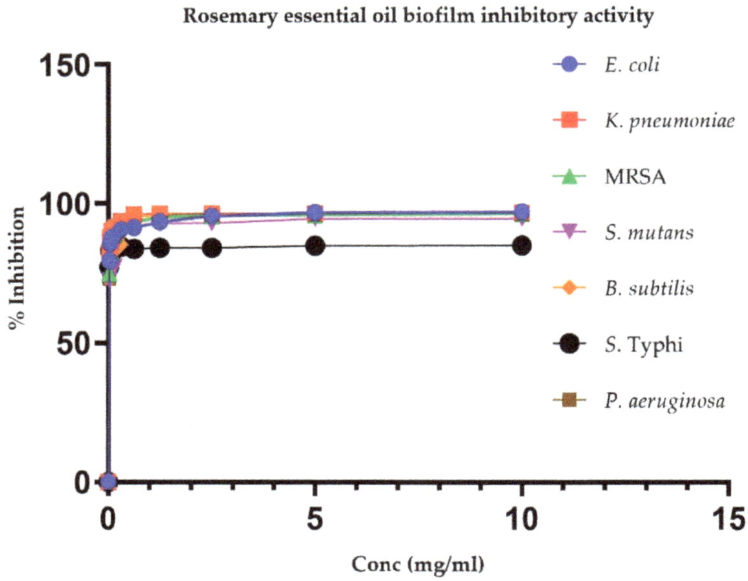

Figure 2. Inhibition of biofilm formation potential of different bacterial strains by rosemary essential oil.

3. Discussion

The increased precariousness of AMR calls for an intensified exploration for newer antimicrobials, especially from plant sources [1,4,5]. To that end, this study investigated the antimicrobial activity of REO extracted from rosemary plants in Ghana, alone and in combination with selected conventional antibiotics, against a spectrum of bacteria, multidrug-resistant ones inclusive.

As previously highlighted, the REO used in the investigation in the current study was mainly composed of eucalyptol and bornanone, with the other constituents of the REO—endo-borneol, α-terpeneol, linalool, bornyl acetate, caryophyllene, 4-terpeneol, and anethole—being in the minority. In contrast, in the studies of Jiang et al. [10], Dhouibi et al. [14], and Murtiastutik et al. [15], 1,8-cineole, camphor, and α-pinene were the dominant constituents. In the study of Becer et al. [16] as well, these three compounds were in the majority, alongside verbenone. Interestingly, none of these studies detected the compounds that dominated in the REO used in the current study, i.e., eucalyptol and bornanone. It is noted, though, that bornyl acetate and caryophyllene, which were detected at lower levels in the current study, were also detected by Jiang et al. [10], Murtiastutik et al. [15], and Becer et al. [16]. These disparities in phytochemical distribution may be accounted for by variations in sources of the REO as well as the extraction method, as alluded to by Melero-Bravo et al. [17].

The diversities in REO phytochemical constituents notwithstanding, significant antibacterial activity of REO was observed against the bacteria tested in this study—*E. coli*, *K. pneumoniae*, MRSA, *S. mutans*, *B. subtilis*, *P. aeruginosa*, and *S.* Typhi—consistent with previous reports on REO. Examples are Alvarez et al.'s [7] and Garcia-Sotelo et al.'s [8] reported significant REO inhibition of *Salmonella* as well as those reported by Puvača et al. [18] against *S. aureus*, Araya et al. [19] against *E. coli* and *S. aureus*, Eid et al. [13] against MRSA, *K. pneumoniae*, and *P. aeruginosa*, Becer et al. [16] against *E. coli*, *K. pneumoniae*, and *S. aureus*, and that of Dhouibi et al. [14] against *E. coli*, *P. aeruginosa*, *Salmonella enterica*, and *S. aureus*. Expectedly, there was a trend of increasing size of the inhibition zone with increasing concentration of REO for these bacteria. Interestingly, even at the lowest concentration of REO tested, MRSA and *P. aeruginosa* were inhibited, which only underscores the promise that REO holds in future antimicrobial chemotherapy against multidrug-resistant pathogens.

The prospects of REO in infectious disease treatment are further deepened by the observed low MIC and MBC values for REO. Similarly, Alvarez et al. [7], Garcia-Sotelo et al. [8], and Puvača et al. [18] also reported low MIC levels of REO against *Salmonella cholerae* and *Listeria monocytogenes*, *Salmonella typhimurium* and *Listeria monocytogenes*, and *S. aureus*, respectively. Moreover, the ratio (R) between the MBC and the MIC, which informs on whether the effect recorded against the bacterial pathogens is bactericidal ($R \leq 4$) or bacteriostatic ($R > 4$), demonstrated the REO to be bactericidal, further increasing its therapeutic value.

Although it is difficult to tell the mechanism of action of REO from the data generated in the current study, it has been noted elsewhere that REO is able to exploit protein transport and ion channels via which it enters the cytoplasm [20]. An alternative mechanism involves disrupting the cell membrane to impede ion transport and cell membrane respiration [20]. Although it can be argued that these mechanisms may be more applicable to fungal pathogens, it goes to reason that the bactericidal effects of REO may be orchestrated through a similar strategy. It may also have demonstrated its antibacterial activity (by virtue of its phytochemicals) through (a) disruption of cell wall synthesis, (b) induction of oxidative stress (such as via protein oxidation, DNA/RNA damage, antioxidant depletion, or reactive oxygen species generation), (c) protein denaturation (for example, via cellular stress, metabolic disruption, structural protein damage, or enzyme inactivation), (d) membrane damage (such as via component leakage, structural integrity loss, increased permeability, or phospholipid bilayer disruption), (e) efflux pump interference, (f) biofilm disruption, (g) quorum sensing interference, or (h) combinations thereof, in the tested bacteria [21–24]. Further analyses on REO can clarify insights on its mechanism(s) of action, as well as its potential acute and sub-chronic toxicity to humans and animals at therapeutic levels.

One welcomed observation in the current study was the demonstrated synergistic effects of REO-conventional antibiotic combinations against most of the bacterial pathogens tested. Although this seems to be the first report suggesting successful synergy between REO and conventional antibiotics, it is noted that synergistic effects between REO and other essential oils have been previously demonstrated [20,25–28]. Of course, such essential oil–essential oil synergy can be complicated by variations in chemical compositions of the given essential oils involved [27]. That said, the synergistic effects observed in this study highlight the potential flexibility of REO use in combination with conventional antibiotics (whose solitary use may have otherwise resulted in treatment failure) in the treatment of infectious diseases. It also reduces the likelihood of imminent AMR development against REO.

Also worth noting is the observed effectiveness of REO in inhibiting biofilms of the test bacterial strains by appreciable dose-dependent concentration of the test extract showing very good IC50s—the lower the IC50s values, the better the biofilm–inhibitory activity. Microbial biofilms are known to cause resistant chronic infections [29]. This activity of the extract in many studies have been attributed to the potential of the active components in the test extract impairing the adhesion of planktonic cells on abiotic surfaces, reducing biofilm metabolic activity, or promoting biomass degradation of mature biofilms as a major breakthrough [30].

This study was limited, albeit negligibly, by the inability of the oil and the broth to evenly mix in the wells, and, hence, the activities recorded may have been underestimated.

4. Materials and Methods

4.1. Materials

Mueller-Hinton broth (Oxoid, CM045), Mueller-Hinton agar (Oxoid CM0337), and nutrient agar (Oxoid, CM0003) were purchased from Oxoid Ltd., Wade Road, Basingstoke, Hants, RG24 8PW, UK. Tetrazolium salt, TTC, was bought from CDH (Central Drug House

(P) Ltd., Cop. Office, 7/28 Vardam House, Daryagang, Delhi-110002, India). Anhydrous sodium sulfate (Daejung Chemicals and Metals CO., Ltd., 186 Seohaean-ro, Siheung-si, Gyeonggi-do, Korea), dimethyl sulfoxide, and MTT dye were purchased from the local vendor Wallart Lab Enterprise (No. 12 Konkonte (Akotex) Street, Kokomlemle, behind Ring Road Central Access Bank, Accra, Ghana). An AKAI high-performance commercial blender was purchased from MELCOM at Stadium Road, Ho, Volta Region, Ghana. Sterile 96-well microtitre plates were purchased from China (Citotest Labware Manufacturing Co., Ltd., Jiangsu, China). Standard antibiotics such as ciprofloxacin, chloramphenicol, streptomycin, tetracycline, and ampicillin were purchased from the local vendor Benburto Enterprise Ltd. (144 Dansoman High St., Sakaman-Accra, Ghana).

4.2. Test Microorganism

Bacterial isolates such as *Escherichia coli* (ATCC 25922), *Pseudomonas aeruginosa* (ATCC 4853), *Klebsiella pneumoniae* (NCTC 13440), methicillin-resistant *S. aureus* (MRSA) (NCTC 12493), *Streptococcus mutans* (ATCC 700610), *Bacillus subtilis* (ATCC 10004), and *Salmonella* Typhi (ATCC 14028) were obtained from the Microbiology Unit of the School of Basic and Biomedical Science Laboratory of the University of Health and Allied Sciences, Ho, Ghana. These microorganisms were sub-cultured for 24 h prior to the experiment, on nutrient agar, at 37 °C.

4.3. Study Site

This study was conducted in the Analytical and Organic Chemistry Laboratory of the Department of Basic Sciences and Microbiology Laboratory of the Department of Biomedical Sciences in the School of Basic and Biomedical Sciences at the University of Health and Allied Sciences, Ho, Volta Region, Ghana.

4.4. Study Design

The study employed an experimental research design. The tests were conducted in duplicates to obtain reliable results, and control groups were also used to validate the results from experimental groups.

4.5. Collection of Samples

Plant samples were bought from the Ho Central Market in the Volta Region of Ghana. Diseased and unfit leaves were not sampled. These samples were authenticated by an experienced botanist and assigned the herbarium voucher number "UHAS/ITAM/2024/L015".

4.6. Extraction of Rosemary Essential Oil

The rosemary leaves were blended into powder using the AKAI high-performance commercial blender; 80 g of the powdered rosemary leaves was suspended in 300 mL of distilled water in a 300 mL round bottom flask and subjected to hydrodistillation for three hours using a Clevenger-type apparatus (Figure 3). The condensed vapors of the oil and water were drained through the delivery tube of the Clevenger-type apparatus and the oil layer separated from the water layer using a 25 mL separating funnel. The separated REO was dried over anhydrous sodium sulfate, transferred into a 10 mL vial, and capped. The vial was wrapped in aluminum foil and then stored at 4 °C until analysis [31].

The percentage yield of REO (2.96 g) from rosemary powder (80.0 g) was calculated to be 3.70% by using the following formula:

$$\text{PercentageYield} = \frac{\text{Mass of extracted rosemary essentialoil, REO (g)}}{\text{Mass of powdered rosemary leaves (g)}} \times 100\%$$

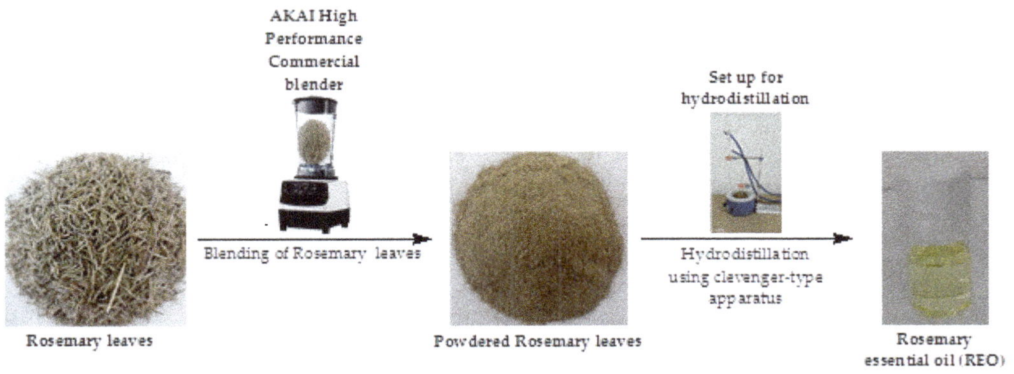

Figure 3. Setup for the extraction of REO using a Clevenger-type apparatus.

4.7. Determination of Stock Concentration and Preparation of Various Concentrations of REO

One milliliter (1.0 mL) of REO was weighed on an analytical balance thrice to determine its stock concentration as 953 mg/mL. The stock REO was used to prepare various diluted concentrations (10–200 mg/mL) by using the dilution formula $C_1V_1 = C_2V_2$, where C_1 is the initial concentration in mg/mL, C_2 is the final concentration in mg/mL, V_1 is the initial volume in ml, and V_2 is the final volume in ml. Dimethyl sulfoxide was employed as the solvent [31].

4.8. Phytochemical Analysis via GC-MS

Aliquots of REO (50 μL) were taken up in hexane (50 μL), mixed and readied. The analysis of REO was performed using a GC Clarus 580 gas chromatograph interfaced with a Clarus SQ 8 mass spectrometer (PerkinElmer Inc., Waltham, MA, USA). The resolution was achieved using a ZB-5HTMS (5% diphenyl/95% dimethyl polysiloxane, Phenomenex Inc, Torrance, CA USA) fused capillary column (30 m length × 0.25 μm ID × 0.25 μm film thickness). The programming was as follows: Initial temperature was 40 °C (isothermal for 2 min), then increased at 10 °C/min to 250 °C, then 20 °C/min to 280 °C, and held for 10 min at 280 °C. Helium gas (99.9999%: Air Liquide, Tema, Ghana) was used as a carrier gas at a constant flow rate of 1 mL/min, and an injection volume of 1 μL was used. The solvent delay was 0 to 3 min, and the total GC/MS running time was 34.5 min. For GC/MS detection, an electron ionisation system was operated in electron impact mode with an ionisation energy of 70 eV. The injector temperature was maintained at 250 °C, and the ion-source temperature was 220 °C. Mass spectra were taken at 70 eV at a scan interval of 1s and fragments from 50 to 450 Da. The mass detector was Turbo-Mass TM, and the software adopted to handle mass spectra and chromatograms was Turbo-Mass ver. 6.1.0. (PerkinElmer Inc.). Compounds were identified according to the NIST 2014 mass spectral library, which is a standard MS reference database released by the National Institute of Standards and Technology (NIST).

4.9. Determination of Antibacterial Susceptibility

Mueller-Hinton agar (20 mL) was aseptically dispensed into Petri dishes and allowed to solidify. The EUCAST (European Committee on Antimicrobial Susceptibility Testing) Standard was followed. Briefly, overnight cultures at a final concentration of 10^8 CFU/mL using a 0.5 McFarland standard were inoculated onto the Mueller-Hinton agar using sterile swab sticks. Each organism was inoculated on a different plate and then labelled accordingly. They were subsequently left to dry for fifteen minutes. Seven wells were bored in each plate using a cork borer having a diameter of 6 mm. Next, 100 μL of rosemary essential oil at concentrations of 200, 100, 50, 20, and 10 (mg/mL) was dispensed into each well on separate plates. One well was filled with 20% DMSO in 0.5% Tween 80 as a negative control. Chloramphenicol (30 μg) was placed in the seventh well as the positive control, owing to its broad-spectrum activity. The extracts were allowed to diffuse for 15 min at room temperature after which they were incubated at 37 °C for 24 h for bacterial activity. After incubation, the plates were checked for the formation of clear zones around the well, which corresponds to the antimicrobial activity of the essential oil; the zones of inhibition (ZOIs) were measured using a rule and recorded in mm [32]. The procedure was performed in duplicates [33,34].

4.10. Determination of Minimum Inhibitory and Bactericidal Concentrations

The minimum inhibitory concentrations (MICs) of the REO against the test organisms were determined by the micro-dilution method [35,36]. All reagents and materials used were placed in a biosafety cabinet. A 100 µL volume each of Mueller-Hinton broth was dispensed into all the 96 wells of the microtitre plates. Aliquots of 100 µL of REO were added in triplicate for each bacterial plate on the first rows (Row A). These were then serially diluted with 100 µL of each of the mixtures discarded from the last row, thus leaving each diluted well with a volume of 100 µL. This was followed by the addition of 100 µL of each of the 0.5 McFarland standardised test organisms on each column, except the last columns (12th wells), which served as the sterile controls (containing 200 µL of broth plus the diluent). The microtitre plates were then incubated in a shaking incubator at 37 °C for 24 h, and the MIC was depicted as the lowest concentration of REO that did not permit the growth of the test organism by the addition of 20 µL of MTT (3-(4,5-dimethylthiazole-2-yl)-2,5-diphenyltetrazolium bromide, 0.2%, *w*/*v*) to each well followed by incubation in a shaking incubator at 37 °C for 30 min. The MTT was prepared by measuring 0.1 g of the MTT dye and dissolving it in 100 mL of sterile distilled water. The least concentration of the mixture that did not show color change from yellow to purple was regarded as the MIC. The MIC was confirmed by spectrophotometry at 490 nm in a microtitre plate reader by recording absorbance values for the estimation of the IC50s [35,37].

In order to confirm if the REO was able to kill the microbial cells (bactericidal effect), the MBC was determined. Aliquots from each well from susceptibility testing assays were transferred to plates containing nutrient agar by streaking and then incubated for 24 h at 37 °C, after which the plates were checked for the presence or absence of growth in the nutrient agar [38].

4.11. Determination of REO Synergy with Conventional Antibiotics

Combinatory effects between the test REO and antibiotics were conducted using the checkerboard against the strains of test microbes with slight modification according to the method reported by da Silva et al. [39], Khodavandi et al. [40], and Dickson et al. [41]. Briefly, solutions with different proportions of each REO:drug (final volume of 200 µL) were prepared from twice the MIC solutions of each test sample and the individual antibiotics (1 mg/mL), and the antimicrobial activity was tested as described for MIC determination. The fractional inhibitory concentration index (FICI) was calculated according to the equation below:

$$\text{FIC index} = \frac{[\text{MIC of antibiotic in combination}]}{[\text{MIC of antibiotic alone}]} + \frac{[\text{MIC of oil in combination}]}{[\text{MIC of oil alone}]}$$

The interaction between the test essential oils and antibiotics was considered synergistic if the FIC index was ≤0.5, partial synergistic if the FIC index was >0.5 and <1, additive if the FIC index was =1, no difference if the FIC index was >1 and ≤4, and antagonistic if the FIC index was >4.0.

4.12. Determination of Antibiofilm Activity of REO

The antibacterial activities of the oil against microbial biofilms under two different treatment options (inhibition of biofilm formation and activity against preformed biofilms) were evaluated using the 96-well microtitre plate of microbial biofilm formation and susceptibility testing, with slight modifications [42,43]. Briefly, for the inhibition of biofilm formation, the double-strength Mueller-Hinton broth (Oxoid Limited, Basingstoke, UK) and the oil extract (100 μL each) were mixed in Column 1 and serially diluted until Column 10 at concentrations ranging from 0.04 to 20 mg/mL. Thereafter, 100 μL of the microbial suspension at a concentration of 1×10^6 cells/mL was added to the wells of Columns 1–11 to arrive at a final volume of 200 μL. To each of these plates, 2 μL of 5% (w/v) sterile-filtered TTC solution (which was used in place of XTT/menadione solution) was added so that the final concentrations of TTC became 0.05% (w/v). The microtitre plates were immediately incubated for 24 h at 37 °C. On the other hand, to determine the inhibition against preformed biofilms, the microbial inoculums (100 μL of a suspension of 1×10^6 cells/mL double-strength Mueller-Hinton broth) were pipetted into each well of a flat-bottom 96-well microplate and subjected to incubation at 37 °C for 24 h to allow for biofilm formation. Subsequently, the mixtures were carefully aspirated not to touch the preformed biofilm, which was then washed with PBS (100 μL) two times to remove planktonic and non-adherent cells. In another microplate, the dilutions of the free extract were prepared from 0.04 to 20 mg/mL and then transferred to the microtitre plate containing the preformed biofilms, which was incubated for an additional 24 h at 37 °C. Then, in the same vein, 2 μL of a TTC, 5% (w/v) sterile-filtered solution was added so that the final concentrations of TTC became 0.05% (w/v) and incubated. After the incubation periods, the liquid in each well of the microplates from both assays was carefully aspirated, and the biofilm was washed with PBS (100 μL) twice in order to remove planktonic and non-adherent cells. The post-processing to measure the metabolic activity after the antimicrobial (oil) treatment was evaluated as previously described [42,43], but by using the TTC reduction assay. Finally, plates were read by spectrophotometry at a modified OD of 492 nm in a microtitre plate reader, and the percentage microbial inhibition obtained by the equation below for the IC50s was subsequently calculated.

$$\%\ \text{biofilm inhibition} = \left(\text{optical density (OD) of control} - \frac{\text{OD of treatment}}{\text{OD of control}}\right) \times 100\%$$

5. Conclusions

Rosemary essential oil had significant bactericidal effects on the bacteria tested (including the multidrug-resistant ones), and its MIC and MBC values were low. Overall, REO was synergistic with known conventional antibiotics and, thus, has encouraging prospects in combination therapy involving conventional antibiotics, even in the treatment of infections with multidrug-resistant bacteria, biofilm-forming ones inclusive. Further authentication of the synergistic effects of REO is, nonetheless, warranted, and these investigations can expand the range of conventional antibiotics tested. Moreover, additional analyses on REO can clarify insights on its mechanism of action, as well as its potential acute and sub-chronic toxicity to humans and animals at therapeutic levels.

Supplementary Materials: The following supporting information can be downloaded at: https://www.mdpi.com/article/10.3390/ph17121653/s1, Figure S1.Zones of Inhibition (in millimeters) of different bacterial strains to Rosemary essential oil; Figure S2. The GC/MS analysis of Rosemary essential oil (REO), Figure S3. The total ion chromatogram (TIC) or mass chromatogram) of Eucalyptol: Scan time = 8.037 min; Figure S4. The total ion chromatogram (TIC) or mass chromatogram) of Linalool: Scan time = 9.430 min; Figure S5. The total ion chromatogram (TIC) or mass chromatogram) of (+)-2-Bornanone: Scan time = 9.944 min; Figure S6. The total ion chromatogram (TIC) or mass chromatogram) of Endo-Borneol: Scan time = 10.641 min; Figure S7. The total ion chromatogram (TIC) or mass chromatogram) of Terpinen-4-ol: Scan time = 10.714 min; Figure S8. The total ion chromatogram (TIC) or mass chromatogram) of α-Terpineol: Scan time = 10.916 min; Figure S9. The total ion chromatogram (TIC) or mass chromatogram) of Bornyl acetate: Scan time = 11.887 min; Figure S10. The total ion chromatogram (TIC) or mass chromatogram) of Anethole: Scan time = 12.052 min; Figure S11. The total ion chromatogram (TIC) or mass chromatogram) of Caryophyllene: Scan time = 13.758 min.

Author Contributions: Conceptualisation, D.E.K.K. and N.T.K.D.D.; methodology, D.E.K.K., D.N., S.E.G., E.K.D., A.D.D. and N.T.K.D.D.; validation, D.E.K.K., D.N., E.K.D., A.D.D., F.C.N.K. and N.T.K.D.D.; formal analysis, D.E.K.K., S.E.G. and F.C.N.K.; investigation, D.E.K.K., D.N., S.E.G., E.K.D., A.D.D. and N.T.K.D.D.; resources, D.E.K.K., D.N., S.E.G., F.C.N.K. and N.T.K.D.D.; data curation, D.E.K.K., D.N., S.E.G., E.K.D., A.A.A. and F.C.N.K.; writing—original draft preparation, D.E.K.K., F.C.N.K. and N.T.K.D.D.; writing—review and editing, D.E.K.K., D.N., S.E.G., E.K.D., A.D.D., A.A.A., F.C.N.K. and N.T.K.D.D.; visualisation, D.E.K.K., S.E.G., E.K.D., A.D.D., A.A.A., F.C.N.K. and N.T.K.D.D.; supervision, D.E.K.K. and N.T.K.D.D.; project administration, D.E.K.K. and N.T.K.D.D.; funding acquisition, N.T.K.D.D. All authors have read and agreed to the published version of the manuscript.

Funding: The APC was funded by the Fleming Fund Fellowship Scheme through the London School of Hygiene and Tropical Medicine and the University of Ghana according to Grant Number RZ07.

Institutional Review Board Statement: Not applicable.

Informed Consent Statement: Not applicable.

Data Availability Statement: All the relevant data are contained in the manuscript.

Acknowledgments: We would like to thank the following individuals: Rita Opoku of the Central Laboratory of Kwame Nkrumah University of Sciences and Technology, who performed the GC-MS analysis on the REO; Shirley Ocloo, and the Ghana Physicians and Surgeons Association, North America (GPSA-NA, N&S Carolina Chapter), who provided funds for furnishing the Organic and Analytical Laboratory used for the work.

Conflicts of Interest: The authors declare no conflicts of interest. The funder had no role in the design of this study; in the collection, analyses, or interpretation of data; in the writing of the manuscript; or in the decision to publish the results.

References

1. Antimicrobial Resistance Collaborators. Global burden of bacterial antimicrobial resistance in 2019: A systematic analysis. *Lancet* **2022**, *399*, 629–655. [CrossRef] [PubMed]
2. O'Neill, J. Antimicrobial resistance: Tackling a crisis for the health and wealth of nations. *Rev. Antimicrob. Resist.* **2014**. Available online: https://www.who.int/news/item/29-04-2019-new-report-calls-for-urgent-action-to-avert-antimicrobial-resistance-crisis (accessed on 11 July 2023).
3. GBD 2021 Antimicrobial Resistance Collaborators. Global burden of bacterial antimicrobial resistance 1990–2021: A systematic analysis with forecasts to 2050. *Lancet* **2024**, *404*, 1199–1226. [CrossRef] [PubMed]
4. Donkor, E.S.; Kotey, F.C.N. Methicillin-resistant *Staphylococcus aureus* (MRSA) in the oral cavity: Its implications for dental care and MRSA surveillance. *Infect. Dis. Res. Treat.* **2020**, *13*, 1178633720976581. [CrossRef]
5. Kotey, F.C.N.; Dayie, N.T.K.D.; Tetteh-Quarcoo, P.B.; Donkor, E.S. *Candida* bloodstream infections: Changes in epidemiology and increase in drug resistance. *Infect. Dis. Res. Treat.* **2021**, *14*, 11786337211026927. [CrossRef]
6. Olmedo, R.H.; Nepote, V.; Grosso, N.R. Preservation of sensory and chemical properties in flavoured cheese prepared with cream cheese base using oregano and rosemary essential oils. *LWT-Food Sci. Technol.* **2013**, *53*, 409–417. [CrossRef]
7. Alvarez, M.V.; Ortega-Ramirez, L.A.; Silva-Espinoza, B.A.; Gonzalez-Aguilar, G.A.; Ayala-Zavala, J.F. Antimicrobial, antioxidant, and sensorial impacts of oregano and rosemary essential oils over broccoli florets. *J. Food Process. Preserv.* **2019**, *43*, e13889. [CrossRef]
8. Garcia-Soteloa, D.; Silva-Espinoza, B.; Perez-Tello, M.; Olivas, I.; Alvarez-Parrilla, E.; González-Aguilar, G.A.; Ayala-Zavala, J.F. Antimicrobial activity and thermal stability of rosemary essential oil: β-cyclodextrin capsules applied in tomato juice. *Lwt* **2019**, *111*, 837–845. [CrossRef]
9. Couto, R.O.; Conceicao, E.C.; Chaul, L.T.; Oliveira, E.M.S.; Martins, F.S.; Bara, M.T.F.; Rezende, K.R.; Alves, S.F.; Paula, J.R. Spraydried rosemary extracts: Physicochemical and antioxidant properties. *Food Chem.* **2012**, *131*, 99–105. [CrossRef]
10. Jiang, Y.; Wu, N.; Fu, Y.J.; Wang, W.; Luo, M.; Zhao, C.J.; Zu, Y.G.; Liu, X.L. Chemical composition and antimicrobial activity of the essential oil of Rosemary. *Environ. Toxicol. Pharmacol.* **2011**, *32*, 63–68. [CrossRef]
11. Cutillas, A.B.; Carrasco, A.; Martinez-Gutierrez, R.; Tomas, V.; Tudela, J. *Rosmarinus officinalis* L. essential oils from Spain: Composition, antioxidant capacity, lipoxygenase and acetylcholinesterase inhibitory capacities, and antimicrobial activities. *Plant Biosyst.* **2018**, *152*, 1282–1292. [CrossRef]
12. Yeddes, W.; Nowacka, M.; Rybak, K.; Boruszewski, P.; Ostrowska-Ligeza, E.; Betlej, I.; Aidi Wannes, W.; Hammami, M.; Jallouli, S.; Horchani-Naifer, K.; et al. Effect of rosemary essential oil and ethanol extract on physicochemical and antibacterial properties of optimized gelatin-chitosan film using mixture design. *J. Food Process. Preserv.* **2021**, *46*, e16059.

13. Eid, A.M.; Jaradat, N.; Issa, L.; Abu-Hasan, A.; Salah, N.; Dalal, M.; Mousa, A.; Zarour, A. Evaluation of anticancer, antimicrobial, and antioxidant activities of rosemary (*Rosmarinus officinalis*) essential oil and its Nanoemulgel. *Eur. J. Integr. Med.* **2022**, *55*, 102175. [CrossRef]
14. Dhouibi, I.; Flamini, G.; Bouaziz, M. Comparative study on the essential oils extracted from Tunisian rosemary and myrtle: Chemical profiles, quality, and antimicrobial activities. *ACS Omega* **2023**, *8*, 6431–6438. [CrossRef]
15. Murtiastutik, D.; Primasari, P.I.; Ervianti, E.; Bintanjoyo, L. Antifungal activity of rosemary essential oil against *Candida* spp. isolates from HIV/AIDS patients with oral candidiasis. *J. Pak. Assoc. Dermatol.* **2023**, *33*, 437–443.
16. Becer, E.; Altundağ, E.M.; Güran, M.; Vatansever, H.S.; Ustürk, S.; Hanoğlu, D.Y.; Başer, K.H.C. Composition and antibacterial, anti-inflammatory, antioxidant, and anticancer activities of *Rosmarinus officinalis* L. essential oil. *South Afr. J. Bot.* **2023**, *160*, 437–445. [CrossRef]
17. Melero-Bravo, E.; Elguea-Culebras, G.O.; Sánchez-Vioque, R.; Fernández-Sestelo, M.; Herraiz-Peñalver, D.; Sánchez-Vioque, R. Variability of essential oil in cultivated populations of *Rosmarinus officinalis* L. in Spain. *Euphytica* **2022**, *218*, 65. [CrossRef]
18. Puvača, N.; Milenković, J.; Galonja Coghill, T.; Bursić, V.; Petrović, A.; Tanasković, S.; Pelić, M.; Ljubojević Pelić, D.; Miljković, T. Antimicrobial activity of selected essential oils against selected pathogenic bacteria: In vitro study. *Antibiotics* **2021**, *10*, 546. [CrossRef]
19. Araya, J.; Esquivel, M.; Jimenez, G.; Navia, D.; Poveda, L. Antimicrobial activity and physicochemical characterization of thermoplastic films based on bitter cassava starch, nanocellulose and rosemary essential oil. *J. Plast. Film Sheeting* **2022**, *38*, 46–71. [CrossRef]
20. Yang, J.; Goksen, G.; Zhang, W. Rosemary essential oil: Chemical and biological properties, with emphasis on its delivery systems for food preservation. *Food Control* **2023**, *154*, 110003. [CrossRef]
21. Jarrar, N.; Abu-Hijleh, A.; Adwan, K. Antibacterial activity of *Rosmarinus officinalis* L. alone and in combination with cefuroxime against methicillin-resistant *Staphylococcus aureus*. *Asian Pac. J. Trop. Med.* **2010**, *3*, 121–123. [CrossRef]
22. Ojeda-Sana, A.M.; van Baren, C.M.; Elechosa, M.A.; Juárez, M.A.; Moreno, S. New insights into antibacterial and antioxidant activities of rosemary essential oils and their main components. *Food Control* **2013**, *31*, 189–195. [CrossRef]
23. Jardak, M.; Elloumi-Mseddi, J.; Aifa, S.; Mnif, S. Chemical composition, anti-biofilm activity and potential cytotoxic effect on cancer cells of *Rosmarinus officinalis* L. essential oil from Tunisia. *Lipids Health Dis.* **2017**, *16*, 190. [CrossRef] [PubMed]
24. de Oliveira, J.R.; Camargo, S.E.A.; de Oliveira, L.D. *Rosmarinus officinalis* L. (rosemary) as therapeutic and prophylactic agent. *J. Biomed. Sci.* **2019**, *26*, 5. [CrossRef] [PubMed]
25. Hossain, F.; Follett, P.; Vu, K.D.; Harich, M.; Salmieri, S.; Lacroix, M. Evidence for synergistic activity of plant-derived essential oils against fungal pathogens of food. *Food Microbiol.* **2016**, *53*, 24–30. [CrossRef]
26. Bajalan, I.; Rouzbahani, R.; Pirbalouti, A.G.; Maggi, F. Antioxidant and antibacterial activities of the essential oils obtained from seven Iranian populations of *Rosmarinus officinalis*. *Ind. Crops Prod.* **2017**, *107*, 305–311. [CrossRef]
27. Boughendjioua, H.; Boughendjioua, Z. Fourier transformed infrared spectroscopy analysis of constituents of *Rosmarinus officinalis* L. essential oil from Algeria. *Inorg. Mater.* **2017**, *14*, 15.
28. Nikkhah, M.; Hashemi, M.; Najafi, M.B.H.; Farhoosh, R. Synergistic effects of some essential oils against fungal spoilage on pear fruit. *Int. J. Food Microbiol.* **2017**, *257*, 285–294. [CrossRef]
29. Joo, H.S.; Otto, M. Molecular basis of in vivo biofilm formation by bacterial pathogens. *Chem. Biol.* **2012**, *19*, 1503–1513. [CrossRef]
30. Wilkins, M.; Hall-Stoodley, L.; Allan, R.N.; Faust, S.N. New approaches to the treatment of biofilm-related infections. *J. Infect.* **2014**, *69*, S47–S52. [CrossRef]
31. Kabotso, D.E.K.; Neglo, D.; Kwashie, P.; Agbo, I.A.; Abaye, D.A. GC/MS Composition and Resistance Modulatory Inhibitory Activities of Three Extracts of Lemongrass: Citral Modulates the Activities of Five Antibiotics at Sub-Inhibitory Concentrations on Methicillin-Resistant *Staphylococcus aureus*. *Chem. Biodivers.* **2022**, *19*, e202200296. [CrossRef] [PubMed]
32. Gaur, P.; Hada, V.; Rath, R.S.; Mohanty, A.; Singh, P.; Rukadikar, A. Interpretation of antimicrobial susceptibility testing using European Committee on Antimicrobial Susceptibility Testing (EUCAST) and Clinical and Laboratory Standards Institute (CLSI) Breakpoints: Analysis of Agreement. *Cureus* **2023**, *15*, e36977. [CrossRef] [PubMed]
33. Irshad, M.; Aziz, S.; Shahid, M.; Ahmed, N.; Minhas, F.A.; Sherazi, T. Antioxidant and antimicrobial activities of essential oil of Skimmea laureola growing wild in the State of Jammu and Kashmir. *J. Med. Plants Res.* **2012**, *6*, 1680–1684. [CrossRef]
34. Neglo, D.; Tettey, C.O.; Essuman, E.K.; Amenu, J.D.; Mills-Robertson, F.C.; Sedohia, D.; Boakye, A.A.; Abaye, D.A. Evaluation of the modulatory effect of *Annona muricata* extracts on the activity of some selected antibiotics against biofilm-forming MRSA. *Evid. -Based Complement. Altern. Med.* **2021**, *2021*, 9342110. [CrossRef]
35. Eloff, J. A Sensitive and quick microplate method to determine the minimal inhibitory concentration of plant extracts for bacteria. *Planta Medica.* **1998**, *64*, 711–713. [CrossRef]
36. Clinical and Laboratory Standards Institute. *Methods for Dilution Antimicrobial Susceptibility Test for Bacteria That Grow Aerobically Document in M07-A9*, 10th ed.; Clinical and Laboratory Standards Institute: Wayne, PA, USA, 2015.
37. Harley, B.K.; Quagraine, A.M.; Neglo, D.; Aggrey, M.O.; Orman, E.; Mireku-Gyimah, N.A.; Amengor, C.D.; Jato, J.; Saaka, Y.; Fleischer, T.C. Metabolite profiling, antifungal, biofilm formation prevention and disruption of mature biofilm activities of Erythrina senegalensis stem bark extract against *Candida albicans* and *Candida glabrata*. *PLoS ONE* **2022**, *17*, e0278096. [CrossRef]

38. Mogana, R.; Adhikari, A.; Tzar, M.N.; Ramliza, R.; Wiart, C.J.B.C.M. Antibacterial activities of the extracts, fractions and isolated compounds from *Canarium patentinervium* Miq. against bacterial clinical isolates. *BMC Complement. Med. Ther.* **2020**, *20*, 55. [CrossRef]
39. da Silva, C.R.; de Andrade Neto, J.B.; Sidrim, J.J.C.; Ângelo, M.R.F.; Magalhães, H.I.F.; Cavalcanti, B.C.; Brilhante, R.S.N.; Macedo, D.S.; de Moraes, M.O.; Lobo, M.D.P.; et al. Synergistic effects of amiodarone and fluconazole on *Candida tropicalis* resistant to fluconazole. *Antimicrob. Agents Chemother.* **2013**, *57*, 1691–1700. [CrossRef]
40. Khodavandi, A.; Alizadeh, F.; Aala, F.; Sekawi, Z.; Chong, P.P. In vitro investigation of antifungal activity of allicin alone and in combination with azoles against *Candida* species. *Mycopathologia* **2010**, *169*, 287–295. [CrossRef]
41. Dickson, R.; Houghton, P.; Hylands, P.; Gibbons, S. Antimicrobial, resistance-modifying effects, antioxidant and free radical scavenging activities of *Mezoneuron benthamianum* Baill., *Securinega virosa* Roxb. &Wlld. and *Microglossa pyrifolia* Lam. *Phytother. Res.* **2006**, *20*, 41–45.
42. Pierce, C.G.; Uppuluri, P.; Tristan, A.R.; Wormley, F.L., Jr.; Mowat, E.; Ramage, G.; Lopez-Ribot, J.L. A simple and reproducible 96-well plate based method for the formation of fungal biofilms and its application to antifungal susceptibility testing. *Nat. Protoc.* **2008**, *3*, 1494–1500. [CrossRef] [PubMed]
43. Pierce, C.G.; Uppuluri, P.; Tummala, S.; Lopez-Ribot, J.L. A 96 well microtiter plate-based method for monitoring formation and antifungal susceptibility testing of *Candida albicans* biofilms. *J. Vis. Exp.* **2010**, *44*, 2287. [CrossRef]

pharmaceuticals

MDPI

Article

Phytochemical Analysis and Evaluation of Antioxidant and Antimicrobial Properties of Essential Oils and Seed Extracts of *Anethum graveolens* from Southern Morocco: In Vitro and In Silico Approach for a Natural Alternative to Synthetic Preservatives

Nadia Hadi [1], Aziz Drioiche [1,*], El Moumen Bouchra [1], Soukayna Baammi [2], Abdelaaty Abdelaziz Shahat [3], Imane Tagnaout [1], Mohamed Radi [1], Fidaous Remok [1], Amal Bouzoubaa [1] and Touriya Zair [1,*]

[1] Research Team of Chemistry of Bioactive Molecules and the Environment, Laboratory of Innovative Materials and Biotechnology of Natural Resources, Faculty of Sciences, Moulay Ismaïl University, B.P. 11201, Zitoune, Meknes 50070, Morocco; nadia.hadi1@gmail.com (N.H.); elmoumen.bouchra4@gmail.com (E.M.B.); ema.tagnaout@gmail.com (I.T.); oncaradi@gmail.com (M.R.); remok.firdaous@gmail.com (F.R.); bouzoubaa.amal@yahoo.fr (A.B.)

[2] Bioinformatics Laboratory, College of Computing, Mohammed VI Polytechnic University, Ben Guerir 43150, Morocco; soukayna.baammi@um6p.ma

[3] Pharmacognosy Department, College of Pharmacy, King Saud University, Riyadh 11451, Saudi Arabia; ashahat@ksu.edu.sa

* Correspondence: a.drioiche@edu.umi.ac.ma (A.D.); t.zair@umi.ac.ma (T.Z.); Tel.: +212-600394841 (A.D.)

Abstract: *Anethum graveolens* is an aromatic plant traditionally used as an antispasmodic and carminative. The objective of this study is to analyze the chemical composition of the essential oils and extracts obtained from seeds gathered in Errachidia, southern Morocco. Additionally, the antioxidant and antimicrobial properties of these oils and extracts will be evaluated. GC-MS analysis of the EO isolated by hydrodistillation revealed that its main compounds were E-anethole (38.13%), estragole (29.32%), fenchone (17.21%), and α-pinene (7.37%). The phenolic components were extracted using the methods of decoction and Soxhlet. The assay of the phenolic compounds showed that *A. graveolens* seeds contained considerable amounts of polyphenols, flavonoids, and condensed tannins, with variable levels depending on the extract analyzed. HPLC/UV-ESI-MS analyses performed on the decoction revealed a structural diversity of the molecules present in this extract, the most important of which were umbelliferone (12.35%), 3-hydroxyflavone (11.23%), rosmanol (8.95%), biotin (8.36%), emmotin H (4.91%), and coumarin (4.21%). The antioxidant activity, as determined by three techniques (DPPH•, FRAP, and CAT), demonstrated that the essential oils (EOs) and extracts had a potent capacity to counteract detrimental free radicals, control the generation of reactive oxygen species, and mitigate oxidative damages. The antimicrobial activity of the Eos and extracts was carried out in a liquid medium against five strains (*E. cloacae*, *K. pneumoniae*, *E. coli*, *S. aureus*, and *S. epidermidis*) and four candidiasis (*C. albicans*, *C. dubliniensis*, *C. tropicalis*, and *C. parapsilosis*) and *Aspergillus niger*. The results showed the effectiveness of the EOs compared to the aqueous, ethanolic, and decoction extracts against most of the microorganisms tested. In addition, the ethanolic extract showed antifungal activity that was distinguished from that of the other extracts. The antimicrobial efficacy of the essential oils under study can primarily be attributed to the synergistic interactions among its three principal constituents (E-anethole, estragole, and fenchone). Furthermore, molecular docking and molecular dynamics simulation results reveal significant interactions and stability between the selected bioactive compounds and different target proteins involved in antimicrobial and antioxidant activities. Compounds like 3-hydroxyflavone, emmotin H, trans-caftaric acid, methyl rosmarinate, 1-caffeoyl-beta-D-glucose, and kaempferol exhibited better binding energies with the explored proteins, indicating their potential as antimicrobial and antioxidant agents. Finally, our findings emphasize the significance of *A. graveolens* seeds as a promising reservoir of advantageous health compounds that can serve as organic substitutes for the presently employed synthetic preservatives.

Keywords: *Anethum graveolens*; GC/MS; HPLC/UV-ESI-MS; polyphenols; flavonoids; antioxidants; antimicrobials

1. Introduction

Foodborne illnesses pose a significant threat to public health worldwide, contributing to substantial socioeconomic impacts, especially in developing countries [1]. The World Health Organization (WHO) has reported that antimicrobial resistance caused 1.27 million deaths globally in 2019 and contributed to 4.95 million deaths in 2023 (WHO). In response to these alarming trends, extensive research is being conducted to develop healthy food products and new antimicrobial agents.

On the other hand, the use of synthetic preservatives such as BHA and BHT to prevent food deterioration has become restricted due to their induction of DNA damage and toxicity [2,3]. From this perspective, consumers are concerned about their adverse effects on human health. This fact has led industries and consumers to search for and consume natural derivatives with antioxidant and antimicrobial properties. Among these natural substances are the essential oils and extracts from medicinal plants. These plants are considered a huge source of active secondary metabolites with medicinal properties. These compounds are primarily involved in defense mechanisms against pathogens, herbivores, and their competitors [4]. Plants have remarkably and diversely contributed to various industries such as pharmaceuticals, agriculture, cosmetics, and industrial raw materials. Indeed, they play two major roles: firstly, providing a pleasant taste to foods; secondly, preserving foods through their antimicrobial and antioxidant potentials, thereby delaying their deterioration. One of the popular plants used in pharmaceutical and agri-food industries is *Anethum graveolens*, commonly known as dill [5]. This plant is a perennial herbaceous species in the *Apiaceae* family, and it is the sole member of the *Anethum* genus. It typically reaches a height of 40 to 60 cm.

Dill, a significant plant, is produced in Eurasia and Mediterranean nations. Its seeds and leaves have been utilized as a herb or spice for flavoring dishes for 5000 years by the Egyptians and Greeks [6]. In traditional medicine, dill is generally employed for alleviating colic in infants and flatulence in young children. Additionally, its seed is used in decoction or infusion mode for the treatment of urinary infections, insomnia, hyposecretion of milk, digestive disorders accompanied by meteorism, and gastrointestinal spasms [6,7]. It is commonly employed as a natural flavor enhancer in many culinary items within the industry, particularly in sauces, salads, soups, shellfish, meats, fries, and pickles. The volatile oil derived from the aboveground portion is utilized as a taste enhancer in culinary and beverage applications owing to its agreeable fragrance. Moreover, the essential oils are employed as a scent to enhance the smell of soaps, detergents, and cosmetics [8,9].

At the scientific level, numerous previous studies have highlighted the biological potential of *Anethum graveolens*, such as anti-inflammatory [10], antidiabetic [11], antimicrobial [12], diuretic [13], insecticidal [14], hepatoprotective [15], anticancer, and antioxidant [16].

Due to its intriguing characteristics, the global economic significance of this species has greatly escalated. In Morocco, this plant holds ecological, socio-economic, and therapeutic significance. However, there is limited information on the chemical composition and biological characteristics of the extracts and essential oils derived from *Anethum graveolens* originating from Morocco. Our study specifically examined the detailed examination of the chemical compounds in the essential oil and extracts of *Anethum graveolens* seeds from the Boulemane area. Moreover, our work aimed to discover naturally occurring chemical compounds with antioxidant capabilities and assess the antioxidant and antibacterial activities of the extracts and essential oils derived from this species using in vitro testing.

Nevertheless, there has been a limited amount of research focused on investigating the chemical composition of extracts derived from *Anethum graveolens* seeds. This study was conducted within the specified context, aiming to contribute to the phytochemical analysis and characterization of chemical families found in *Anethum graveolens* seeds gathered from the Boulemane region. Additionally, it entails the assessment of the antibacterial and antioxidant properties of the essential oils and extracts by in vitro and in silico methods in order to uncover their potential as antioxidants and antimicrobials.

2. Results & Discussion

2.1. Quality Control of Plant Material

The quality control findings of the examined plant material are displayed in Table 1. The seeds of *A. graveolens* had a moisture content of around 15.80%, which was within the typical range for seeds. The plant extract had a pH that was somewhat acidic, which aligned with its mineral content of 15.03%. This pH level meets the quality criteria set by AFNOR (NF ISO 5984).

Table 1. Analysis and quality control of *A. graveolens* seeds.

MC (%)	pH	Ash (%)	Organic Matter (%)
15.80	5.2	15.03	84.97

Medicinal plants, despite their health advantages, frequently become polluted by different agents or poisonous compounds during their cultivation and processing. Out of these, heavy metals are particularly worrisome since they can disrupt the proper operation of the central nervous system, liver, lungs, heart, kidneys, and brain. This disruption can result in hypertension, stomach aches, skin rashes, intestinal ulcers, and different types of cancer. In order to tackle this problem, we utilized atomic absorption spectrophotometry to analyze the concentration of six specific heavy metals: chromium (Cr), lead (Pb), cadmium (Cd), iron (Fe), antimony (Sb), and titanium (Ti).

According to the results shown in Table 2, Aneth seeds exhibit a high content of iron (Fe) at 0.5858 mg/L, followed by antimony (Sb) with a content of 0.0087 mg/L. Regarding the other detected heavy metals, it is noteworthy that they all fall within the allowable range set by FAO/WHO regulatory standards. Consequently, the studied plant is suitable for direct consumption, as an ingredient in food processing, or for repackaging if necessary.

Table 2. Heavy metal concentration (mg/L) and maximum limit FAO/WHO (2009).

Element	Heavy Metal Content (mg/L)	Maximum Limit
Chromium (Cr)	0.0008	2
Antimony (Sb)	0.0134	1
Lead (Pb)	0.0034	3
Cadmium (Cd)	<0.0001	0.3
Iron (Fe)	0.5858	20
Titanium (Ti)	0.0082	-

2.2. Physical-Chemical Properties and Extraction Yield of Essential Oils

The data reported in Table 3 indicate that the essential oils (EOs) obtained from the seeds of *A. graveolens* gathered in the Errachidia region during full bloom were characterized by an aromatic scent, a yellowish hue, and a yield of 2.73 ± 0.12%.

Table 3. Essential Oil Yield of *A. graveolens*.

Properties	Yield (%)	Color	Odor	Density (g/mL)
Results	2.73 ± 0.12	Yellowish	Aromatic	0.9362 ± 0.0032

Notably, this result was, on the one hand, significant compared to those from other origins: in Egypt 1.88% [17], in India 1.5% [9], in Iran (0.04–1.86%) [18], and also within the same country 1.92% [19]. On the other hand, it was lower than those reported elsewhere: in southern Morocco (3.5%) [20] and in China (6.7%) [21]. Based on the literature results and those obtained in this study, the variation in EO yield is attributed to various genetic, ecological, and environmental factors (plant age, climatic conditions, soil type, growth stage of the species, part used, harvest time, drying process, harvest period and environment, and cultural practices) as well as the extraction method used.

The plant under investigation yielded essential oils with a density of 0.9362 ± 0.0732 g/mL. Based on the AFNOR standard (2005), essential oils are advised to have a density ranging from 0.906 g/mL, which indicates lesser grade oils, to 0.990 g/mL, which is suggestive of oils of extremely high quality. The measurement indicates that the density of our essential oil is comfortably within the allowed range, indicating a quality that meets or exceeds the normal standards for essential oil density. This discovery suggests that the essential oil extracted from this plant possesses a praiseworthy quality that meets the standards set by the industry.

2.3. Chemical Composition of EO

The chemical profile (Supplementary Figure S1) revealed the presence of 29 chemical compounds for the total chemical composition of this essential oil. These results are summarized in Table 4.

Table 4. Chemical Composition of *Anethum graveolens* Essential Oil.

N°	Compounds	KI *	RA%	Formula
1	α-Pinene	939	7.37	$C_{10}H_{16}$
2	Camphene	954	0.08	$C_{10}H_{16}$
3	Sabinene	975	0.13	$C_{10}H_{16}$
4	β-Pinene	979	0.35	$C_{10}H_{16}$
5	Myrcene	990	0.76	$C_{10}H_{16}$
6	α-Phellandrene	1002	0.17	$C_{10}H_{16}$
7	α-Terpinene	1017	0.02	$C_{10}H_{16}$
8	Limonene	1029	1.24	$C_{10}H_{16}$
9	β-Phellandrene	1029	0.37	$C_{10}H_{16}$
10	Z-β-Ocimene	1037	0.16	$C_{10}H_{16}$
11	1,8-Cineole	1031	0.11	$C_{10}H_{18}O$
12	γ-Terpinene	1059	0.66	$C_{10}H_{16}$
13	Terpinolene	1088	0.05	$C_{10}H_{16}$
14	**Fenchone**	**1086**	**17.21**	$C_{10}H_{16}O$
15	Linalool	1096	2.68	$C_{10}H_{18}O$
16	trans-Pinene hydrate	1122	0.03	$C_{10}H_{18}O$
17	Camphor	1146	0.35	$C_{10}H_{16}O$
18	Terpinen-4-ol	1177	0.13	$C_{10}H_{18}O$
19	**Estragole**	**1196**	**29.32**	$C_{10}H_{12}O$
20	Carvone	1243	0.01	$C_{10}H_{14}O$
21	Z-Anethole	1252	0.06	$C_{10}H_{12}O$
22	ρ-Anis aldehyde	1250	0.05	$C_8H_8O_2$
23	**E-Anethole**	**1284**	**38.13**	$C_{10}H_{12}O$

Table 4. *Cont.*

N°	Compounds	KI *	RA%	Formula
24	α-Copaene	1376	0.02	$C_{15}H_{24}$
25	Z-Isoeugenol	1407	0.02	$C_{10}H_{12}O_2$
26	Methyleugenol	1403	0.34	$C_{11}H_{14}O_2$
27	Germacrene D	1481	0.09	$C_{15}H_{24}$
28	δ-Cadinene	1523	0.03	$C_{15}H_{24}$
29	E-Methylisoeugenol	1492	0.06	$C_{11}H_{14}O_2$
	% Hydrogenated Monoterpenes			**11.36**
	% Oxygenated Monoterpenes			**20.57**
	% Phenylpropanoids			**67.93**
	% Hydrogenated Sesquiterpenes			**0.14**
	Total			**100**

* RA: Relative abundance (%); KI: Kovats index.

The analysis of the chemical composition revealed that phenylpropanoids constituted the most abundant group of all identified compounds in the essential oil of *Anethum graveolens*, accounting for 67.93%, followed by monoterpenes divided between oxygenated monoterpenes (20.57%) and hydrogenated monoterpenes (11.36%). Hydrogenated sesquiterpenes were also identified but with a low percentage (0.14%).

Furthermore, the chemical composition of the *A. graveolens* essential oil was rich in ethers (68.04%), followed by ketones with a percentage of 17.57%. We also note the presence of hydrocarbons (11.5%) and alcohols (2.84%). However, aldehydes were nearly absent (0.05%) (Figure 1).

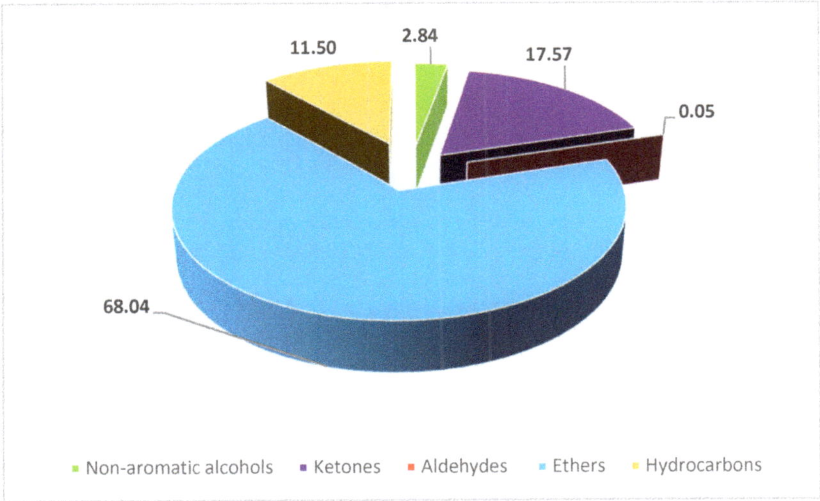

Figure 1. Distribution of the main chemical groups in the essential oil of *A. graveolens*.

The essential oil extracted from the seeds of *A. graveolens* was mainly composed of (E)-anethole (38.13%), estragole (29.32%), fenchone (17.21%), and α-pinene (7.37%), while other compounds were present in smaller amounts, such as linalool (2.68%) and limonene (1.24%) (Table 4 and Supplementary Figure S2).

An analysis of the data revealed that the chemical composition of our *A. graveolens* essential oil differs from that reported in previous studies of other origins, with qualitative and quantitative differences in individual components being identified. Indeed, we observed that the studied plant exhibited an interesting chemical polymorphism.

In Morocco, few studies have focused on the chemical profile of dill essential oil. Znini et al. [20] identified 12 compounds representing 98% of the essential oil extracted from seeds from southern Morocco, with carvone (43.5%), dillapiole (26.7%), and limonene (15.4%) being the major compounds. Furthermore, chromatographic and spectrophotometric analyses conducted by El-Sayed et al. [17] on the essential oil extracted from Egyptian seeds revealed the following major compounds as the major constituents of dill essential oil: dillapiole (44.01%), D-limonene (19.47%), and carvotanacetone (13.03%). Meanwhile, in Tunisia, Snuossi et al. [22] reported carvone (27%), piperitone (25.7%), limonene (20.6%), dillapiole (8%), trans-dihydrocarvone (4.9%), and camphor (4.4%).

In Europe, French dill essential oil is mainly composed of limonene (48.05%), carvone (37.94%), cis-dihydrocarvone (3.5%), and trans-carvone (1.07%) [23]. Kostić et al. [24] reported the dominant presence of oxygenated monoterpenes (52.79%) and the total absence of phenylpropanoids in the composition of dill essential oil from Serbia. The latter contained a large quantity of carvone (42.47%), limonene (29.04%), and α-phellandrene (13.12%). Meanwhile, in Asia and Saudi Arabia, Aati et al. [25] found that the essential oil extracted from seeds, using the solid-phase microextraction method Headspace, was rich in monoterpenes (65.1%).

Moreover, its major compounds were anethole (33.3%), limonene (30.8%), carvone (17.7%), and trans-dihydrocarvone (12.2%). A study conducted reported that Iranian dill essential oil contains linalool (63.41%), δ-terpinene (4.27%), β-pinene (3.97%), p-cymene (3.35%), geranyl acetate (3.32%), octyl butyrate (3.3%), and α-pinene (3.23%) [26]. However, in the same country, Najafzadeh et al. [14] found that phellandrene (34.19%), carvone (23.67%), limonene (21.47%), α-terpineol (5.58%), and para-cymene (5.50%) were the main constituents of this species. In China, the major constituents of this studied essential oil are D-carvone (40.36%), D-limonene (19.31%), apiole (17.50%), α-pinene (6.43%), 9-octadecenoic acid (9.00%), and 9,12-octadecadienoic acid (2.44%) [21]. Similarly, in India, Kaur et al. [9] reported carvone (41.15%), limonene (23.11%), camphor (9.25%), and dihydrocarvone (3.75%) as the main compounds, while butyl acetate (2.65%), myrcene (2.365%), anethole (1.65%), α-pinene (1.06%), and aneth ether (1.02%) as the minor compounds in the essential oil of this species.

The various components reported by different studies also depend on the different growth stages of the plant, the cultivation area, and the specific part of the plant used.

2.4. Phytochemical Screening

Phytochemical tests were conducted on various extracts prepared from *A. graveolens* seeds using specific revealing reagents. The results of phytochemical screening are reported in Table 5.

This species was rich in primary metabolites, including polysaccharides, reducing sugars (glucose and fructose), proteins, and lipids at variable concentrations. Similarly, the presence of secondary metabolites, including flavonoids, tannins, mucilages, leucoanthocyanins, oses and holosides, sterols, and triterpenes, were confirmed. However, saponins and alkaloids were found to be absent.

Our results are consistent with those of El Mansouri et al. [27], who revealed the abundant presence of tannins and flavonoids, as well as the absence of saponins in dill seeds from Southern Morocco. Similarly, Kaur et al. [9] demonstrated the presence of phenolic compounds, flavonoids, tannins, and terpenoids.

Table 5. Results of phytochemical tests conducted on extracts of *A. graveolens* seeds.

Chemical Group		*A. graveolens*
Polysaccharide		starch
Reducing sugars		+
Protein	Biuret reaction	+
	Xanthoprotein reaction	+
Lipids (Lieberman Burchard reaction)		+++
Tannins		+++
Catechic tannins		++
Gallic tannins		++
Flavonoids		++
Leucoanthocyanins		++
Saponosides		-
Alkaloids		-
Reducing Compounds		++
Oses and holosides		++
Mucilages		++
Sterols and triterpenes		++

+++ Very abundant; ++: abundant; + weak; - absent.

2.5. Phenolic Compound Yields of Extracts

We were able to determine the yield of several phenolic compounds found in the plant under investigation by extracting them. The extracts included ethanol, aqueous, and decocted extracts. The yield was calculated as a percentage relative to 30 g of the plant material that had been dried and powdered. The findings are depicted in Figure 2.

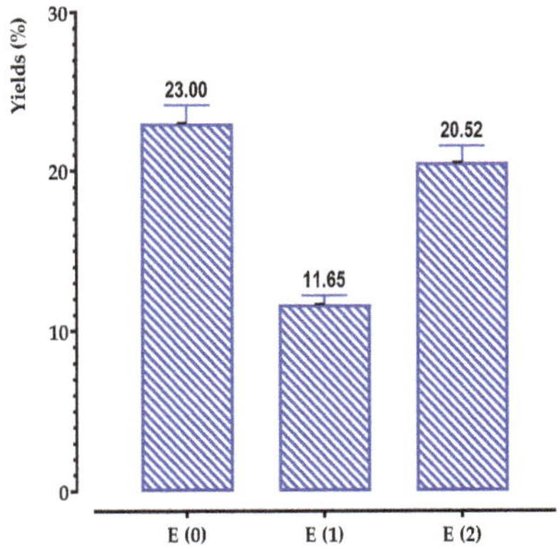

Figure 2. Yields of extracts obtained from *A. graveolens*.

The results obtained showed that extraction yields depended both on the extraction solvent and the extraction method. Indeed, the average extraction yields of phenolic compounds were more or less variable and were higher in the decocted (23.00% ± 0.04) and aqueous extracts (20.52% ± 0.006) than in the ethanol extract (11.65% ± 0.003).

We observed a propensity for water to extract a greater number of chemicals compared to ethanol. This phenomenon may be attributed to the inherent property of water as a highly polar solvent, which has the ability to selectively extract a diverse array of molecules. This includes a substantial quantity of non-phenolic substances, such as sugars and proteins.

2.6. Content of Phenolic Compounds, Flavonoids, and Condensed Tannins

Figure 3 displays the outcomes acquired through the use of a UV–visible spectrophotometer pertaining to the concentrations of total phenolic components and flavonoids in extracts derived from *A. graveolens* seeds. Based on the observed data, it seemed that the amounts of these compounds exhibited significant variation between different extracts. The ethanolic extract recorded the highest quantities of phenolic compounds, flavonoids, and tannins at approximately 52.65 ± 0.22 mg GAE/g of extract, 35.58 ± 2.79 mg QE/g of extract, and 0.090 mg CE/g of extract, respectively, followed by the aqueous extract noting values of 39.72 ± 0.00 mg GAE/g of extract, 13.79 ± 0.63 mg QE/g of extract, and 0.075 ± 0.002 mg CE/g of extract. Meanwhile, the decoction procedure produced the lowest quantities of the tested molecules; notably, 23.35 ± 0.66 mg GAE/g of extract for phenolic compounds, 9.40 ± 0.51 mg QE/g of extract for flavonoids, and 0.046 ± 0.003 mg CE/g of extract for tannins. The results we obtained are significantly higher than those published by El Mansouri et al. [27]. Our research showed that the decoction had higher quantities of phenolic compounds and flavonoids but a somewhat reduced tannin content compared to a previous study. El Mansouri et al. [27], reported that the dill seed decoction had polyphenol and tannin concentrations of 6.16 mg GAE/g of extract and 0.21 mg CE/g of extract, respectively. This discrepancy underscores the fluctuation in phytochemical composition caused by factors such as geographic source, extraction procedure, and analytical methodologies.

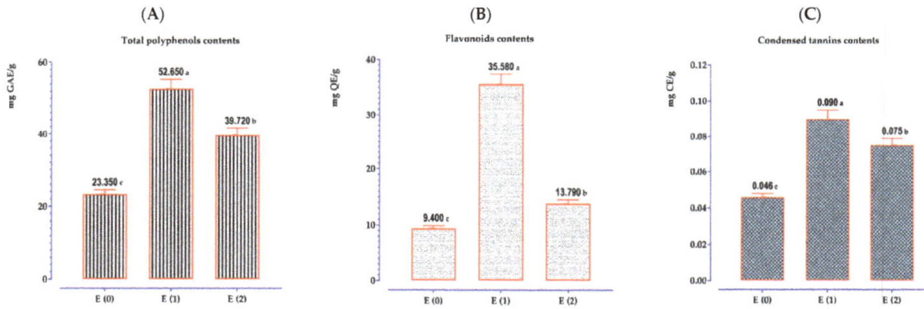

Figure 3. Contents of total polyphenols (**A**), flavonoids (**B**), and condensed tannins (**C**) in extracts from *A. graveolens* seeds. The values are means ± SD. Results with different superscripts are significantly different from each other ($p < 0.05$).

2.7. Chromatographic Analysis by HPLC/UV-ESI-MS of the Extracts

The chromatographic profile, depicted below (Supplementary Figure S3), illustrates the peaks of compounds derived from the decoction of *A. graveolens* seeds, along with their retention times and relative abundances.

Using analytical and spectral data in negative and positive modes, we identified 38 compounds whose names and molecular formulas are presented in Table 6.

Analysis of the results obtained from the decoction revealed a structural diversity of molecules constituting the dill extract. Indeed, we detected the presence of several compounds, the most significant of which were two coumarins, umbelliferone (12.35%) and coumarin (4.21%), a 3-hydroxyflavone flavonoid (11.23%), a diterpene rosmanol (8.95%), a vitamin B7 biotin (8.36%), and a sesquiterpenoid emmotin H (4.91%).

ESI-MS, which stands for electrospray ionization-mass spectrometry, is a crucial technique for identifying the structure of compounds. It allows for the analysis of each component by fragmentation in both negative and positive ion modes.

The ESI-MS spectrum of umbelliferone showed that this molecule underwent ionization, resulting in the loss of a proton (H^-), forming the $[M-H]^-$ ion, observable at $m/z = 161$ and detected at 8.96 min in the mass spectrometer. Furthermore, the predominant fragments identified at $m/z = 133$ and 106 corresponded respectively to the separation of an acetate (CH_3CO) group and a carbon monoxide (CO) group, thus characterizing the typical fragmentation of the coumarin structure. In a similar context, 3-hydroxyflavone ($C_{15}H_{10}O_3$, M = 238) presented an $[M-H]^-$ ion at m/z = 237, appearing at 9.91 min, accompanied by major fragments at m/z = 237, 135, and 101 that reflects the fragmentation of the flavonoid skeleton, including the release of a CO group and a $C_5H_4O_2$ fragment. Moreover, rosmanol revealed an $[M-H]^-$ ion at m/z = 345, observed at 10.15 min, with major fragments at m/z = 243 and 197, indicating the characteristic fragmentation of its polyphenolic structure.

Table 6. List of compounds identified by HPLC/UV-ESI-MS in the decoction E (0) of *A. graveolens* seeds.

N°	RT	Area (%)	Molecules	Structure	Classes	Exact Weights	$[M-H]^-$ (m/z)	$[M+H]^+$ (m/z)	Fragment Ions (m/z)
1	4.05	1.8	Medioresinol	$C_{21}H_{23}O_7$	Flavonoid	388	387		207-179
2	4.23	1.75	Caffeic acid	$C_9H_8O_4$	Phenolic acid	180		181	181-163-145-139-114
3	4.33	2.47	Cinnamic acid	$C_9H_8O_2$	Phenolic acid	148	147		119-103-93
4	4.51	1.21	Scopoletin	$C_{10}H_8O_4$	Coumarin	192	191		176-148-104
5	4.75	3.58	Pimelic acid	$C_7H_{12}O_4$	Fatty acid	160	159		115-97
6	5.34	0.53	Retusin	$C_{19}H_{18}O_7$	Flavonoid	358	357		357-342-327-312-297
7	8.39	0.60	Syringic acid	$C_9H_{10}O_5$	Phenolic acid	198	197		179-135-123
8	8.53	1.30	Carnosic acid	$C_{20}H_{27}O_4$	Diterpene	332		333	333-287
9	8.96	12.35	Umbelliferone	$C_9H_6O_3$	Coumarin	162	161		133-106
10	9.00	8.36	Biotin	$C_{10}H_{16}N_2O_3S$	Vitamin	244		243	297-228-174-130
11	9.24	4.21	Coumarin	$C_9H_6O_2$	Coumarin	146		147	147-103
12	9.48	1.34	Kaempferide	$C_{16}H_{12}O_6$	Flavonoid	300	299		217-149-107
13	9.91	11.23	3-Hydroxyflavone	$C_{15}H_{10}O_3$	Flavonoid	238	237		237-135-101
14	10.15	8.95	Rosmanol	$C_{20}H_{26}O_5$	Polyphenol	346	345		243-197-147
15	10.78	3.40	Homovanillic acid	$C_9H_{10}O_4$	Other	182	181		137-123-108
16	11.08	3.35	kaempferol	$C_{15}H_{10}O_6$	Flavonoid	286	285		201-165-151-117
17	11.37	3.56	Methyl rosmarinate	$C_{19}H_{18}O_8$	Polyphenol	374		375	375-181-137
18	11.55	0.98	Chlorogenic acid	$C_{16}H_{18}O_9$	Phenolic acid	354	353		191-179
19	12.33	0.55	Apigenin 7-rhamnoside	$C_{21}H_{20}O_9$	Flavonoid	416		417	417-271-243-229
20	12.71	1.02	Quercitine 7-glucuronide	$C_{21}H_{18}O_{13}$	Flavonoid	478	477		431-301-175
21	12.99	0.42	Epicatechin gallate	$C_{22}H_{18}O_{10}$	Polyphenol	442	441		289-169-125
22	13.72	1.26	Rhamnetin	$C_{16}H_{12}O_7$	Flavonoid	316	315		300-179-165-151
23	13.92	0.42	Riboflavin	$C_{17}H_{20}N_4O_6$	Vitamin	376	375		375-255-243-241
24	14.11	1.29	Quercetin-3-O-galactoside	$C_{21}H_{20}O_{12}$	Flavonoid	464		465	465-427-303-91
25	14.80	1.29	Quercetin 3-O-rhamnoside	$C_{21}H_{20}O_{11}$	Flavonoid	448	447		301-300-284
26	15.25	1.67	δ-tocopherol	$C_{27}H_{46}O_2$	Vitamin	402	401		385-135
27	15.73	3.85	trans-caftaric acid	$C_{13}H_{12}O_9$	Phenolic acid	312	311		249-203-179-149
28	16.10	1.03	3-Feruloylquinic acid	$C_{17}H_{20}O_9$	Phenolic acid	368	367		293-209-193-173
29	16.60	0.56	Quercetin 3,3′-dimethyl ether	$C_{17}H_{14}O_7$	Flavonoid	330	329		314-301-285-270
30	17.35	1.62	Rosmarinic acid	$C_{18}H_{16}O_8$	Phenolic acid	360		361	181-163-145-135-117
31	19.06	1.23	Apigenin	$C_{15}H_{10}O_5$	Flavonoid	270	269		227-159-121-105
32	20.26	0.78	Apigenin-7-glucoside	$C_{21}H_{20}O_{10}$	Flavonoid	432	431		431-385-268-240-151-107
33	20.41	0.80	Folic acid	$C_{19}H_{19}N_7O_6$	Vitamin	441			311-267-224-175
35	21.43	4.91	Emmotin H	$C_{15}H_{16}O_3$	Sesquiterpenoid	244	243		243-228-200-184
36	23.74	0.47	caffeoyl-feruloyltartaric acid	$C_{23}H_{20}O_{12}$	Phenolic acid	488	487		487-443-293
37	25.35	3.37	1-Caffeoyl-beta-D-glucose	$C_{15}H_{18}O_9$	Polyphenol	342	341		341-179-135
38	25.76	0.45	Ascorbyl palmitate	$C_{22}H_{38}O_7$	Other	414		415	415-371-115

Furthermore, biotin was detected by an $[M+H]^+$ ion at m/z = 243, which appeared at 9.00 min, accompanied by fragments at m/z = 297, 228, 174, and 130 that testify to its specific fragmentation. The ion at m/z = 297 could result from the loss of a part of the biotin's side structure, potentially involving the disappearance of a valerate group or a section of the imidazole. The fragment at m/z = 228 could result from the loss of a C_3H_8NS group, including a portion of the thiol group and the nitrogen. Finally, the ion at m/z = 174 could result from the loss of a $C_4H_6NO_2$ group, likely associated with a section of the valeric acid or the imidazole.

Similarly, emmotin H ($C_{15}H_{16}O_3$, M = 244) presented an $[M-H]^-$ ion at m/z = 243, detected at 21.43 min, accompanied by fragments at m/z = 243, 228, 200, and 184, characteristic of the fragmentation-specific to its sesquiterpenoid structure. The ion at m/z = 243 corresponded to the parent $[M-H]^-$ ion of the emmotin H molecule, revealing a loss of a proton during ionization, consistent with negative mass spectrometry processes. The fragment at m/z = 228 could result from the dissociation of a CH_2 (methylene) group, a frequent observation in sesquiterpenoids. Furthermore, the fragment at m/z = 200 could indicate a more substantial loss in the carbon chain, possibly associated with the cleavage of an alkene group or another functional group. Finally, the ion at m/z = 184 could result from additional fragmentation of the sesquiterpenoid skeleton, likely involving the loss of a less complex structure.

Lastly, coumarin ($C_9H_6O_2$, M = 146) showed an $[M+H]^+$ ion at m/z = 147, identified at 9.24 min, accompanied by a principal fragment at m/z = 103, marking the distinctive fragmentation of its structure by the loss of a CO group.

Our results align with previous studies that have highlighted the richness of dill seeds in these molecules. Bota et al. [28] reported the presence of umbelliferone, kaempferol, and quercetin in hydromethanolic extracts of dill seeds from Romania. Similarly, Mashraqi et al. [29] observed the presence of phenolic acids and flavonoids such as chlorogenic acid, cinnamic acid, caffeic acid, rosmarinic acid, quercetin, and apigenin in dill from Saudi Arabia. In addition to these compounds, Erdogan et al. [30] revealed the presence of vanillic acid and the abundance of rosmarinic acid in dill seeds from Turkey. Furthermore, a bibliographic review by Meena et al. [31] noted the presence of vitamins B1 and B2 in dill seeds.

The pharmacological properties of coumarins are already well-documented in the literature, especially umbelliferone [32]. This coumarin is utilized as a sunscreen agent and possesses anti-inflammatory, antioxidant, antimicrobial, antihyperglycemic, molluscicidal, and antitumor activities [33].

Regarding flavonoids, apigenin, kaempferol, and quercetin, known for their various pharmacological effects, are used as dietary supplements due to their high antioxidant activity. Numerous preclinical studies have demonstrated their wide range of biological activities, including anti-inflammatory, antimicrobial, anticancer, and cardioprotective effects [34–37].

Clinical investigations have demonstrated that phenolic acids have beneficial effects on several significant pathological illnesses, including cancer, cardiovascular diseases, hepatotoxicity, neurotoxicity, and viral infections [38–41].

The chemical profile of the dill seed extract studied in our research explains, on the one hand, its numerous pharmacological properties proven by these cited studies, and on the other hand, confirms its use in traditional medicine. The chemical structures of the primary chemicals found in *A. graveolens* seeds are displayed in Supplementary Figure S4.

2.8. Antioxidant Activity of A. graveolens Essential Oil and Extracts

2.8.1. Antioxidant Activity of Essential Oil Using DPPH

The results obtained showed a concentration-dependent variation in the inhibition of DPPH* radicals by the *A. graveolens* essential oil. According to the IC_{50} values grouped in Figure 4, the standard antioxidant power of butylated hydroxytoluene (BHT) exceeded that of Dill. Indeed, the latter was considered less effective in reducing free radicals with an IC_{50} equal to 9.02 mg/mL.

This observation has been reported in several previous studies. For instance, Kaur et al. [9] identified through the DPPH method that Indian dill essential oil, mainly composed of carvone (41.15%), limonene (23.11%), camphor (9.25%), and dihydrocarvone (3.75%), exhibits low antioxidant activity (IC_{50} = 0.65 mg/mL) compared to the standard ascorbic acid (IC_{50} = 0.04 mg/mL). These authors attributed this antioxidant power to the presence of polar compounds. Similarly, Osanloo et al. [42] observed the low antioxidant activity of Iranian dill essential oil, whose major constituents are α-phellandrene (26.75%), p-cymene (24.81%), carvone (10.77%), dill ether (9.78), and cis-sabinol (3.61%), using the DPPH method. A study conducted in Serbia showed that dill essential oil, composed of limonene (45.24%) and carvone (45.90%), has higher antiradical activity than anise composed mainly of anethole (96.40%) [43]. Stanojević et al. [44] reported that dill essential oil from Serbia, primarily composed of carvone (85.9%), limonene (5.1%), and cis-dihydrocarvone (3.0%), inhibited 79.62% of DPPH radicals at a concentration of 29 mg/mL for 60 min.

The antioxidant activity of essential oils is determined by the collective interaction of their chemical components, which can operate either antagonistically or synergistically. Eos that include volatile phenolic compounds have potent antioxidant action as a result of their heightened reactivity with peroxyl radicals. Furthermore, in our work, the studied EO of dill was composed primarily of phenylpropanoids (67.93%). As a result, several previous studies have reported the antioxidant capacity of phenylpropanoids [45]. Additionally, the studied EO, composed of trans-anethole (38.13%), estragole (29.32%), and fenchone (17.21%), exhibited slight antioxidant activity. This low antioxidant activity has already been noted by Donati et al. [46]. These researchers have evaluated the antioxidant activity of trans-anethole and estragole using the DPPH and FRAP methods, and they have found their moderate antioxidant power. Moreover, another study conducted by Senatore et al. [47] has shown the low ability of anethole to scavenge DPPH free radicals and reduce ferric ions compared to the Trolox standard.

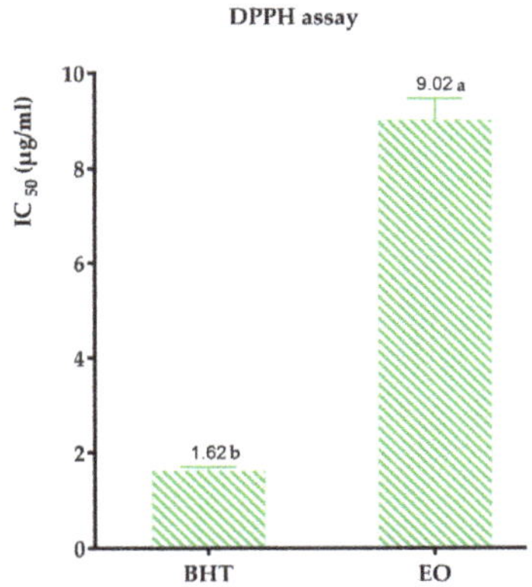

Figure 4. IC_{50} values of *A. graveolens* and the standard antioxidant BHT using the DPPH method. The results with different letters are significantly different from each other ($p < 0.001$).

Moreover, Luís et al. [48] have tested the antioxidant activity of the EO of *I. Verum*, composed primarily of phenylpropanoids (92.2%), using the DPPH method. Crucially, these authors found that this EO, rich in trans-anethole (88.5%), has an IC_{50} (3.46%) that is nearly seventeen times higher than that of gallic acid (0.20%). Consequently, this suggests that the antioxidant potential of the *I. verum* EO is significantly lower compared to the standard gallic acid.

Furthermore, the antioxidant activity of the Indian dill essential oil was studied using DPPH (1,1-diphenyl-2-picrylhydrazyl) tests. Notably, the results have shown moderate antioxidant activity with inhibition percentages ranging from 26.1% to 43.62% for concentrations varying from 5 to 25 µL [49]. Additionally, Coêlho et al. [50] have revealed the antioxidant potential of estragole using DPPH and ABTS methods, but it remains lower than that of Trolox. Regarding fenchone, the work of El Omari et al. [51] has found, using the FRAP method, that it possesses a more pronounced reducing power than camphor and the essential oil of *Lavandula stoechas*. Similarly, Singh et al. [52] have highlighted the antioxidant effect of fenchone. Although these previous studies have demonstrated the antioxidant potential of trans-anethole, estragole, and fenchone, the moderate antioxidant activity of the studied dill EO is also attributed to the minor compounds, which may either strengthen or weaken its antioxidant activity through synergistic or antagonistic effects.

2.8.2. Antioxidant Activity of Extracts

Based to the results presented in Figure 5, the antioxidant effects of extracts from *A. graveolens* are shown. The IC_{50} values noted for ascorbic acid and BHA, used as reference compounds by the DPPH and FRAP methods, were significantly lower than those of the extracts, indicating a high antioxidant activity of the standards.

Additionally, we can observe that the nature of the extraction solvent significantly affects the antioxidant activity. Notably, the ethanolic extract, which has shown high contents of polyphenols, flavonoids, and condensed tannins, has proven to be the most active, possessing a powerful antioxidant potential compared to the aqueous extract and decoction.

Moreover, all the tests have allowed us to highlight higher anti-radical ferric and molybdenum ion-reducing activities in the ethanolic extract than in the aqueous extract and decoction. Specifically, the IC_{50} value of this extract reaches 46.90 ± 0.73 µg/mL via the DPPH method, an EC_{50} equal to 161.33 ± 6.18 µg/mL via the FRAP method, and a total antioxidant capacity of 72.97 ± 0.71 mg EAA/g E.

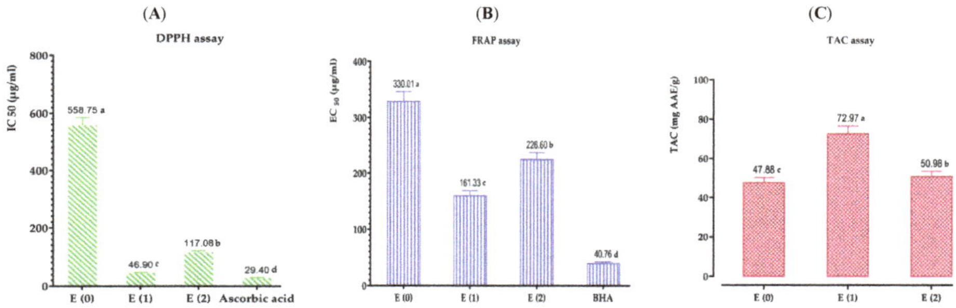

Figure 5. Antioxidant effects of extracts of *A. graveolens* by DPPH (**A**), and FRAP methods (**B**), and CAT (**C**). Mean values ± standard deviations of determinations performed in triplicate are reported; Means are significantly different ($p < 0.001$).

Furthermore, for the aqueous extract, its ability to scavenge DPPH free radicals is superior to that of the decoction. This fact is confirmed by a lower IC_{50} of the aqueous extract (IC_{50} = 117.08 ± 0.16 µg/mL) compared to that of the decoction (IC_{50} = 558.75 ± 4.07 µg/mL). Similarly, for the FRAP and TAC methods, the aqueous extract indicated a higher capacity to reduce ferric and molybdenum ions than the decoction; the EC_{50} value was 226.60 ± 11.73 µg/mL, and the total antioxidant capacity reached 50.98 ± 0.2 mg EAA/g E. In contrast, the decoction had an EC_{50} of 330.01 ± 3.09 µg/mL and a total antioxidant capacity of 47.88 ± 1.73 mg EAA/g E.

Moreover, the difference in the antioxidant activity of the extracts is primarily related to the contents of polyphenols, flavonoids, and other aromatic compounds present. Based on our analysis of the phenolic compound assay results, we have discovered that the examined extracts contain substantial quantities of phenolic compounds. The ethanolic extract exhibits the highest levels of polyphenols, flavonoids, and condensed tannins, surpassing the aqueous extract and the commonly used decoction in traditional medicine.

Furthermore, with the help of the results from the chromatographic analyses conducted using HPLC/UV-ESI-MS for the decoction of dill seeds, we have identified a diverse chemical richness in its chemical profile, reflected by the presence of several chemical families such as coumarins, flavonoids, phenolic acids, and terpenoids. Its main compounds are umbelliferone (12.35%), 3-hydroxyflavone (11.23%), rosmanol (8.95%), vitamin B7 biotin (8.36%), emmotin H (4.91%), and coumarin (4.21%).

The antioxidant potential of *A. graveolens* seeds has been verified by several researchers in the literature. Specifically, Basavegowda et al. [53] have observed strong antioxidant activities of the methanolic extract of dill seeds from India. They have indicated, via the three radical scavenging methods of DPPH, hydroxyl, and nitric oxide, IC_{50} values of 19 ± 0.94, 28 ± 0.36, and 36 ± 0.64 µg/mL, respectively. Moreover, Al-oqail et al. [16] have shown, using the DPPH and hydrogen peroxide radical scavenging methods, that the methanolic extract of Saudi dill seeds has a considerable antioxidant capacity, with IC_{50} values of 225 and 126.3 µg/mL, respectively. Additionally, these researchers have found, using the FRAP method, that the maximum absorbance of this extract is 1.387 at a concentration of 1 mg/mL. Similarly, the study by El Mansouri et al. [27] has revealed the antioxidant power of the aqueous extract of Moroccan dill seeds using the DPPH, ABTS, and hydroxyl radical scavenging methods, as well as the reducing power using FRAP.

2.9. Correlation between Phenolic Compound Content and Antioxidant Activity of Extracts

The entirety of the previously obtained results highlights the relationship between the phenolic compounds and the antioxidant activity of *A. graveolens*. With this in mind, the linear correlation coefficients were calculated (Table 7).

The coefficients varied between 0.686 and 0.990. The total polyphenol contents of the extracts correlated strongly with the DPPH (R^2 = 0.970), FRAP (R^2 = 0.990), and CAT (R^2 = 0.762) tests. Similarly, a positive correlation was observed between the flavonoids and the anti-radical activity, reducing activity, and total antioxidant capacity, with Pearson coefficients of $R^2 = 0.982$, $R^2 = 0.957$, and $R^2 = 0.964$, respectively. The antioxidant activity recorded in our extracts is attributed to their richness in phenolic compounds. However, the condensed tannins are an exception. Although the ethanolic, aqueous, and decoction extracts did not possess high contents, there was a significant correlation in the case of FRAP ($R^2 = 0.969$), DPPH ($R^2 = 0.938$), and CAT ($R^2 = 0.686$). This leads us to deduce that, while the quantity of condensed tannins is an important factor, it is not always sufficient, and there is another criterion related to condensed tannins that must be considered when interpreting antioxidant power, which is the quality criterion. Additionally, there was a positive linear correlation between the three evaluated antioxidant activities, either by the DPPH test and the CAT test for $R^2 = 0.896$, between the DPPH test and the FRAP test for $R^2 = 0.995$, or between the CAT test and the FRAP test for $R^2 = 0.845$. This observation likely indicates that in the three extracts, the polyphenols, flavonoids, and condensed tannins are the major compounds involved in the anti-radical activity, reducing activity, and total antioxidant capacity.

Table 7. Correlation coefficients (R^2) between polyphenol (PC),flavonoid (FC), tannin content (TC) and antioxidant activity of *A. graveolens* extract.

	PC	FC	TC	DPPH	FRAP	CAT
PC	1	0.907	0.994	0.970	0.990	0.762
FC	0.907	1	0.856	0.982	0.957	0.964
TC	0.994	0.856	1	0.938	0.969	0.969
DPPH	0.970	0.982	0.938	1	0.995	0.896
FRAP	0.990	0.957	0.969	0.995	1	0.845
CAT	0.762	0.964	0.686	0.896	0.845	1

2.10. Antimicrobial Activity

Tables 8 and 9 present the minimum inhibitory concentrations (MICs), minimum fungicidal concentrations (MFCs), and minimum bactericidal concentrations (MBCs) expressed in mg/mL for the extracts and in µL/mL for the essential oil of *Anethum graveolens* against the tested microorganisms.

Table 8. MICs and MBCs (mg/mL) of *A. graveolens* EO and extracts (ethanolic, aqueous, and decocted).

Bacterial Strains	E (0)			E (1)			E (2)			EO		
	MIC	MBC	MBC/MIC	MIC	MBC	MBC/MIC	MIC	MBC	MBC/MIC	MIC	MBC	MBC/MIC
E. cloacae	50	50	1	>50	>50	-	50	50	1	25	25	1
K. pneumoniae	50	50	1	50	50	1	50	50	1	25	25	1
E. coli	>50	>50	-	>50	>50	-	>50	>50	-	25	25	1
S. aureus	50	50	1	50	50	1	50	50	1	25	50	2
S. epidermidis	>50	>50	-	>50	>50	-	>50	>50	-	50	50	1

Table 9. MIC and MFC of *A. graveolens* EO and extracts (ethanolic, aqueous, and decocted).

Fungal Strains	E (0)			E (1)			E (2)			EO		
	MIC	MFC	MFC/MIC	MIC	MFC	MFC/MIC	MIC	MFC	MFC/MIC	MIC	MFC	MFC/MIC
C. albicans	>50	>50	-	50	50	1	50	50	1	3.125	6.25	2
C. dubliniensis	>50	>50	-	6.25	6.25	1	12.5	12.5	1	3.125	3.125	1
C. tropicalis	>50	>50	-	12.5	12.5	1	25	25	1	6.25	6.25	1
C.parapsilosis	>50	>50	-	12.5	12.5	1	12.5	12.5	1	6.25	6.25	1
A. niger	>50	>50	-	0.78	0.78	1	25	25	1	3.125	3.125	1

According to the obtained results, the dill extracts and essential oil tested against the four fungi have revealed a promising antifungal activity, except for the decoction, which is inactive. For the ethanolic and aqueous extracts, the MICs and MFCs ranged between 0.78 and 50 mg/mL. Notably, the fungus *Aspergillus niger* was the most sensitive, with MICs and MFCs of 0.78 mg/mL. The highest MICs and MFCs were 50 mg/mL, which were obtained against *C. albicans*. Regarding *C. parapsilosis*, the ethanolic and aqueous extracts exerted fungistatic and fungicidal effects at the same concentration of 12.5 mg/mL. Furthermore, we also observed that the ethanolic extract exhibited a higher antifungal power compared to the other tested extracts. This high activity can be directly attributed to its elevated contents of polyphenols and flavonoids.

Regarding the essential oil, the MICs and MFCs ranged between 3.125 and 6.25 μL/mL. Notably, the fungi *A. niger* and *C. dubliniensis* were the most sensitive, with MICs and MFCs of 3.13 μL/mL. The highest MICs and MFCs of 50 μL/mL were observed in *Candida tropicalis* and *Candida parapsilosis.*

Regarding the antibacterial activity, the dill extracts and essential oil appeared to be sensitive to various bacterial strains to varying degrees. Specifically, the aqueous and decoction extracts presented bacteriostatic and bactericidal actions at a concentration of 50 mg/mL on *K. pneumoniae* and *S. aureus*. Moreover, the ethanolic extract exhibited a similar action on all the tested bacterial strains except for the *Enterobacter cloacae* strain, where it was inactive. Additionally, the three tested extracts did not exert any power on wild-type *E. coli* and *S. epidermidis*. In contrast, the essential oil inhibited and destroyed the *E. cloacae*, *K. pneumoniae*, and wild-type *E. coli* strains at a concentration of 25 μL/mL. Meanwhile, *S. aureus* and *S. epidermidis* appeared to be less sensitive, with higher MBCs of 50 μL/mL.

These results corroborate those found by Kaur et al. [54]. These authors have highlighted the antibacterial potential of the aqueous extract of Indian dill seeds against *E. coli* and *S. aureus*, noting MICs of 40 and 20 mg/mL, respectively. Additionally, another study has revealed the antimicrobial potential of the essential oils extracted from different parts: the leaves, stems, flowers, and seeds of *A. graveolens* from Saudi Arabia. Furthermore, this study indicated that the essential oil of the seeds, composed of dillapiole (33.3%), limonene (30.8%), carvone (17.7%), and trans-dihydrocarvone (12.2%), exhibited a higher antimicrobial power than the essential oils from the other parts against *S. aureus*, *C. albicans*, and *C. parapsilosis* [25]. Basavegowda et al. [53] have reported the antibacterial effect of the methanolic extract of dill seeds from India against *E. coli*, *K. pneumoniae*, and *S. aureus*, with MICs of 1250, 833, and 125 μg/mL, respectively. Generally, the observed antimicrobial power of the essential oil is closely linked to its chemical composition. Moreover, Mota et al. [55] have attributed the distinguished antibacterial activity of the essential oil of *Foeniculum vulgare* seeds to the synergistic effects of the major compounds present in an equivalent percentage, namely, (E)-anethole (37.2%), estragole (31.1%), and fenchone (28.5%).

Accordingly, in our study, the analyzed essential oil contained three main compounds in an almost equivalent percentage, namely, (E)-anethole (38.13%), estragole (29.32%), and fenchone (17.21%). Consequently, we can attribute the antimicrobial effect to the synergistic effects among the principal compounds present in this complex mixture. Furthermore, the observed antimicrobial potential can also be related to the richness of the studied essential oil in ethers (68.04%) and the presence of ketones (17.57%).

2.11. Prediction of PASS Activity, ADME, Toxicity (ProTox II), and Efficacy for Potentially Active Compounds Isolated from the Essential Oil and Aqueous Extract of A. graveolens Seeds

Examining the physicochemical features of the candidate compounds is crucial for developing therapeutic agents and confirming the effectiveness of *A. graveolens* as a nutraceutical preservative agent, in addition to its biological qualities. Therefore, an analysis was conducted on the chemicals found in the essential oil and aqueous extract of *A. graveolens* seeds to determine their pharmacokinetic and physicochemical characteristics, as well as their similarity to medications.

The main compounds of the EO (E-anethole, estragole, fenchone, and α-pinene) and the aqueous extract (umbelliferone, 3-Hydroxyflavone, rosmanol, biotin, emmotin H, coumarin, trans-caftaric acid, pimelic acid, methyl rosmarinate, homovanillic acid, 1-caffeoyl-beta-D-glucose, and kaempferol) of *A. graveolens* were selected for PASS and ADMET (absorption, distribution, metabolism, excretion, and toxicity) prediction studies.

The SMILES formats of these molecules were generated utilizing the ChemBio-Draw web tool [56], and subsequently simulated with the PASS web prediction tool [57] and the

SwissADME and pkCSM [58] web tools. The outcomes of the PASS and ADMET prediction studies are presented in Table 10.

The efficiency of antioxidant and antibacterial properties of the major components extracted from the EO and aqueous extract of *A. graveolens* seeds was evaluated using PASS predictions.

Based on our projections, all the important chemicals had substantial "Pa" values for different activities, including antioxidant (0.150–0.856), antifungal (0.267–0.717), and antibacterial potential (0.216–0.587) (Table 10). Moreover, these compounds had highly favorable antioxidant characteristics, a potent antifungal impact, and commendable antibacterial activities.

The pkCSM and SwissADME websites are useful for analyzing the pharmacokinetic properties and the similarity of certain compounds to drugs. The lipophilicity indices of all the selected compounds indicate that they are quite water-soluble (Table 10).

The chosen substances present favorable values of skin permeability (log Kp) and high Caco-2 permeability values. Consequently, most of the studied compounds show excellent intestinal absorption (HIA > 30%), except for trans-caftaric acid.

The P-glycoprotein, or P-gp, plays a crucial role in the distribution and absorption of drugs. None of the chemical compounds of the studied essential oil act as inhibitors of P-gp I and P-gp II, and the main constituents of the essential oil are also not P-gp substrates. In contrast, for the studied compounds in the aqueous extract, we observed that compounds such as 3-hydroxyflavone, rosmanol, methyl rosmarinate, homovanillic acid, 1-caffeoyl-beta-D-glucose, and kaempferol can be P-gp substrates. Additionally, only rosmanol could act as an inhibitor of P-gp I.

The majority of the isolated compounds studied, eight out of a total of sixteen, obtained an SNC score greater than -3.0, suggesting that they easily cross the blood-brain barrier (BBB). However, certain exceptions were noted, particularly for biotin, emmotin H, coumarin, trans-caftaric acid, pimelic acid, methyl rosmarinate, homovanillic acid, and 1-caffeoyl-beta-D-glucose, which did not reach this threshold. Among the compounds with weak penetration into the central nervous system (log BB > 0.3), we found the compounds from the studied essential oils as well as 3-hydroxyflavone from the aqueous extract. Their volume of distribution in tissues (logVDss) ranged from -1.533 L/kg to 1.274 L/kg.

The main constituents of the essential oil and the aqueous extract examined are unlikely to have negative effects when taken orally due to drug interactions; however, cytochrome P450 (CYP) enzymes and molecular interactions play a crucial role in the elimination of drugs. The retinal organic cation transporters 2 (OCT2) and the total clearance of hepatic and renal substrates (CLTOT) were represented in log mL/min/kg to predict the excretion pathway. All the studied phytochemical compounds presented good overall clearance values and were excreted according to the data.

In order to evaluate the potentially harmful effects of the essential oil and aqueous extract of *A. graveolens* seeds, various aspects such as AMES, hERG channel inhibition, skin sensitization, immunotoxicity, hepatotoxicity, carcinogenicity, mutagenicity, and cytotoxicity were examined. The analysis focused on the main phytochemical constituents, as shown in Table 11. The data indicated the absence of significant toxic effects, except for certain molecules. Among these compounds, Biotin may have minimal hepatic effects; (E)-anethole, estragole, umbelliferone, 3-hydroxyflavone, and coumarin may have minimal carcinogenic effects. However, rosmanol, trans-caftaric acid, methyl rosmarinate, and 1-Caffeoyl-beta-D-glucose may present immunotoxicity effects. Finally, umbelliferone, also known as 7-hydroxycoumarin, is a natural organic compound widely distributed in the coumarin family with an LD_{50} of 10,000 mg/kg, classified in the predicted toxicity class 6. This compound is one of the main constituents of the aqueous extract of the studied *A. graveolens* seeds. These findings indicate that as long as the suggested doses are followed, the essential oil and aqueous extracts obtained from *A. graveolens* seeds from southern Morocco can be considered safe for oral consumption as nutraceuticals and/or as natural substitutes for synthetic preservatives. However, further research, including rigorous clinical trials, would be necessary to conclusively verify that there are no long-term risks to consumers.

Table 10. In Silico Analysis of PASS, ADME of Compounds from the Essential Oil, and Decoction of *A. graveolens* Seeds.

Prediction	Parameters	EO 1	EO 2	EO 3	EO 4	D 1	D 2	D 3	D 4	D 5	D 6	D 7	D 8	D 9	D 10	D 11	D 12
PASS Prediction (Pa/Pi)																	
Antioxidant	Antioxidant	0.337/0.018			0.563/0.005	0.641/0.004	0.551/0.005	0.150/0.103	0.286/0.026	0.389/0.013	0.711/0.004	0.260/0.033	0.483/0.007	0.321/0.020	0.751/0.004	0.856/0.003	0.337/0.018
Antimicrobial	Antifungal	0.425/0.045	0.267/0.097	0.439/0.042	0.519/0.027	0.367/0.058	0.639/0.014	0.494/0.032	0.504/0.030	0.440/0.041	0.544/0.024	0.363/0.059	0.474/0.035	0.292/0.084	0.717/0.009	0.495/0.031	0.425/0.045
	Antibacterial	0.264/0.075	0.219/0.102	0.326/0.051	0.398/0.030	0.331/0.049	0.569/0.011	0.357/0.041	0.301/0.060	0.344/0.045	0.303/0.059	0.292/0.063	0.218/0.102	0.216/0.104	0.587/0.010	0.395/0.031	0.264/0.075
ADME Prediction																	
Physiochemical Properties	TPSA (Å^2)	9.23	9.23	17.07	0.00	50.44	50.44	86.99	103.73	54.37	30.21	161.59	74.60	133.52	66.76	156.91	111.13
	Molar Refractivity	47.83	47.04	45.64	45.22	44.51	69.94	93.99	69.34	70.37	42.48	70.60	39.31	95.72	46.50	79.13	76.01
Drug Likeness Prediction	Bioavailability Score	0.55	0.55	0.55	0.55	0.55	0.55	0.55	0.56	0.55	0.55	0.11	0.85	0.55	0.85	0.55	0.55
	Synthetic accessibility	1.47	1.28	3.22	4.44	2.56	2.93	5.07	3.38	3.03	2.74	3.45	1.37	3.52	1.49	4.47	3.14
Absorption Parameters Prediction	Water solubility	−2.936	−2.874	−3.097	−3.733	−2.131	−3.683	−3.606	−2	−3.366	−1.517	−2.541	−1.088	−3.17	−2.453	−1.869	−3.04
	Caco2 permeability	1.669	1.41	1.501	1.38	1.206	1.263	1.015	0.698	1.267	1.649	−0.801	0.598	−0.562	0.265	0.05	0.032
	Intestinal absorption (human)	95.592	94.536	95.813	96.041	94.551	94.776	93.407	71.182	96.41	97.344	9.399	72.877	64.776	86.286	50.517	74.29
	Skin Permeability	−1.139	−1.739	−1.872	−1.827	−2.6	−2.775	−2.772	−2.727	−2.93	−1.921	−2.735	−2.735	−2.735	−2.722	−2.74	−2.735
	P-glycoprotein substrate	No	No	No	No	No	Yes	Yes	No	No	No	No	No	Yes	Yes	No	Yes
	P-glycoprotein I inhibitor	No	No	No	No	No	No	Yes	No	No	No	No	No	No	No	No	No
	P-glycoprotein II inhibitor	No	No	No	No	No	No	No	No	No	No	No	No	No	No	No	No
Distribution Parameters Prediction	VDss (human)	0.343	0.401	0.341	0.667	0.032	0.214	0.653	−0.933	0.161	−0.143	−0.919	−1.429	0.75	−1.533	0.141	1.274
	Fraction unbound (human)	0.266	0.213	0.423	0.425	0.432	0.151	0.109	0.58	0.3	0.367	0.472	0.543	0.229	0.467	0.609	0.178
	BBB permeability	0.529	0.601	0.624	0.791	−0.278	0.462	−0.581	−0.679	0.291	−0.007	−1.233	−0.21	−1.454	−0.312	−1.081	−0.939
	CNS permeability	−1.659	−1.74	−1.988	−2.201	−2.741	−1.733	−2.101	−3.541	−2.784	−1.926	−3.93	−3.042	−3.358	−2.723	−3.982	−2.228
Metabolism Parameters Prediction	CYP2D6 substrate	No	No	No	No	No	No	No	No	No	No	No	No	No	No	No	No
	CYP3A4 substrate	No	No	No	No	No	Yes	No	No	No	No	No	No	Yes	No	No	No
	CYP1A2 inhibitor	Yes	Yes	No	No	Yes	Yes	No	No	Yes	Yes	No	No	No	No	No	Yes
	CYP2C19 inhibitor	No	No	No	No	No	Yes	No	No	No	No	No	No	No	No	No	No
	CYP2C9 inhibitor	No	No	No	No	No	No	No	No	No	No	No	No	No	No	No	No
	CYP2D6 inhibitor	No	No	No	No	No	No	No	No	No	No	No	No	No	No	No	No
	CYP3A4 inhibitor	No	No	No	No	No	No	No	No	No	No	No	No	No	No	No	No
Excretion	Total Clearance	0.268	0.332	0.085	0.043	0.706	0.233	0.289	0.368	0.19	0.97	0.449	0.565	0.187	0.246	0.059	0.477
	Renal OCT2 substrate	No	No	No	No	No	No	No	No	No	No	No	No	No	No	No	No

EO1: E-Anethole; EO2: Estragole; EO3: Fenchone; EO4: α-Pinene; D1: Umbelliferone; D2: 3-hydroxyflavone; D3: Rosmanol; D4: Biotine; D5: Emmotin H; D6: Coumarin; D7: trans-Caftaric acid; D8: pimelic acid; D9: Methyl rosmarinate; D10: Homovanillic Acid; D11: 1-Caffeoyl-beta-D-glucose; D12: Kaempferol.

Table 11. In silico analysis of the predictive toxicity (ProTox II) of Compounds from the Essential Oil and Decoction of *A. graveolens* Seeds.

Compounds	AMES Toxicity	hERG I Inhibitor	hERG II Inhibitor	Skin Sensitization	Minnow Toxicity	LD_{50} (mg/kg)	Predicted Toxicity Class	Hepatotoxicity	Carcinogenicity	Immunotoxicity	Mutagenicity	Cytotoxicity
EO1	No	No		Yes	0.869	150	3	Inactive	Active (0.57)		Inactive	
EO2	Yes			Yes	1.398	1230	4		Active (0.51)			
EO3	No			Yes	1.366	775	4		Inactive			
EO4	No			No	1.159	3700	5		Inactive			
D1	No	No	No	No	1.714	10,000	6	Inactive	Active (0.64)	Inactive	Inactive	Inactive
D2	Yes		No		1.205	2500	5	Inactive	Inactive	Inactive		Inactive
D3	No		Yes		0.285	450	4	Inactive	Inactive	Active (0.95)		Inactive
D4	No		No		2.183	4000	5	Active (0.41)	Inactive	Inactive		Inactive
D5	No		No		1.329	1600	4	Inactive	Inactive	Inactive		Inactive
D6	No		No		1.555	196	3	Inactive	Active (0.83)	Inactive		Active (0.55)
D7	No		No		4.872	3800	5	Inactive	Inactive	Active (0.97)		Inactive
D8	No		No		2.006	900	4	Inactive	Inactive	Inactive		Inactive
D9	No		No		1.92	5000	5	Inactive	Inactive	Active (0.93)		Inactive
D10	No		No		2.106	1123	4	Inactive	Inactive	Inactive		Inactive
D11	No		No		5.989	5000	5	Inactive	Inactive	Active (0.95)		Inactive
D12	No		No		2.885	3919	5	Inactive	Inactive	Inactive		Inactive

EO1: E-Anethole; EO2: Estragole; EO3: Fenchone; EO4: α-Pinene; D1: Umbelliferone; D2: 3-hydroxyflavone; D3: Rosmanol; D4: Biotine; D5: Emmotin H; D6: Coumarin; D7: trans-Caftaric acid; D8: pimelic acid; D9: Methyl rosmarinate; D10: Homovanillic Acid; D11: 1-Caffeoyl-beta-D-glucose; D12: Kaempferol.

2.12. Molecular Docking

Considering the much-increased in vitro bioactivities shown in the EO and aqueous extract of *A. graveolens* in this work, the compounds discovered using GC/MS and HPLC/UV-ESI-MS were chosen for in silico molecular docking experiments.

The antioxidant, antifungal, and antibacterial activities of the compounds, as well as their potential mechanism of action, were deduced through molecular docking experiments. These deductions were based on the molecular interactions at the atomic level between the compounds and their respective target proteins (1JZQ, 1KZN, 2CAG, 2VEG, 2ZDQ, 3SRW, 3UDI, 4URN, 2CDU, 1OG5, and 3NRZ). The molecular docking study was mostly concentrated on assessing factors such as Van der Waals (VDW) interactions, hydrogen bonds, binding free energy, and carbon–hydrogen (C–H) bonds. The stability of the ligands (chosen molecules) and the docked receptor is determined by the C–H bonds and Pi-sigma interactions, whereas the binding interactions are influenced by hydrogen bonds and Van der Waals (VDW) interactions. Table 12 displays the docking energy binding scores for the binding sites of the target proteins involved in antibacterial activities (1JZQ, 1KZN, 2CAG, 2VEG, 2ZDQ, 3SRW, 3UDI, and 4URN), as well as antioxidant activities (2CDU, 1OG5, and 3NRZ). This study analyzed the Van der Waals interactions, hydrogen bonds, and C–H bonds involving the amino acids found in the binding sites of the selected proteins.

Table 12. Details of the Binding Affinities of Antimicrobial and Antioxidant Target Proteins with Selected Ligands.

Ligands\Targets	1JZQ	1KZN	2CAG	2VEG	2ZDQ	3SRW	3UDI	4URN	2CDU	1OG5	3NRZ
EO1	−5.1	−5.6	−7.1	−4.8	−7.1	−5.8	−4.7	−5.5	−5.6	−5.4	−7.5
EO2	−5.2	−5.6	−6.7	−4.5	−7.0	−5.5	−4.6	−5.3	−5.5	−5.3	−7.0
EO3	−5.6	−4.8	−6.5	−4.6	−6.6	−5.9	−5.0	−4.7	−5.3	−6.0	−6.2
EO4	−5.5	−4.6	−6.0	−4.6	−6.2	−5.6	−4.5	−4.6	−5.0	−5.5	−5.1
D1	−6.0	−6.7	−8.1	−5.8	−8.2	−6.4	−5.8	−6.2	−6.4	−6.3	−8.8
D2	−7.6	−7.7	−9.4	−7.0	−8.4	−8.1	−7.4	−7.5	−7.5	−7.9	−8.8
D3	−8.2	−8.0	−7.2	−7.0	−6.5	−8.6	−8.2	−7.7	−7.3	−8.9	−6.2
D4	−6.3	−6.2	−7.5	−5.3	−7.3	−7.0	−6.0	−6.2	−6.1	−7.1	−7.0
D5	−7.5	−7.5	−9.0	−6.2	−10.0	−8.0	−7.6	−6.3	−7.6	−8.0	−6.2
D6	−5.8	−6.6	−7.7	−5.5	−7.9	−6.3	−5.6	−5.8	−6.4	−6.6	−8.1
D7	−6.8	−7.3	−8.9	−6.8	−9.1	−7.8	−7.2	−6.5	−7.9	−7.3	−7.6
D8	−4.9	−5.2	−5.9	−4.5	−5.8	−4.9	−4.9	−4.9	−5.1	−5.4	−6.6
D9	−7.8	−8.4	−10.2	−7.8	−9.2	−8.4	−8.3	−7.3	−8.0	−8.4	−9.8
D10	−5.5	−6.1	−7.1	−5.4	−7.0	−6.0	−5.5	−5.5	−6.1	−6.0	−7.4
D11	−7.6	−7.6	−9.5	−6.7	−9.8	−8.0	−7.4	−7.0	−7.7	−7.9	−10.0
D12	−8.1	−8.2	−10.0	−6.6	−9.0	−8.5	−8.3	−7.9	−7.7	−8.6	−7.8

EO1: E-Anethole; EO2: Estragole; EO3: Fenchone; EO4: α-Pinene; D1: Umbelliferone; D2: 3-hydroxyflavone; D3: Rosmanol; D4: Biotine; D5: Emmotin H; D6: Coumarin; D7: trans-Caftaric acid; D8: pimelic acid; D9: Methyl rosmarinate; D10: Homovanillic Acid; D11: 1-Caffeoyl-beta-D-glucose; D12: Kaempferol.

The results of our study reveal that among the tested compounds, 3-hydroxyflavone, emmotin H, trans-caftaric acid, methyl rosmarinate, 1-caffeoyl-beta-D-glucose, and kaempferol presented the greatest binding energies with the exploratory proteins. These compounds demonstrated significant interactions with different target proteins involved in antimicrobial and antioxidant activities. In particular, 3-Hydroxyflavone exhibited a marked affinity with the 2CAG protein (−9.4 Kcal/mol) for antimicrobial activity. Similarly, Emmotin H manifested substantial binding energy with the 2ZDQ protein in this same context (−10 Kcal/mol). Moreover, Caftaric <trans> acid also displayed a strong affinity with the 2ZDQ protein (−9.1 Kcal/mol) for antimicrobial activity.

On the other hand, Methyl rosmarinate revealed significant binding energies with the 2CAG (−10.2) and 2ZDQ (−9.2 Kcal/mol) proteins for antimicrobial activity, as well as with the 3NRZ (−9.8 Kcal/mol) protein for antioxidant activity. Similarly, 1-Caffeoyl-beta-D-glucose presented high affinity with the 2CAG (−9.5 Kcal/mol) and 2ZDQ (−9.8 Kcal/mol) proteins for antimicrobial activity, as well as with the 3NRZ (−10 Kcal/mol) protein for antioxidant activity. Finally, Kaempferol also demonstrated substantial binding energy with the 2CAG protein (−10 Kcal/mol) for antimicrobial activity. These results highlight the promising potential of these bioactive compounds as antimicrobial and antioxidant agents, thus paving the way for future research in the fields of pharmaceutical chemistry and natural products.

The study of interaction types using Discovery Studio revealed that the interactions of 3-Hydroxyflavone with Catalase were associated with hydrogen bonds, Pi-alkyl, Pi-cation, and Pi–Pi-stacked with each of these residues (HIS341, PHE313, VAL125, ALA112, ALA340, ARG51, HIS54, and TYR337, respectively) (Figure 6).

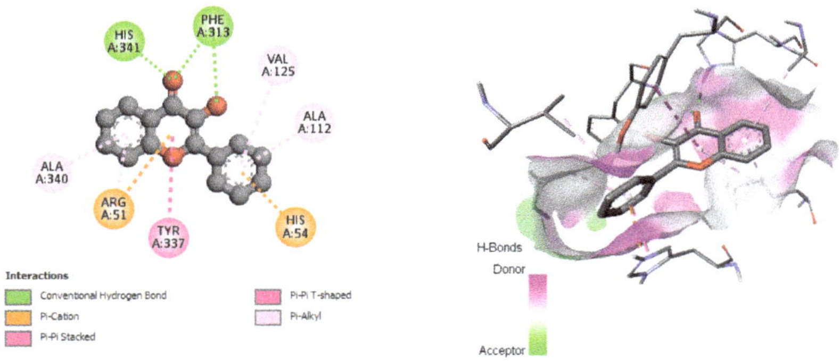

Figure 6. 2D and 3D Interactions of 3-Hydroxyflavone with the 2CAG Target Protein.

This interaction study revealed that in the case of the D-alanine ligase protein, Emmotin H developed hydrogen bonds, Pi–Pi stacking, and Pi–alkyl interactions with each of the residues (LYS153, PHE151, VAL195, and ALA191, respectively) at their binding site on the D-Alanine Ligase (Figure 7).

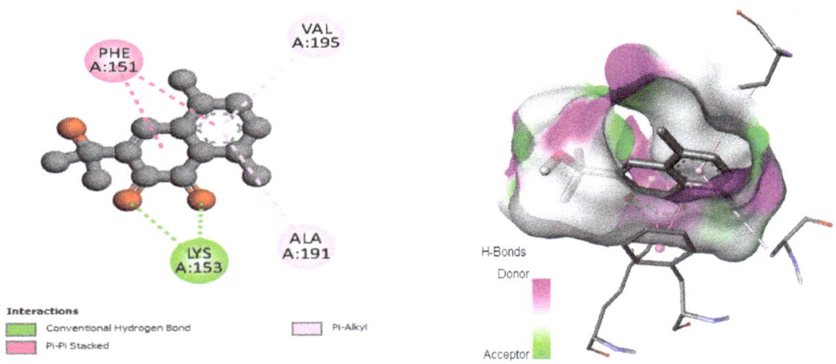

Figure 7. 2D and 3D interaction of Emmotin H with D-Alanin Ligase protein.

Furthermore, in the case of trans-caftaric acid, hydrogen bonds and Pi–Pi stacking interactions were observed with each of the residues (GLU189, ASN281, GLU197, ASP270, GLU282, LYS228, SER160, PHE272, and PHE151) (Figure 8).

For each of these catalytic residues (ARG344, PHE313, HIS341, ARG91, ARG51, TYR337, HIS54, VAL125, ALA340, and ALA112), the interaction of Methyl rosmarinate with them involved hydrogen bonds, carbon–hydrogen bonds, Pi–Pi stacked interactions, and Pi–alkyl interactions (Figure 9). On the other hand, the interactions of this molecule with D-Alanine ligase were associated with hydrogen bonds, carbon–hydrogen bonds, Pi–cation, Pi–anion, and Pi–Pi stacked interactions with each of the involved residues (GLU199, ARG268, LYS190, LEU192, LYS228, SER160, THR157, GLU282, ASP270, PHE151, and PHE272) (Figure 9). Finally, the interactions of Methyl rosmarinate with 3NRZ were characterized by hydrogen bonds, carbon–hydrogen bonds, Pi–Pi stacked, Pi–Pi-shaped, and Pi–alkyl interactions with each of the concerned proteins (SER1082, GLY799, GLN767, ALA1079, THR1010) (Figure 9).

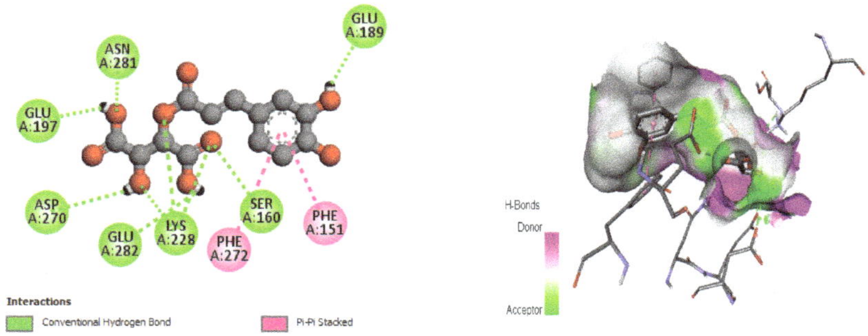

Figure 8. 2D and 3D Interactions of trans-caftaric Acid with the 2ZDQ Protein.

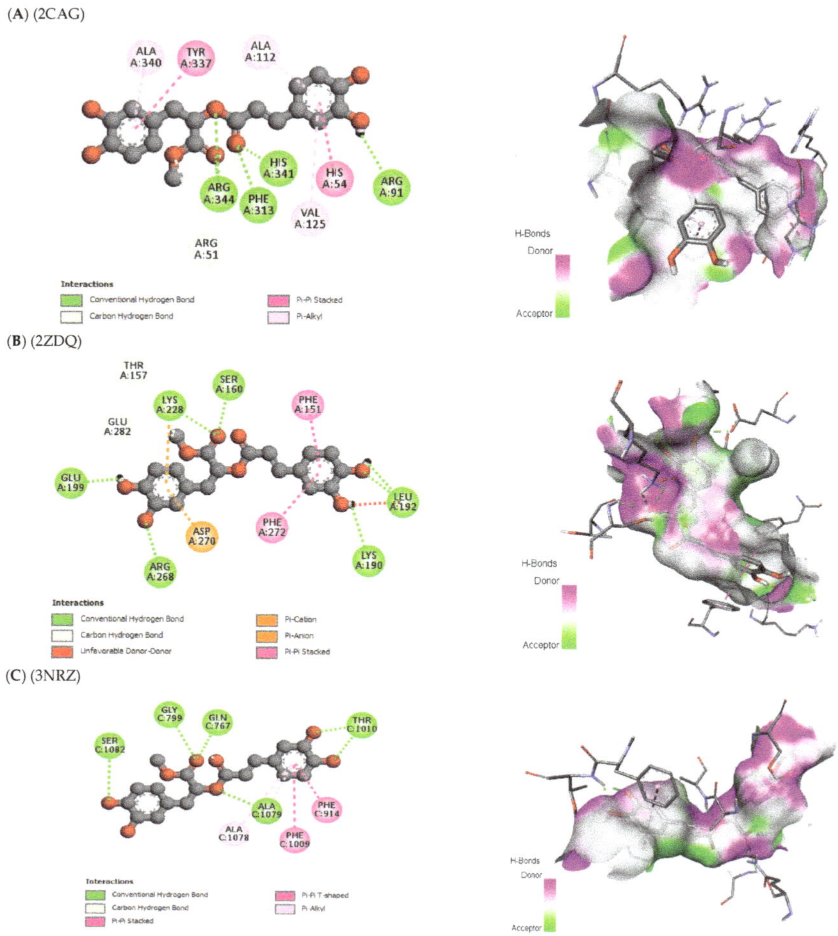

Figure 9. 2D and 3D interaction of methyl rosmarinate with target proteins: (**A**) 2CAG, (**B**) 2ZDQ, and (**C**) 3NRZ.

For each protein (OMT53, ARG344, PHE312, GLY126, ALA312, TYR337, ALA112, HIS54, and VAL125), the interaction of 1-Caffeoyl-beta-D-glucose with catalase was associated with hydrogen bonds, carbon–hydrogen bonds, Pi–sigma interactions, Pi–Pi stacked interactions, and Pi–alkyl interactions (Figure 10). Furthermore, the interactions of 1-Caffeoyl-beta-D-glucose with D-Alanine ligase were characterized by hydrogen bonds, carbon–hydrogen bonds, Pi–Pi stacked interactions, and Pi–alkyl interactions with each of the involved proteins (LYS190, GLU189, ASN281, LYS228, TYR223, ASP270, LYS116, PHE151, PHE272, LEU192, and VAL195) (Figure 10). Finally, the interactions of 1-Caffeoyl-beta-D-glucose with bovine xanthine oxidase were associated with hydrogen bonds, carbon–hydrogen bonds, Pi–Pi stacked, Pi–Pi-shaped, and Pi–alkyl interactions with each of the concerned proteins (PHE798, GLY799, SER1080, GLU802, THR1010, ALA1079, THR1077, ALA1078, PHE914, and PHE1009) (Figure 10).

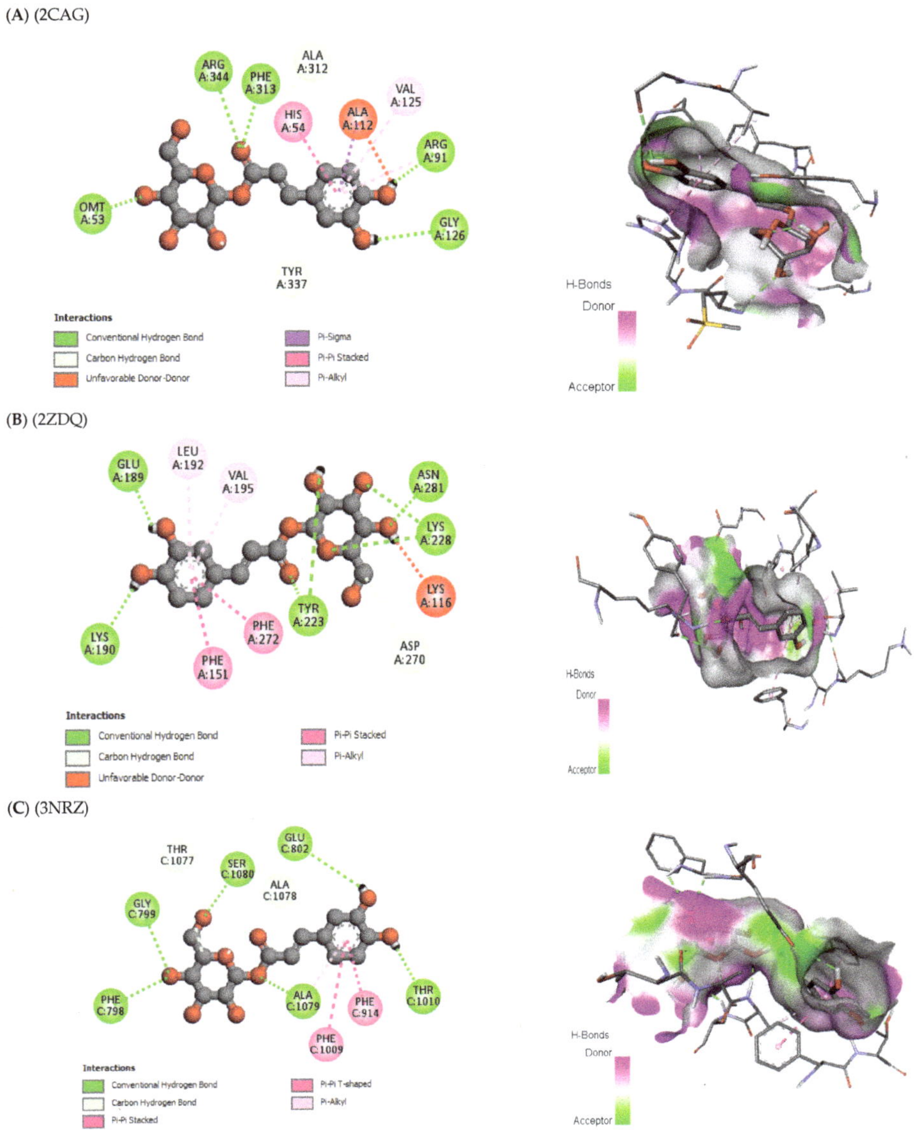

Figure 10. 2D and 3D interaction of 1-Caffeoyl-beta-D-glucose with target proteins: (**A**) 2CAG, (**B**) 2ZDQ, and (**C**) 3NRZ.

In conclusion, the interaction analysis has highlighted that the interactions of Kaempferol with the catalase protein were characterized by hydrogen bonds, carbon–hydrogen bonds, Pi–sigma interactions, Pi–Pi stacked interactions, and Pi–alkyl interactions with each of the protein residues (ARG344, HIS341, PHE313, ALA112, HIS54, ALA340, ARG51, and ARG91, respectively) (Figure 11).

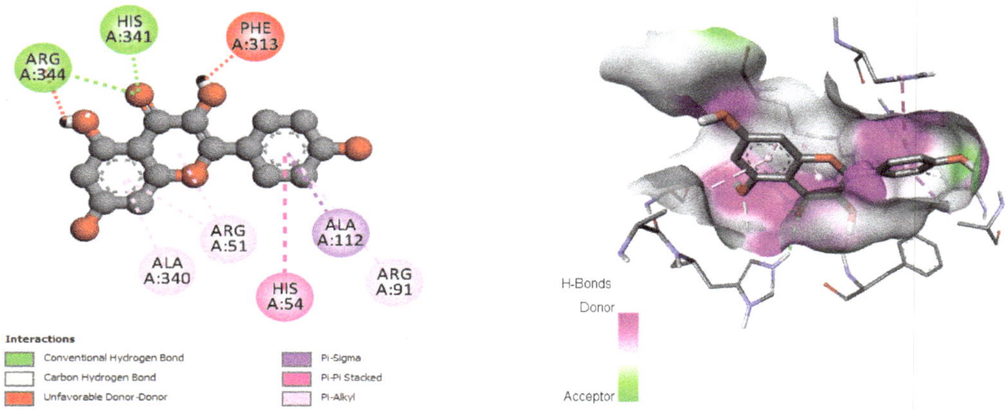

Figure 11. Interaction of 2CAG with kaempferol.

2.13. *Molecular Dynamics Simulation*

It is worth noting that during an interaction with a drug molecule, a protein target can undergo significant conformational changes. Molecular dynamics simulation (MDS) serves as an effective tool for understanding internal motions, conformational alterations, and the stability of protein–ligand complexes. Analyzing MDS trajectories for the ten complexes, with two complexes in the case of 3NRZ, four complexes in the case of 2CAG, and four complexes in the case of 2ZDQ, allows for the computation of parameters such as root-mean-square deviation (RMSD), root-mean-square fluctuation (RMSF), radius of gyration (Rg), number of hydrogen bonds, and binding free energy. These analyses provide insights into the structural stability, binding modes, and binding strengths of the complexes.

2.13.1. Structural Dynamics of 3NRZ

Our study employed molecular dynamics simulations to investigate the complex structural dynamics of protein 3NRZ when interacting with methyl-rosmarite and 1-Caffeoyl-beta-D-glucose ligands. We aimed to understand the subtle effects of ligand binding on the stability of the protein's conformation. We focused on various measures to comprehend how the protein and ligands interact dynamically. Upon examining the RMSD graph displayed in Figure 12, it can be observed that all the protein–ligand entities had a reduced variation in their spectrum. This indicates that there was a minimal disturbance in their conformational dynamics over the whole simulation. The RMSF analysis investigated ligand binding effects on protein dynamics over 100 ns, revealing decreased flexibility and lower potential conformational changes within protein–ligand complexes. This suggests that all complexes have a minimal impact on receptor flexibility, as depicted in Figure 12. Furthermore, examination of the Radius of Gyration (RG) profiles demonstrated consistent trends in both complexes, suggesting the maintenance of a stable conformation. Notably, hydrogen bonding analysis unveiled the formation of multiple hydrogen bonds in both complexes, underscoring their pivotal role in maintaining stability, even amidst ligand dissociation.

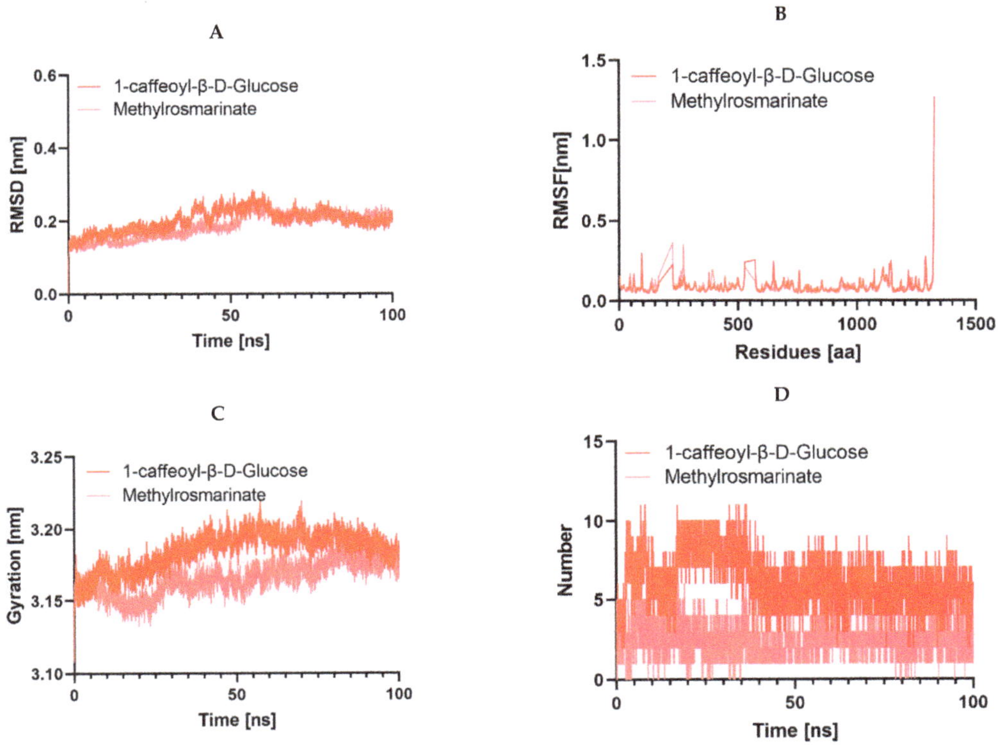

Figure 12. Structural dynamics of the 3NRZ protein: (**A**) RMSD and (**B**) RMSF. (**C**) Total number of intramolecular hydrogen bonds. (**D**) Radius of gyration.

2.13.2. Structural Dynamics of 2CAG

In this study, we delved into the structural dynamics of 2CAG through molecular dynamics simulations, focusing on their interaction with various ligands (Figure 13). Our analysis covered four different ligands (3-hydroxyflavone, Methylrosmarinate, 1-caffeoyl-β-D-Glucose, and Kaempferol), shedding light on their effects on protein conformation and dynamics. Notably, we observed strikingly similar RMSD profiles across the protein-ligand complexes, indicating minimal conformational changes upon ligand binding, except for Kaempferol, which displayed a notably higher RMSD. This suggests that while 3-hydroxyflavone, Methylrosmarinate, and 1-caffeoyl-β-D-Glucose induce negligible structural rearrangements in the protein backbone, Kaempferol triggers more pronounced changes, possibly reflecting a distinct binding mode or affinity. Further analysis of RMSF patterns revealed consistent dynamics among complexes 2CAG/3-hydroxyflavone, 2CAG/Methylrosmarinate, 2CAG/1-caffeoyl-β-D-Glucose, while the 2CAG/Kaempferol complex exhibited heightened flexibility, implying differential impacts of the ligands on protein flexibility. Examination of protein compactness using the radius of gyration (Rg) showed that 3-hydroxyflavone, Methylrosmarinate, and 1-caffeoyl-β-D-Glucose led to higher protein compactness compared to Kaempferol, correlating with the RMSD findings and suggesting tighter binding of the protein structure. Additionally, simulations unveiled the formation of hydrogen bonds between 3-hydroxyflavone, Methylrosmarinate, and 1-caffeoyl-β-D-Glucosethe target proteins over a 100 ns period, indicative of significant molecular interactions conducive to stable binding. However, Kaempferol formed fewer hydrogen bonds, implying weaker or less favorable interactions with the protein.

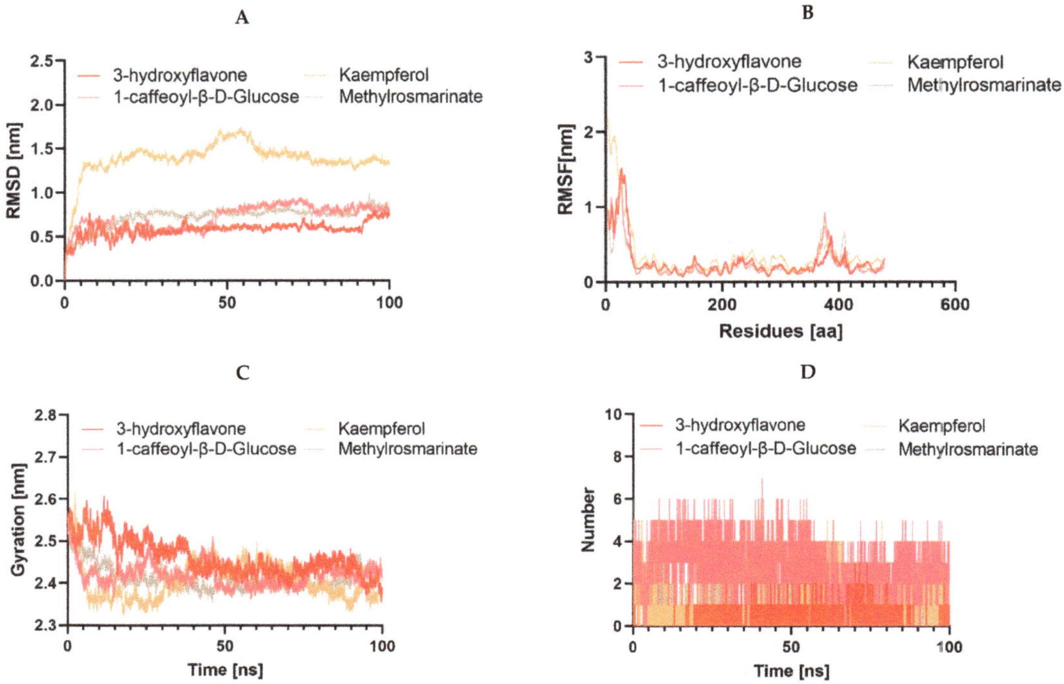

Figure 13. Structural dynamics of the 2CAG protein: (**A**) RMSD and (**B**) RMSF. (**C**) Total number of intramolecular hydrogen bonds. (**D**) Radius of gyration.

2.13.3. Structural Dynamics of 2ZDQ

In this case, we explored the structural dynamics of 2ZDQ via molecular dynamics simulations, with a specific focus on how it interacts with four distinct ligands: emmotin H, trans-caftaric acid, methyl rosmarinate, and 1-caffeoyl-β-D-glucose. This investigation sheds light on their effects on protein conformation and dynamics. Notably, we observed strikingly similar RMSD profiles across the protein–ligand complexes, indicating minimal conformational changes upon ligand binding, except for emmotin H, which displayed a notably higher RMSD. This suggests that while trans-caftaric acid, methyl rosmarinate, and 1-caffeoyl-β-D-glucose induce negligible structural rearrangements in the protein backbone, emmotin H triggers more pronounced changes, possibly reflecting a distinct binding mode or affinity. Further analysis of RMSF patterns showed that complexes formed with trans-caftaric acid, methyl rosmarinate, or 1-caffeoyl-β-D-glucose had similar dynamics. However, the emmotin H-2ZDQ complex showed increased flexibility, suggesting that the ligands had varied effects on the flexibility of the protein. Next, we investigated the changes in the protein's structural compactness resulting from its interaction with these various compounds. To achieve this, we computed the radius of gyration (Rg) over time (Figure 14). Consistent with the results of the RMSD analysis of the protein backbone, the examination of protein compactness using the Rg showed that trans-caftaric acid, Methyl rosmarinate, and 1-caffeoyl-β-D-Glucose led to higher protein compactness compared to emmotin H. Furthermore, simulations revealed the establishment of hydrogen bonds over 100 ns between trans-caftaric acid, methyl rosmarinate, or 1-caffeoyl-β-D-glucose and the target protein, indicating substantial molecular interactions favorable for persistent binding. However, emmotin H created fewer hydrogen bonds, which suggests that its interactions with the protein were weaker or less advantageous.

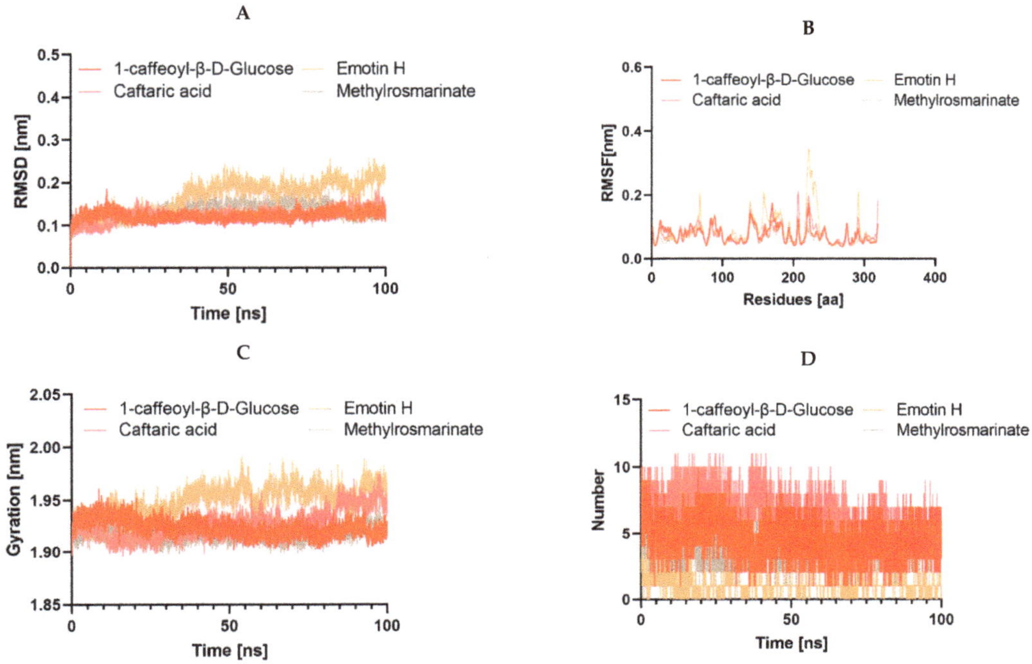

Figure 14. Structural dynamics of the 2ZDQ protein: (**A**) RMSD and (**B**) RMSF. (**C**) Total number of intramolecular hydrogen bonds. (**D**) Radius of gyration.

To design therapeutic agents and support the efficacy of the chemical composition of *A. graveolens* as a nutraceutical preservative, it is essential to analyze in detail the physicochemical characteristics of potential compounds, as well as the pharmacokinetic and physicochemical properties of the substances identified in the essential oil (EO) and aqueous extract (E_0) of *A. graveolens* seeds, comparing them to drugs. The predictive PASS and ADMET evaluations of the main constituents of the EO and aqueous extract (AE) of *A. graveolens* revealed significant values for various activities, such as antioxidant, antifungal, and antibacterial properties.

Previous research, particularly that of Najaran et al. [59], Noumi et al. [23], as well as the work of Madhuri [60], confirm the antioxidant and antimicrobial capabilities of the compounds contained in *A. graveolens*, thus suggesting their potential as therapeutic agents for various ailments. These findings highlight the exceptional qualities of the compounds identified in the EO and aqueous extract (E_0) of *A. graveolens*, which exhibit notable antioxidant, antifungal, and antibacterial activities.

The main phenolic, flavonoid, and terpenoid compounds extracted from *A. graveolens* seeds offer a wide range of pharmacological and biological applications. These compounds demonstrate promising antimicrobial, antioxidant, and anticancer properties in preclinical studies. These molecules, such as methyl rosmarinate, trans-caftaric acid, 1-caffeoyl-beta-D-glucose, kaempferol, and 3-hydroxyflavone, are currently being investigated for their biological activity. Methyl rosmarinate stands out for its antioxidative properties and antifungal activities.

It exhibits inhibitory activities against tyrosinase, α-glucosidase, and matrix metallo-pro
teinase-1 (MMP-1) [61–64]. Trans-caffeic acid shows promise in antioxidant, anti-inflammatory, antimutagenic, anticarcinogenic, hepatoprotective, antidiabetic, antihypertensive, anti-obesity, and metabolic syndrome, as well as neuroprotective effects [65]. 1-Caffeoyl-beta-D-glucose,

kaempferol, and 3-hydroxyflavone display a variety of pharmacological activities, suggesting a significant role in several therapeutic areas [66,67].

The results of our molecular docking reveal significant interactions between several bioactive compounds and various target proteins involved in antimicrobial and antioxidant activities. Among these compounds, 3-hydroxyflavone, emmotin H, trans-caftaric acid, methyl rosmarinate, 1-caffeoyl-beta-D-glucose, and kaempferol exhibited the highest binding energies with the explored proteins. These compounds have demonstrated a strong affinity with specific proteins, such as 2CAG, 2ZDQ, and 3NRZ, indicating their potential as antimicrobial and antioxidant agents. Furthermore, the study of molecular interactions using 3-hydroxyflavone revealed hydrogen bonds, Pi–alkyl bonds, Pi–cation interactions, and Pi–Pi-shaped interactions with specific catalase residues. Similarly, emmotin H formed hydrogen bonds, Pi–Pi stacking, and Pi–alkyl interactions with D-Alanine ligase residues, while trans-caftaric acid formed hydrogen bonds and Pi–Pi stacking with the latter's residues.

These specific interactions highlight the diversity of the action modes of the bioactive compounds on the target proteins. Furthermore, the analysis of catalytic residues involved in interactions with Methyl rosmarinate revealed the presence of hydrogen bonds, carbon–hydrogen bonds, Pi–Pi stacked interactions, and Pi–alkyl interactions. Additionally, interactions of this molecule with D-Alanine ligase were characterized by hydrogen bonds, carbon–hydrogen bonds, Pi–cation interactions, Pi–anion interactions, and Pi–Pi stacked interactions. Finally, interactions with 3NRZ showed hydrogen bonds, carbon-hydrogen bonds, Pi–Pi-stacked interactions, Pi–Pi-shaped interactions, and Pi–alkyl interactions. Regarding 1-Caffeoyl-beta-D-glucose, its interactions with catalase, D-Alanine ligase, and bovine xanthine oxidase were associated with different bonds, such as hydrogen bonds, carbon–hydrogen bonds, Pi–sigma interactions, Pi–Pi stacked interactions, and Pi–alkyl interactions.

Furthermore, the analysis of structural dynamics using molecular dynamics simulations provided insights into conformational changes and the stability of protein–ligand complexes [68]. These simulations revealed similar dynamic behaviors among certain complexes, as well as significant differences, suggesting distinct interaction modes and variable effects on protein flexibility and stability.

These results underscore the diversity of molecular interactions between bioactive compounds and target proteins, thus paving the way for future research in the fields of pharmaceutical chemistry and natural products.

Ultimately, despite their promising therapeutic potential, these compounds still require FDA approval for medical use, highlighting the need for further research, particularly clinical trials, to assess their efficacy and safety in patients in combating oxidative stress. These molecules are being explored for their antioxidant potential and could act as scavengers of free radicals, thereby protecting cells against oxidative stress-induced damage by modulating the expression of specific cytokines and enzymes such as SOD, dehydratase, CAT, GST, GSH, GPx, and GRd.

The antioxidant activity of *A. graveolens* essential oil, as determined by the DPPH technique and quantified by an IC_{50} value of 9.02 mg/mL, might potentially be elucidated by the findings of molecular docking investigations. Hence, compounds like trans-anethole and fenchone, which have exhibited substantial interactions with specific proteins associated with antioxidant processes, such as superoxide dismutases or catalases, may be accountable for the reported antiradical activity in laboratory settings. These compounds have electrical and structural features that are advantageous for neutralizing free radicals. This is mainly due to their phenolic or terpenic groups, which may efficiently remove reactive oxygen species.

The antifungal and antibacterial activities of the extracts and essential oils were observed to have minimum inhibitory concentrations (MICs) and minimum bactericidal concentrations (MBCs) ranging from 0.78 to 50 mg/mL and 3.125 to 6.25 µL/mL, respectively. These activities can be attributed to binding energies and interactions, such as hydrogen bonding and Van der Waals forces, which were identified in molecular docking studies. The strong attraction between emmotin H, a phenolic compound found in the hydro-ethanolic extract, and the proteins 2ZDQ and 2CAG, which are crucial enzymes in fungi and bacteria, may account for the potent antimicrobial effects of this extract against *Aspergillus niger* and *Candida albicans*. The binding energies between emmotin H and these proteins are −10 and −9.4 kcal/mol, respectively. Undoubtedly, this type of selective molecular interaction is likely to disturb the overall structure and functional stability of these specific proteins, resulting in the suppression of the metabolic processes and development of microorganisms.

3. Materials and Methods

3.1. Plant Material

Anethum graveolens belongs to the *Apiaceae* family, commonly known as dill. The sample under study was collected from a cultivated population in the Errachidia area. Table 13 provides information on the collection location, the component harvested, and the origin. This species was identified at the Laboratory of Botany and Plant Ecology of the Scientific Institute of Rabat, Department of Botany.

Table 13. Harvesting Site, Parts Used, Habitat, and Harvesting Season for *A. graveolens*.

Scientific Name	Part Collected	Harvesting Area					Harvest Period
		Region	Location	Latitude (x)	Longitude (y)	Altitude (m)	
Anethum graveolens	Seeds	Errachidia	Annif	31°06′54″ N	5°09′38″ W	905	June 2022

3.2. Microbiological Materials

In this study, the antimicrobial activity of the essential oil (EO) and extracts of *A. graveolens* seeds was evaluated against five bacterial and five fungal strains. These microorganisms are pathogens commonly encountered in various human diseases (Table 14). These strains were isolated from the hospital environment of the Mohamed V Provincial Hospital, Meknes. All strains were stored in a 20% glycerol stock at −80 °C, rejuvenated in Mueller–Hinton and Sabouraud broths, and subcultured before use.

Table 14. List of tested bacterial and fungal strains used for antimicrobial tests.

Strains			Abbreviations
Bacteria	Gram-negative bacilli	*Enterobacter cloacae*	*E. cloacae*
		Klebsiella pneumoniae	*K. pneumoniae*
		Escherichia coli	*E. coli*
	Gram-positive cocci	*Staphylococcus aureus*	*S. aureus*
		Staphylococcus epidermidis	*S. epidermidis*
Fungi	Yeasts	*Candida albicans*	*C. albicans*
		Candida dubliniensis	*C. dubliniensis*
		Candida tropicalis	*C. tropicalis*
		Candida parapsilosis	*C. parapsilosis*
	Mold	*Aspergillus niger*	*A. niger*

3.3. Quality Control of Plant Material

3.3.1. Moisture Content

The approach used to determine the moisture content complied with the AFNOR standard (NF-V03-402 1985) [69]. A total of 5 g of plant samples were measured using pre-dried and pre-weighed crucibles. The crucibles, which held the plant material, were thereafter placed in an oven and exposed to a temperature ranging from 103 to 105 °C for a duration of 24 h. Subsequently, the samples were subjected to cooling in a desiccator and subsequently weighed. The moisture content was calculated using the Formula (1). The experiment was repeated three times.

$$\mathbf{MC\%} = \left(\frac{\mathbf{m_0 - m_1}}{\mathbf{m_0}}\right) \times \mathbf{100} \quad (1)$$

With m_0 as the initial mass of the plant in (g) and m_1 as the mass after drying in (g). The result is expressed as a percentage of dry matter.

3.3.2. Ash Content

The ash content refers to the amount of mineral materials that remain after the organic matter was destroyed by high-temperature incineration in a furnace. A total of 5 g of ground samples were put in a muffle furnace at a temperature of 550 °C until all charred particles were destroyed and whitish ashes were obtained, which had a consistent weight (according to NF ISO 5984) [70]. The organic matter content was determined by employing the subsequent Formula (2):

$$\mathbf{OM\%} = \left(\frac{\mathbf{m_1 - m_2}}{\mathbf{TE}}\right) \times \mathbf{100} \quad (2)$$

OM%: Organic Matter
m_1: Weight of the capsule and sample before calcination
m_2: Weight of the capsule and sample after calcination
TE: Test portion
The ash content was calculated as follows (Formula (3)):

$$\mathbf{Ash\ \% = 100 - OM\%} \quad (3)$$

3.3.3. Heavy Metal Analysis: Inductively Coupled Plasma Atomic Emission Spectrometry (ICP-AES)

The analysis of the heavy metals in *A. graveolens* seeds was conducted using the technique of Inductively Coupled Plasma Atomic Emission Spectrometry according to the standardized mineralization protocol [71].

This method involved first preparing the sample for analysis in liquid form by mixing 0.1 g of plant powder with 3ml of aqua regia prepared from 1 mL of nitric acid HNO_3 (99%) and 2 mL of hydrochloric acid HCl (37%), all placed in a reflux setup at 200 °C for two hours to ensure the complete dissolution of residual metal particles. Following the process of chilling and decantation, the liquid remaining above the sediment was gathered. It was then passed through a filter with a pore size of 0.45 µm and brought to a volume of 15 mL by adding distilled water. The concentrations of the heavy metals including arsenic (As), cadmium (Cd), chromium (Cr), iron (Fe), lead (Pb), antimony (Sb), and titanium (Ti) were quantified using an Inductively Coupled Plasma Atomic Emission Spectrometer (Ultima 2 Jobin Yvon) at the laboratory of UATRS (Technical Support Unit for Scientific Research) at CNRST in Rabat.

3.4. Phytochemical Screening

This is a qualitative analysis that allows for the identification of primary and secondary metabolites present in *A. graveolens* seeds. These tests were based on the visual observation of color changes, and formation of precipitates and complexes, while other tests included the examination of the samples under UV light. The detection of chemical compound groups was carried out according to protocols described in previous studies [72–77].

3.5. Extraction and Quality Control of Essential Oils

3.5.1. Extraction and Determination of Essential Oil Yields

The extraction of essential oils from *A. graveolens* seeds was carried out by hydrodistillation. A total of 100 g of dried dill seeds were immersed in a 2 L flask containing 1 L of water, topped with a Clevenger apparatus and a ball-type condenser. The mixture was brought to a boil for 3 h. The oils obtained were subsequently dehydrated using anhydrous sodium sulfate (Na_2SO_4) and kept in a sealed brown glass container at a temperature of 4 °C until they were ready for use. The extraction yield of the essential oil was quantified as the volume of essential oil obtained per unit mass of plant material (v/m), using Formula (4) [78].

$$\%\ \text{Yield} = \left[\frac{\text{V}}{\text{m}_0 - (\text{m}_0 \times \%\ \text{MC})} \times 10^4\right] \mp \text{Standard Deviation} \quad (4)$$

MC (%): Percentage of moisture in the plant material (moisture content).
m_0: Mass of distilled plant material
V: Volume of collected essential oil (in mL).

3.5.2. Analysis and Identification of the Chemical Composition of Essential Oils

The chromatographic analysis of essential oils was performed on a gas chromatograph of the Thermo Electron type (Trace GC Ultra) coupled with a mass spectrometer of the Thermo Electron Trace MS system (Thermo Electron: Trace GC Ultra; Polaris Q MS), with fragmentation carried out by electron impact at a 70 eV intensity. The chromatograph is equipped with a DB-5 type column (5% phenyl-methyl-siloxane) (30 m × 0.25 mm × 0.25 μm film thickness) and a flame ionization detector (FID) powered by an H2/Air gas mixture. The column temperature was programmed to increase by 4 °C/min from 50 to 200 °C for 5 min. The injection mode was split (leak ratio: 1/70, flow rate mL/min), and the carrier gas used was nitrogen at a flow rate of 1 mL/min.

The identification of the chemical composition of essential oils was performed by comparing their calculated Kovats indices (IK) with those of Adams and known reference products in the literature [79–81]. This was accomplished by conducting a comparison of the retention indices and mass spectra with those found in the mass spectral libraries of the National Institute of Standards and Technologies (NIST). Additionally, the experimental retention indices were compared with those available in the NIST online data collection at https://webbook.nist.gov/chemistry/name-ser/ (accessed on 10 April 2024). The proportions of each component were automatically determined using the total ion count observed by the GC-MS and represented as a percentage composition.

3.6. Extraction of Phenolic Compounds

To begin with, in order to isolate the phenolic compounds, two extraction methods were employed: decoction and solid–liquid extraction using the Soxhlet apparatus. The decoction procedure consisted of adding 30 g of the sample to 600 mL of distilled water and heating and bringing the mixture to a boil for one hour at 80 °C. After a five-minute decantation, the mixture was filtered under reduced pressure, and the decocted extract was recovered. This extract was then dried in an oven at 70 °C and subsequently stored in a glass vial.

As for the solid–liquid extraction, it was carried out using the Soxhlet apparatus on two additional samples weighing 30 g each. Two extraction solvents were used: pure water and an ethanol/water mixture in a ratio of 70/30. The extracts were concentrated using a rotary evaporator after several extraction cycles. These extracts were then identified, as indicated in Table 15.

Table 15. Coding of *A. graveolens* extracts.

Extraction Methods	Solvents	Coding
Decoction	Water	E (0)
Soxhlet	Ethanol/water (70/30; *v*/*v*)	E (1)
	Water	E (2)

3.7. *Quantification of Phenolic Compounds*

The total phenolic content of the different extracts was determined using the Folin–Ciocalteu method described by Singleton and Rossi [82]. This method is based on the reduction in the basic medium of the mixture of phosphotungstic acid $H_3P(W_3O_{10})_4$ and phosphomolybdic acid $H_3PMO_{12}O_4$ by the oxidizable groups of phenolic compounds present in various *A. graveolens* extracts. The chemical compounds tungsten oxide (W_8O_{23}) and molybdenum oxide (Mo_8O_3), which have a blue tint, were examined using colorimetry and optical density measurement. The absorbance measurement was acquired using a UV mini-1240 spectrophotometer configured at a wavelength of 760 nm and then compared to a blank sample, which consisted of a reaction mixture without the extract. A calibration curve was created in parallel, using the same working conditions, with a concentration range of 0.05 to 50 µg/mL of gallic acid as a positive control. The total phenolic content was determined by applying the calibration curve equation (Y = 0.095X + 0.003; R^2 = 0.998), and the results were expressed in milligrams of gallic acid equivalent per gram of extract (mg GAE/g). The experiment was replicated thrice.

3.8. *Quantification of Flavonoids*

The method by Djeridane and colleagues was used to determine the flavonoid content of our samples using aluminum trichloride as a reagent [83]. The technique is based on the oxidation of flavonoids by this reagent, leading to the formation of a stable yellowish flavonoid–aluminum complex, detectable in the visible range at 433 nm. The flavonoid content in our samples was determined from a calibration range established with increasing concentrations of quercetin ranging from 5 to 30 µg/mL, with the linear regression equation of Y = 0.073X − 0.081 and a determination coefficient R^2 equal to 0.995. The flavonoid content was expressed in milligrams of quercetin equivalent per gram of extract (mg EQ/g). Each test was repeated three times.

3.9. *Quantification of Condensed Tannins*

The vanillin method was employed to evaluate the concentrations of condensed tannins [84]. During this process, a solution containing vanillin dissolved in methanol at a concentration of 4% *w*/*v* was combined with 20 µL portions of the extracts or a solution of (+)-catechin at a concentration of 2 mg/mL. Subsequently, the mixes were manually agitated. Subsequently, each concentration was transferred to a test tube containing 1.5 milliliters of hydrochloric acid. The reaction mixture was allowed to stand at ambient temperature for a duration of 20 min. The measurement of absorbance was conducted at a wavelength of 499 nm using a UV–visible spectrophotometer, with a reference to a blank sample. The content of condensed tannins in the samples was calculated from the catechin calibration curve used as a standard (Y = 0.7421X + 0.0318; R^2 = 0.998). The tannin content was expressed in milligrams of catechin equivalent per gram of extract (mg EC/g).

3.10. *HPLC/UV ESI-MS Analysis of A. graveolens Seed Extracts*

The phenolic components of *A. graveolens* in the decoction were analyzed using High-performance liquid Chromatography combined with a Q Exactive Plus mass spectrometer and electrospray ionization as the molecular ionization method (HPLC/UV-ESI-MS). The analysis was performed on an UltiMate 3000 HPLC system (Thermo Fisher Scientific, Sunnyvale, CA, USA) with an autosampler maintained at 5 °C. The HPLC system employed a reverse-phase C18 column with a column temperature of 40 °C (Lichro CART, Lichrospher,

Merck, Darmstadt, Germany, 250 × 4 mm, ID 5 µm). The mobile phase was composed of solvent A, which was a mixture of 0.1% formic acid in water (*v*/*v*), and solvent B, which was a mixture of 0.1% formic acid in acetonitrile (*v*/*v*). The gases were eliminated from the mobile phase using the process of sonication. The description of the gradient's composition may be found in Supplementary Table S1. The rate of flow was 1 milliliter per minute, and the amount injected was 20 µL. After negative electrospray ionization, broadband collision-induced dissociation (bbCID) detection was carried out using a Maxis Impact HD instrument (Bruker Daltonik, Bremen, Germany). The UV detection in the range of 190 to 600 nm and acquisition of three wavelengths from 280 to 320 to 360 nm were performed using a diode array detector L-2455 (Merck-Hitachi, Darmstadt, Germany). The parameters used were a capillary voltage of 3000 V, drying gas temperature of 200 °C, dry gas flow rate of 8 L/min, nebulizer gas pressure of 2 bars, and offset voltage of 500 V. Nitrogen was used as both the nebulizer and desolvation gas. The m/z range of the MS data was from 100 to 1500.

The process of gathering and examining data was conducted using Thermo Scientific's Chromeleon 7.2 chromatography data system (CDS). The eluted chemicals were analyzed by studying the mass spectra of the isolated molecules.

3.11. Antioxidant Activity

3.11.1. Radical Scavenging Activity by DPPH• Test

The antioxidant activity of the essential oils (EO) and extracts of *A. graveolens* was assessed using the 2,2-diphenyl-1-picrylhydrazyl (DPPH) radical, following the procedure outlined by [85]. A total of 200 µL of *A. graveolens* extract or EO was applied to test tubes containing 100% ethanol. Afterward, 2.8 mL of a solution of DPPH• in ethanol (24 µg/mL, *w*/*v*) was added to the mixture and allowed to incubate for 30 min in the absence of light. The measurement of absorbance was conducted at a wavelength of 515 nm using a UV–Vis spectrophotometer. The experiments were replicated thrice. The reference standard utilized was butylated hydroxytoluene (BHT) at varying concentrations. The results were quantified as a percentage of DPPH• decrease, denoted as AA% (Formula (5)):

$$\mathbf{AA\%} = \frac{\mathbf{A_{control}} - \mathbf{A_{Sample}}}{\mathbf{A_{control}}} \times \mathbf{100} \tag{5}$$

AA%: Percentage of antioxidant activity.

$A_{\_control}$: Absorbance of the solution containing only the DPPH• radical solution.

$A_{\_sample}$: Absorbance of the test sample solution in the presence of DPPH•.

The 50% inhibitory concentration of the DPPH• free radicals (IC_{50}) for BHT or our extracts was determined from a graph of antioxidant activity variation with concentration.

3.11.2. Ferric Reducing Antioxidant Power (FRAP) Method

The capacity of the phenolic extracts from *A. graveolens* to convert ferric iron (Fe^{3+}) in the potassium ferricyanide complex to ferrous iron (Fe^{2+}) was assessed using the technique outlined by Oyaizu [86]. The experiment consisted of combining 1 mL of the plant extract being investigated with 2.5 mL of a phosphate buffer solution (0.2 M, pH 6.6) and 2.5 mL of a potassium ferricyanide solution ($K_3Fe(CN)_6$ at a concentration of 1%). The resultant mixture was subjected to incubation in a water bath maintained at a temperature of 50 °C for a duration of 20 min. Next, 2.5 mL of a solution containing 10% trichloroacetic acid was introduced to halt the progress of the reaction. The solution was subjected to centrifugation at a speed of 3000 revolutions per minute for a duration of 10 min. Ultimately, 2.5 mL of the liquid remaining after centrifugation from each concentration was combined with 2.5 mL of pure water and 0.5 mL of a solution containing 0.1% $FeCl_3$ dissolved in water. The absorbance of the reaction medium was measured at a wavelength of 700 nm using a UV–Vis spectrophotometer. A blank sample was generated in the same way, but distilled water was used instead of the aqueous extract for calibration reasons. The positive control was represented by a solution of a standard antioxidant, BHA (Butylated Hydroxyanisole), for which the absorbance was measured under the same conditions as the samples. All tests were repeated three times. The graph of the variation in reducing power as a function of BHT concentration or our extracts allowed the determination of the concentration corresponding to an absorbance of 0.5 (EC_{50}).

3.11.3. Total Antioxidant Capacity

The phosphomolybdenum test described by Khiya et al. [87] was used to screen the total antioxidant capacity of *A. graveolens* extracts. This test is based on the reduction of molybdenum Mo^{6+} (VI) to molybdenum Mo^{5+} (V) in the presence of extracts, leading to the formation of a green complex, phosphate/Mo^{5+} (V) at acidic pH with a maximum absorbance at 695 nm.

In a test tube, a volume of 3 mL of the reactive solution (0.6 M sulfuric acid, 28 mM sodium phosphate, and 4 mM ammonium molybdate) was added to a volume of extract. The tubes were shaken and left in an incubator at 95 °C for 90 min and then normalized to room temperature. After cooling, the absorbance of the solutions was measured at 695 nm. Ascorbic acid was used as a standard. The results were expressed in milligrams of ascorbic acid equivalents per gram of extract (mg AAE/g).

3.12. Antimicrobial Activity

The Minimum Inhibitory Concentration (MIC) represents the lowest concentration of essential oil or extract capable of completely inhibiting the growth of a microorganism. The determination of the MIC was performed using the microdilution method [88]. Initially, a stock solution of essential oil, prepared in 10% DMSO, was subjected to a series of dilutions to obtain concentrations ranging from 5 to 0.93×10^{-2} mg/mL for the essential oil. As for the extracts, a stock solution was prepared beforehand and then diluted to achieve the desired concentrations, expressed in μg/mL. The dilutions of essential oil and extracts were carried out in a Mueller–Hinton broth for bacteria and Sabouraud broth for fungi, with a final volume of 100 μL for each concentration.

Afterwards, 100 μL of the microbial inoculum, with a final concentration of 10^6 CFU/mL for bacteria and 10^4 CFU/mL for fungus, were added to the various concentrations of the dilution series. Following a 24 h incubation period at a temperature of 37 °C, 10 μL of resazurin was introduced into each well as a means of detecting bacterial proliferation. After a further incubation period of 2 h at a temperature of 37 °C, the presence of microbial growth was indicated by a shift in hue from violet to pink. The minimum inhibitory concentration (MIC) is defined as the lowest concentration of a substance that effectively blocks the observed color shift of resazurin. The 11th and 12th wells in each series were designated as the growth control and sterility control, respectively. This technique was replicated twice for both the oil and extracts.

To determine the Minimum Bactericidal Concentration (MBC) or Minimum Fungicidal Concentration (MFC), 10 μL was taken from each well without visible growth and inoculated on Mueller–Hinton agar (MH) for bacteria or Sabouraud agar for fungi. The plates were incubated for 24 h at 37 °C. The MBC and MFC were defined as the lowest concentration of the samples analyzed, which resulted in a 99.99% reduction in CFU/mL compared to the control. The ratio of MBC/MIC or MFC/MIC was calculated to assess the antimicrobial power. A ratio less than 4 indicated a bactericidal/fungicidal effect of the essential oil, while a ratio greater than 4 indicated a bacteriostatic/fungistatic effect of the sample.

3.13. PASS, ADMET, Pro-Tox, and Prediction of the Efficacy of Potentially Active Compounds Isolated from the Essential Oil and Aqueous Extract of A. graveolens Seeds

The main constituents of the essential oil (EO) and aqueous extract derived from *A. graveolens* seeds examined were selected for ADMET (absorption, distribution, metabolism, excretion, and toxicity) tests and PASS prediction tests. To choose the SMILES format of these chemical substances, ChemBioDraw (PerkinElmer Informatics, Waltham, MA, USA, v13.0) [56] was used. Subsequently, simulations were conducted using the PASS-Way2Drug online prediction tool [57], as well as the online tools SwissADME and pkCSM for ADMET prediction [58]. The potential activity (Pa) and probable inactivity (Pi) of "drug-like" substances were designated by the PASS acronym [89].

ProTox II, a useful tool created specifically for this purpose, was used to examine toxicity levels and gather relevant data on several toxicological parameters, including LD50 and the toxicity class [90]. The ADMET software, consisting of SwissADME, pkCSM, and ProTox II, was employed to assess the chosen ligands. This allowed for the prediction of their physicochemical properties, lipophilicity, water solubility, pharmacokinetics, drug-likeness, medicinal chemistry, and toxicological features. The utilization of these methodologies and analytical instruments enabled reliable observations on the possible therapeutic uses and negative consequences linked to the primary chemical constituents found in the EO and aqueous extract of *A. graveolens* seeds being studied.

3.14. Molecular Docking

The protein targets' three-dimensional structures, as indicated in Table 16, were acquired from the Protein Data Bank RCSB, which may be accessed at the URL https://www.rcsb.org/ (accessed on 10 April 2024). The visualization of protein structure was conducted using UCSF Chimera. The protein structures were constructed as suitable docking targets using Autodock Tools (version 1.5.6, The Scripps Research Institute, La Jolla, CA, USA). Before analysis, the protein structures underwent preprocessing steps, including the removal of water molecules, heteroatoms (hetatm), unwanted protein chains, and co-crystallized ligands. Subsequently, polar hydrogen atoms and Gesteiger charges were added, and the resulting structures were converted to pdbqt format for further analysis.

The three-dimensional structures of the sixteen compounds were represented using their respective structures, collected from PubChem, and then subjected to structural energy minimization. The ligands were then processed using the Prescription Virtual Screening Python script (AutoDock Vina 1.2.0), where their SDF files were converted into pdbqt formats.

The compound docking process utilized the scoring function of AutoDock Vina. After selecting the protein and ligand molecules for docking in the Vina control, a grid box was overlaid onto the protein structure. The grid box size could be adjusted based on the chosen active site residues before launching the AutoDock Vina program for the docking process. The search space was bounded by the grid box, whose size and position were determined by coordinates to precisely align with the active binding site (Table 16). The resulting data for docked molecules, expressed in free binding energy values, were recorded, and the analysis of ligand-protein binding features was conducted using PyMOL.

Subsequently, we proceeded with redocking, a method representing a reliable approach to validate the molecular docking process. This method involves separating the crystallized ligand from the protein, followed by a new docking analysis in the same region where the ligand was initially located. This approach allows us to accurately assess whether the docked ligand effectively overlaps with the crystallized ligand by closely examining the RMSD parameter value using specialized software such as PyMOL 2.5.0. In summary, redocking offers rigorous validation of the molecular docking process by confirming the consistency of the results obtained.

Table 16. Protein targets and molecular docking parameters.

Protein	PDB ID	Grid Box Center Coordinates	Grid Box Size
Isoleucyl-tRNA synthetase	1JZQ	center_x = −27.803	size_x = 34
		center_y = 6.619	size_y = 22
		center_z = −28.722	size_z = 21
DNA gyrase	1KZN	center_x = 18.325	size_x = 23
		center_y = 30.783	size_y = 38
		center_z = 36.762	size_z = 38

Table 16. *Cont.*

Protein	PDB ID	Grid Box Center Coordinates	Grid Box Size
Catalase compound II	2CAG	center_x = 60.017	size_x = 28
		center_y = 14.760	size_y = 22
		center_z = 15.935	size_z = 34
Dihydropteroate synthase	2VEG	center_x = 31.404	size_x = 24
		center_y = 48.530	size_y = 24
		center_z = 0.204	size_z = 23
D-Alanine ligase	2ZDQ	center_x = 47.378	size_x = 21
		center_y = 12.782	size_y = 26
		center_z = 5.730	size_z = 32
Dihydrofolate reductase	3SRW	center_x = -4.701	size_x = 20
		center_y = -31.536	size_y = 26
		center_z = 6.341	size_z = 26
Penicillin-binding protein 1a PBP1a	3UDI	center_x = 34.198	size_x = 24
		center_y = −1.249	size_y = 22
		center_z = 12.715	size_z = 28
Crystal structure of Staph ParE 24 kDa	4URN	center_x = -31.684	size_x = 28
		center_y = 8.021	size_y = 40
		center_z = −4.598	size_z = 42
NADPH oxidase	2CDU	center_x = 18.26	size_x = 22
		center_y = −6.35	size_y = 24
		center_z = −1.53	size_z = 28
Cytochrome P450 2C9	1OG5	center_x = −20.236	size_x = 21
		center_y = 86.761	size_y = 23
		center_z = 38.657	size_z = 20
Xanthine dehydrogenase/oxidase	3NRZ	center_x = 37.526	size_x = 20
		center_y = 19.929	size_y = 20
		center_z = 17.643	size_z = 20

3.15. Molecular Dynamics Simulation

The GROMACS 2019.3 software was employed to perform molecular dynamics simulations in order to evaluate the stability of the protein–ligand complex [91]. The protein was subjected to the all-atom CHARMM36 force field, and the topologies of the ligands were generated using the CGenFF service. The systems were rendered neutral by introducing ions to counterbalance the overall charges after the immersion of all complexes in a rectangular container filled with TIP3P water molecules. The steepest descent strategy was used to achieve both the least energy and maximum force by selecting a force threshold (Fmax) of 1000 kJ/mol/nm. The ensembles were maintained at constant NVT (number of atoms, volume, and temperature) and NPT (number of atoms, pressure, and temperature) for molecular dynamics simulation investigations. Subsequently, every molecule underwent molecular dynamics simulations lasting 100 ns. Analyzed output trajectories yielded a comprehensive understanding of protein behavior.

3.16. Statistical Analysis

The outcomes are presented as the average, and the measure of variability is known as the standard deviation. The data were evaluated using GraphPad Prism 8 software (version 8.0.2, San Diego, CA, USA) by the use of a one-way ANOVA test and Tukey's post-test. Significance was attributed to P values below 0.05. The relationship between the phenolic compounds and antioxidant activity content was assessed using the Pearson correlation coefficient. A difference was considered statistically significant when the P-value was less than 0.05.

4. Conclusions

This study emphasized the abundance of phytochemicals in the seeds of *Anethum graveolens*. The essential oil was analyzed by GC-MS, which showed that (E)-anethole was the most abundant compound at 38.13%, followed by estragole at 29.32%, fenchone at 17.21%, and α-pinene at 7.37%. The seeds furthermore possessed secondary metabolites, including tannins, flavonoids, sterols, triterpenes, and mucilage.

This quantitative study revealed substantial concentrations of polyphenols, flavonoids, and condensed tannins. The use of HPLC/UV-ESI-MS analysis enabled the detection and identification of 38 prominent compounds, such as umbelliferone (12.35%), hydroxyflavone (11.23%), rosmanol (8.95%), biotin (8.36%), Emmotin H (4.91%), and coumarin (4.21%).

The essential oils and extracts exhibited significant antioxidant activity as demonstrated by the DPPH˙, FRAP, and CAT tests. They were able to effectively neutralize free radicals and bind metal ions. The antimicrobial tests demonstrated that the essential oil exhibited more efficacy compared to the aqueous, ethanolic, and decoction extracts against the majority of the bacteria tested. This enhanced effectiveness can be attributed to the synergistic effects of its primary constituents.

The docking and molecular dynamics simulations validated substantial connections and enduring stability between certain bioactive chemicals and diverse target proteins.

The findings indicate that *A. graveolens* exhibits a significant therapeutic promise for a range of human diseases and has the ability to serve as a natural preservative in the food business.

Supplementary Materials: The following supporting information can be downloaded at https://www.mdpi.com/article/10.3390/ph17070862/s1, Figure S1. GC-MS chromatogram of the essential oil from *A. graveolens*; Figure S2. Structures of the main compounds identified in *A. graveolens* EO; Figure S3. HPLC chromatogram of compounds from the decocted extract of *A. graveolens*; Figure S4. Structures of the majority of compounds identified in extract E (0) of *A. graveolens*; Table S1. Gradient mobile phase elution.

Author Contributions: Conceptualization, N.H. and A.D.; methodology, N.H. and A.A.S.; software, M.R.; validation, T.Z. and A.B.; formal analysis, S.B.; investigation, N.H. and F.R.; resources, T.Z.; data curation, E.M.B.; writing—original draft preparation, N.H. and A.D.; writing—review and editing, N.H., A.A.S. and A.D.; visualization, I.T.; supervision, A.B.; project administration, T.Z.; funding acquisition, A.A.S. All authors have read and agreed to the published version of the manuscript.

Funding: This research was funded by Researchers supporting project number (RSPD2024R1057), King Saud University, Riyadh, Saudi Arabia.

Institutional Review Board Statement: Not applicable.

Informed Consent Statement: Not applicable.

Data Availability Statement: Data are contained within this article.

Acknowledgments: Authors are thankful to the Researchers supporting project number (RSPD2024R1057), King Saud University, Riyadh, Saudi Arabia.

Conflicts of Interest: The authors declare that they have no known competing financial interests or personal relationships that could have appeared to influence the work reported in this paper.

References

1. Mathers, C.; Ma Fat, D.; Boerma, J.T.; World Health Organization. *The Global Burden of Disease: 2004 Update*; World Health Organization: Geneva, Switzerland, 2008; ISBN 978-92-4-156371-0.
2. Zhang, X.-J.; Diao, M.; Zhang, Y.-F. A Review of the Occurrence, Metabolites and Health Risks of Butylated Hydroxyanisole (BHA). *J. Sci. Food Agric.* **2023**, *103*, 6150–6166. [CrossRef]
3. Ito, N.; Hirose, M.; Fukushima, S.; Tsuda, H.; Shirai, T.; Tatematsu, M. Studies on Antioxidants: Their Carcinogenic and Modifying Effects on Chemical Carcinogenesis. *Food Chem. Toxicol.* **1986**, *24*, 1071–1082. [CrossRef]

4. Lopez-Romero, J.C.; González-Ríos, H.; Borges, A.; Simões, M. Antibacterial Effects and Mode of Action of Selected Essential Oils Components against Escherichia Coli and Staphylococcus Aureus. *Evid. Based Complement. Altern. Med.* **2015**, *2015*, 795435. [CrossRef]
5. Paven, C.S.J.; Radu, D.; Alexa, E.; Pintilie, S.; Rivis, A. *Anethum graveolens*—An Important Source of Antioxidant Compounds for Food Industry. *Adv. Biotechnol.* **2018**, *18*, 11–18. [CrossRef]
6. Jana, S.; Shekhawat, G. *Anethum graveolens*: An Indian Traditional Medicinal Herb and Spice. *Pharmacogn. Rev.* **2010**, *4*, 179–184. [CrossRef]
7. Brinsi, C.; Selmi, H.; Jedidi, S.; Sebai, H. Enquête Ethno-Pharmacologique Sur l' Usage Traditionnel de l'Aneth (*Anethum graveolens* L.) Dans Le Nord-Ouest de La Tunisie. *Rev. Marocaine Des Sci. Agron. Et Vétérinaires* **2022**, *10*, 282–286.
8. Jirovetz, L.; Buchbauer, G.; Stoyanova, A.S.; Georgiev, E.V.; Damianova, S.T. Composition, Quality Control, and Antimicrobial Activity of the Essential Oil of Long-Time Stored Dill (*Anethum graveolens*, L.) Seeds from Bulgaria. *J. Agric. Food Chem.* **2003**, *51*, 3854–3857. [CrossRef]
9. Kaur, N.; Chahal, K.K.; Kumar, A.; Singh, R.; Bhardwaj, U. Antioxidant Activity of *Anethum graveolens*, L. Essential Oil Constituents and Their Chemical Analogues. *J. Food Biochem.* **2019**, *43*, e12782. [CrossRef]
10. Nam, H.H.; Nan, L.; Choo, B.K. Anti-Inflammation and Protective Effects of *Anethum graveolens* L. (Dill Seeds) on Esophageal Mucosa Damages in Reflux Esophagitis-Induced Rats. *Foods* **2021**, *10*, 2500. [CrossRef]
11. Goodarzi, M.T.; Khodadadi, I.; Tavilani, H.; Abbasi Oshaghi, E. The Role of *Anethum graveolens*, L. (Dill) in the Management of Diabetes. *J. Trop. Med.* **2016**, *2016*, 1098916. [CrossRef]
12. Ozliman, S.; Yaldiz, G.; Camlica, M.; Ozsoy, N. Chemical Components of Essential Oils and Biological Activities of the Aqueous Extract of *Anethum graveolens*, L. Grown under Inorganic and Organic Conditions. *Chem. Biol. Technol. Agric.* **2021**, *8*, 1–16. [CrossRef]
13. Mahran, G.H.; Kadry, H.A.; Isaac, Z.G.; Thabet, C.K.; Al-Azizi, M.M.; El-Olemy, M.M. Investigation of Diuretic Drug Plants. 1. Phytochemical Screening and Pharmacological Evaluation of *Anethum graveolens*, L., *Apium graveolens*, L., *Daucus carota*, L. and *Eruca sativa* Mill. *Phytother. Res.* **1991**, *5*, 169–172. [CrossRef]
14. Najafzadeh, R.; Ghasemzadeh, S.; Mirfakhraie, S. Effect of Essential Oils from Nepeta Crispa, *Anethum graveolens* and *Satureja hortensis* Against the Stored-Product Insect "*Ephestia kuehniella* (Zeller)". *J. Med. Plants By-Prod.* **2019**, *2*, 163–169.
15. Rabeh, N.M.; Aboraya, A.O. Hepatoprotective Effect of Dill (*Anethum graveolens*, L.) and Fennel (*Foeniculum vulgare*) Oil on Hepatotoxic Rats. *Pak. J. Nutr.* **2014**, *13*, 303–309. [CrossRef]
16. Al-Oqail, M.M.; Farshori, N.N. Antioxidant and Anticancer Efficacies of *Anethum graveolens* against Human Breast Carcinoma Cells through Oxidative Stress and Caspase Dependency. *BioMed Res. Int.* **2021**, *2021*, 5535570. [CrossRef]
17. El-Sayed, K.K.; El-Sheikh, E.-S.A.; Sherif, R.M.; Gouhar, K.A. Chemical Composition and Bio-Efficacy of Essential Oils Isolated from Seeds of *Anethum graveolens*, L., Leaves of *Thymus vulgaris*, L., and Nuts of *Myristica fragrans* Houtt. Against *Callosobruchus maculatus* (Fab.) (Coleoptera: Bruchidae). *J. Essent. Oil Bear. Plants* **2021**, *24*, 1402–1414. [CrossRef]
18. Farmanpour Kalalagh, K.; Mohebodini, M.; Fattahi, R.; Beyraghdar Kashkooli, A.; Davarpanah Dizaj, S.; Salehifar, F.; Mokhtari, A.M. Drying Temperatures Affect the Qualitative–Quantitative Variation of Aromatic Profiling in *Anethum graveolens*, L. Ecotypes as an Industrial–Medicinal–Vegetable Plant. *Front. Plant Sci.* **2023**, *14*, 1137840. [CrossRef] [PubMed]
19. Mehdizadeh, T.; Mojaddar Langroodi, A.; Shakouri, R.; Khorshidi, S. Physicochemical, Microbiological, and Sensory Characteristics of Probiotic Yogurt Enhanced with *Anethum graveolens* Essential Oil. *J. Food Saf.* **2019**, *39*, e12683. [CrossRef]
20. Znini, M.; Ansari, A.; Costa, J.; Senhaji, O.; Paolini, J.; Majidi, L. Experimental, Quantum Chemical and Molecular Dynamic Simulations Studies on the Corrosion Inhibition of C38 Steel in 1M HCl by *Anethum graveolens* Essential Oil. *Anal. Bioanal. Electrochem* **2019**, *11*, 1426–1451.
21. Li, H.; Zhou, W.; Hu, Y.; Mo, H.; Wang, J.; Hu, L. GC-MS Analysis of Essential Oil from *Anethum graveolens* L (Dill) Seeds Extracted by Supercritical Carbon Dioxide. *Trop. J. Pharm. Res.* **2019**, *18*, 1291–1296. [CrossRef]
22. Snuossi, M.; Trabelsi, N.; Ben Taleb, S.; Dehmeni, A.; Flamini, G.; De Feo, V. Laurus Nobilis, Zingiber Officinale and *Anethum graveolens* Essential Oils: Composition, Antioxidant and Antibacterial Activities against Bacteria Isolated from Fish and Shellfish. *Molecules* **2016**, *21*, 1414. [CrossRef] [PubMed]
23. Noumi, E.; Ahmad, I.; Adnan, M.; Merghni, A.; Patel, H.; Haddaji, N.; Bouali, N.; Alabbosh, K.F.; Ghannay, S.; Aouadi, K.; et al. GC/MS Profiling, Antibacterial, Anti-Quorum Sensing, and Antibiofilm Properties of *Anethum graveolens*, L. Essential Oil: Molecular Docking Study and In-Silico ADME Profiling. *Plants* **2023**, *12*, 1997. [CrossRef] [PubMed]
24. Kostić, I.; Lazarević, J.; Šešlija Jovanović, D.; Kostić, M.; Marković, T.; Milanović, S. Potential of Essential Oils from Anise, Dill and Fennel Seeds for the Gypsy Moth Control. *Plants* **2021**, *10*, 2194. [CrossRef] [PubMed]
25. Aati, H.Y.; Perveen, S.; Aati, S.; Orfali, R.; Alqahtani, J.H.; Al-Taweel, A.M.; Wanner, J.; Aati, A.Y. Headspace Solid-Phase Microextraction Method for Extracting Volatile Constituents from the Different Parts of Saudi *Anethum graveolens*, L. and Their Antimicrobial Activity. *Heliyon* **2022**, *8*, e09051. [CrossRef] [PubMed]
26. Anvar, N.; Nateghi, L.; Shariatifar, N.; Mousavi, S.A. The Effect of Essential Oil of *Anethum graveolens*, L. Seed and Gallic Acid (Free and Nano Forms) on Microbial, Chemical and Sensory Characteristics in Minced Meat during Storage at 4 °C. *Food Chem. X* **2023**, *19*, 100842. [CrossRef] [PubMed]
27. El Mansouri, L.; Bousta, D.; Balouiri, M.; Ouedrhiri, W.; Elyoubi-El Hamsas, A. Antioxidant Activity of Aqueous Seed Extract of *Anethum graveolens*, L. *Int. J. Pharm. Sci. Res.* **2016**, *7*, 1219–1223. [CrossRef]

28. Bota, S.R.; Stanasel, O.D.; Blidar, C.F.; Serban, G. Phenolic Constituents of *Anethum graveolens* Seed Extracts: Chemical Profile and Antioxidant Effect Studies. *J. Pharm. Res. Int.* **2021**, *33*, 168–179. [CrossRef]
29. Mashraqi, A. Induction Role of Chitosan Nanoparticles to *Anethum graveolens* Extract against Food-Borne Bacteria, Oxidant, and Diabetic Activities In Vitro. *Front. Microbiol.* **2023**, *14*, 1209524. [CrossRef] [PubMed]
30. Erdogan Orhan, I.; Senol, F.S.; Ozturk, N.; Celik, S.A.; Pulur, A.; Kan, Y. Phytochemical Contents and Enzyme Inhibitory and Antioxidant Properties of *Anethum graveolens*, L. (Dill) Samples Cultivated under Organic and Conventional Agricultural Conditions. *Food Chem. Toxicol.* **2013**, *59*, 96–103. [CrossRef]
31. Meena, S.S.; Lal, G.; Dubey, P.N.; Meena, M.D.; Ravi, Y. Medicinal and Therapeutic Uses of Dill (*Anethum graveolens* L.)—A Review. *Int. J. Seed Spices* **2019**, *9*, 14–20.
32. Sharifi-Rad, J.; Cruz-Martins, N.; López-Jornet, P.; Lopez, E.P.F.; Harun, N.; Yeskaliyeva, B.; Beyatli, A.; Sytar, O.; Shaheen, S.; Sharopov, F.; et al. Natural Coumarins: Exploring the Pharmacological Complexity and Underlying Molecular Mechanisms. *Oxidative Med. Cell. Longev.* **2021**, *2021*, 6492346. [CrossRef]
33. Mazimba, O. Umbelliferone: Sources, Chemistry and Bioactivities Review. *Bull. Fac. Pharm. Cairo Univ.* **2017**, *55*, 223–232. [CrossRef]
34. Chen, S.; Wang, X.; Cheng, Y.; Gao, H.; Chen, X. A Review of Classification, Biosynthesis, Biological Activities and Potential Applications of Flavonoids. *Molecules* **2023**, *28*, 4982. [CrossRef]
35. Thomas, S.D.; Jha, N.K.; Jha, S.K.; Sadek, B.; Ojha, S. Pharmacological and Molecular Insight on the Cardioprotective Role of Apigenin. *Nutrients* **2023**, *15*, 385. [CrossRef]
36. Abid, R.; Ghazanfar, S.; Farid, A.; Sulaman, S.M.; Idrees, M.; Amen, R.A.; Muzammal, M.; Shahzad, M.K.; Mohamed, M.O.; Khaled, A.A.; et al. Pharmacological Properties of 4′,5,7-Trihydroxyflavone (Apigenin) and Its Impact on Cell Signaling Pathways. *Molecules* **2022**, *27*, 4304. [CrossRef]
37. Maneesai, P.; Potue, P.; Khamseekaew, J.; Sangartit, W.; Rattanakanokchai, S.; Poasakate, A.; Pakdeechote, P. Kaempferol Protects against Cardiovascular Abnormalities Induced by Nitric Oxide Deficiency in Rats by Suppressing the TNF-α Pathway. *Eur. J. Pharmacol.* **2023**, *960*, 176112. [CrossRef]
38. Deng, H.; Xu, Q.; Guo, H.Y.; Huang, X.; Chen, F.; Jin, L.; Quan, Z.S.; Shen, Q.K. Application of Cinnamic Acid in the Structural Modification of Natural Products: A Review. *Phytochemistry* **2023**, *206*, 113532. [CrossRef]
39. Ruwizhi, N.; Aderibigbe, B.A. Cinnamic Acid Derivatives and Their Biological Efficacy. *Int. J. Mol. Sci.* **2020**, *21*, 5712. [CrossRef]
40. Babaeenezhad, E.; Nouryazdan, N.; Nasri, M.; Ahmadvand, H.; Moradi Sarabi, M. Cinnamic Acid Ameliorate Gentamicin-Induced Liver Dysfunctions and Nephrotoxicity in Rats through Induction of Antioxidant Activities. *Heliyon* **2021**, *7*, e07465. [CrossRef] [PubMed]
41. Koczurkiewicz-Adamczyk, P.; Klaś, K.; Gunia-Krzyżak, A.; Piska, K.; Andrysiak, K.; Stępniewski, J.; Lasota, S.; Wójcik-Pszczoła, K.; Dulak, J.; Madeja, Z.; et al. Cinnamic Acid Derivatives as Cardioprotective Agents against Oxidative and Structural Damage Induced by Doxorubicin. *Int. J. Mol. Sci.* **2021**, *22*, 6217. [CrossRef] [PubMed]
42. Osanloo, M.; Ghanbariasad, A.; Taghinezhad, A. Antioxidant and Anticancer Activities of *Anethum graveolens*, L., *Citrus limon* (L.) Osbeck and *Zingiber officinale* Roscoe Essential Oils. *Tradit. Integr. Med.* **2021**, 333–347. [CrossRef]
43. Gladikostić, N.; Ikonić, B.; Teslić, N.; Zeković, Z.; Božović, D.; Putnik, P.; Bursać Kovačević, D.; Pavlić, B. Essential Oils from Apiaceae, Asteraceae, Cupressaceae and Lamiaceae Families Grown in Serbia: Comparative Chemical Profiling with In Vitro Antioxidant Activity. *Plants* **2023**, *12*, 745. [CrossRef]
44. Stanojević, L.P.; Radulović, N.S.; Djokić, T.M.; Stanković, B.M.; Ilić, D.P.; Cakić, M.D.; Nikolić, V.D. The Yield, Composition and Hydrodistillation Kinetics of the Essential Oil of Dill Seeds (*Anethi Fructus*) Obtained by Different Hydrodistillation Techniques. *Ind. Crop. Prod.* **2015**, *65*, 429–436. [CrossRef]
45. Galicka, A.; Krętowski, R.; Nazaruk, J.; Cechowska-Pasko, M. Anethole Prevents Hydrogen Peroxide-Induced Apoptosis and Collagen Metabolism Alterations in Human Skin Fibroblasts. *Mol. Cell Biochem.* **2014**, *394*, 217–224. [CrossRef] [PubMed]
46. Donati, M.; Mondin, A.; Chen, Z.; Miranda, F.M.; do Nascimento, B.B., Jr.; Schirato, G.; Pastore, P.; Froldi, G. Radical Scavenging and Antimicrobial Activities of Croton Zehntneri, Pterodon Emarginatus and Schinopsis Brasiliensis Essential Oils and Their Major Constituents: Estragole, Trans-Anethole, β-Caryophyllene and Myrcene. *Nat. Prod. Res.* **2015**, *29*, 939–946. [CrossRef]
47. Senatore, F.; Oliviero, F.; Scandolera, E.; Taglialatela-Scafati, O.; Roscigno, G.; Zaccardelli, M.; De Falco, E. Chemical Composition, Antimicrobial and Antioxidant Activities of Anethole-Rich Oil from Leaves of Selected Varieties of Fennel [*Foeniculum vulgare* Mill. Ssp. *vulgare* Var. *azoricum* (Mill.) Thell]. *Fitoterapia* **2013**, *90*, 214–219. [CrossRef]
48. Luís, Â.; Sousa, S.; Wackerlig, J.; Dobusch, D.; Duarte, A.P.; Pereira, L.; Domingues, F. Star Anise (*Illicium verum* Hook. f.) Essential Oil: Antioxidant Properties and Antibacterial Activity against *Acinetobacter baumannii*. *Flavour Fragr. J.* **2019**, *34*, 260–270. [CrossRef]
49. Singh, S.; Das, S.; Singh, G.; Perotti, M.; Schuff, C.; Catalan, C. Comparative Studies of Chemical Composition, Antioxidant and Antimicrobial Potentials of Essential Oils and Oleoresins Obtained from Seeds and Leaves of *Anethum graveolens*, L. *Toxicol. Open Access* **2017**, *3*, 2–9.
50. Coêlho, M.L.; Islam, M.T.; Laylson da Silva Oliveira, G.; Oliveira Barros de Alencar, M.V.; Victor de Oliveira Santos, J.; Campinho dos Reis, A.; Oliveira Ferreira da Mata, A.M.; Correia Jardim Paz, M.F.; Docea, A.O.; Calina, D.; et al. Cytotoxic and Antioxidant Properties of Natural Bioactive Monoterpenes Nerol, Estragole, and 3,7-Dimethyl-1-Octanol. *Adv. Pharmacol. Pharm. Sci.* **2022**, *2022*, e8002766. [CrossRef]

51. El Omari, N.; Balahbib, A.; Bakrim, S.; Benali, T.; Ullah, R.; Alotaibi, A.; Naceiri El Mrabti, H.; Goh, B.H.; Ong, S.-K.; Ming, L.C.; et al. Fenchone and Camphor: Main Natural Compounds from *Lavandula stoechas*, L., Expediting Multiple In Vitro Biological Activities. *Heliyon* **2023**, *9*, e21222. [CrossRef]
52. Singh, A.; Raja, W. Assessment of Antioxidant Activity of Foeniculum Vulgare Seed Extract Using Fenton Reaction. *Res. J. Med. Plants Ayurveda* **2020**, *1*, 1–7.
53. Basavegowda, J.; Raveesha, K.A.R.; Amruthesh, K.N. Bioactivity and Phytochemical Studies of Seed Extracts of *Anethum graveolens* Linn. *Lett. Appl. NanoBioScience* **2022**, *11*, 3560–3572. [CrossRef]
54. Kaur, G.J.; Arora, D.S. Antibacterial and Phytochemical Screening of *Anethum graveolens*, Foeniculum Vulgare and Trachyspermum Ammi. *BMC Complement. Altern. Med.* **2009**, *9*, 30. [CrossRef]
55. Mota, A.S.; Rosário Martins, M.; Arantes, S.; Lopes, V.R.; Bettencourt, E.; Pombal, S.; Gomes, A.C.; Silva, L.A. Antimicrobial Activity and Chemical Composition of the Essential Oils of Portuguese Foeniculum Vulgare Fruits. *Nat. Prod. Commun.* **2015**, *10*, 673–676. [CrossRef]
56. Li, Z.; Wan, H.; Shi, Y.; Ouyang, P. Personal Experience with Four Kinds of Chemical Structure Drawing Software: Review on ChemDraw, ChemWindow, ISIS/Draw, and ChemSketch. *J. Chem. Inf. Comput. Sci.* **2004**, *44*, 1886–1890. [CrossRef]
57. Filimonov, D.A.; Lagunin, A.A.; Gloriozova, T.A.; Rudik, A.V.; Druzhilovskii, D.S.; Pogodin, P.V.; Poroikov, V.V. Prediction of the Biological Activity Spectra of Organic Compounds Using the Pass Online Web Resource. *Chem. Heterocycl. Comp.* **2014**, *50*, 444–457. [CrossRef]
58. Daina, A.; Michielin, O.; Zoete, V. SwissADME: A Free Web Tool to Evaluate Pharmacokinetics, Drug-Likeness and Medicinal Chemistry Friendliness of Small Molecules. *Sci. Rep.* **2017**, *7*, 42717. [CrossRef]
59. Najaran, Z.T.; Hassanzadeh, M.K.; Nasery, M.; Emami, S.A. Dill (*Anethum graveolens*, L.) Oils. In *Essential Oils in Food Preservation, Flavor and Safety*; Preedy, V.R., Ed.; Academic Press: San Diego, CA, USA, 2016; pp. 405–412. ISBN 978-0-12-416641-7.
60. Madhuri, J.V. Bioactivity of *Anethum graveolens*–An in Silico Approach. *New Vis. Biol. Sci.* **2022**, *13*, 85.
61. Suriyarak, S.; Bayrasy, C.; Schmidt, H.; Villeneuve, P.; Weiss, J. Impact of Fatty Acid Chain Length of Rosmarinate Esters on Their Antimicrobial Activity against Staphylococcus Carnosus LTH1502 and Escherichia Coli K-12 LTH4263. *J. Food Prot.* **2013**, *76*, 1539–1548. [CrossRef] [PubMed]
62. Lin, L.; Dong, Y.; Zhao, H.; Wen, L.; Yang, B.; Zhao, M. Comparative Evaluation of Rosmarinic Acid, Methyl Rosmarinate and Pedalitin Isolated from Rabdosia Serra (MAXIM.) HARA as Inhibitors of Tyrosinase and α-Glucosidase. *Food Chem.* **2011**, *129*, 884–889. [CrossRef] [PubMed]
63. Yuan, H.; Lu, W.; Wang, L.; Shan, L.; Li, H.; Huang, J.; Sun, Q.; Zhang, W. Synthesis of Derivatives of Methyl Rosmarinate and Their Inhibitory Activities against Matrix Metalloproteinase-1 (MMP-1). *Eur. J. Med. Chem.* **2013**, *62*, 148–157. [CrossRef] [PubMed]
64. Woo, E.-R.; Piao, M.S. Antioxidative Constituents from Lycopus Lucidus. *Arch. Pharm. Res.* **2004**, *27*, 173–176. [CrossRef] [PubMed]
65. Koriem, K.M.M. Caftaric Acid: An Overview on Its Structure, Daily Consumption, Bioavailability and Pharmacological Effects. *Biointerface Res. Appl. Chem* **2020**, *10*, 5616–5623.
66. Parveen, S.; Bhat, I.U.H.; Bhat, R. Kaempferol and Its Derivatives: Biological Activities and Therapeutic Potential. *Asian Pac. J. Trop. Biomed.* **2023**, *13*, 411. [CrossRef]
67. Tambe, V.; Ditani, A.; Rajpoot, K.; Tekade, R.K. Chapter 4—Pharmacokinetics Aspects of Structural Modifications in Drug Design and Therapy. In *Biopharmaceutics and Pharmacokinetics Considerations*; Tekade, R.K., Ed.; Advances in Pharmaceutical Product Development and Research; Academic Press: Cambridge, MA, USA, 2021; Volume 1, pp. 83–108. ISBN 978-0-12-814425-1.
68. Hirano, Y.; Okimoto, N.; Fujita, S.; Taiji, M. Molecular Dynamics Study of Conformational Changes of Tankyrase 2 Binding Subsites upon Ligand Binding. *ACS Omega* **2021**, *6*, 17609–17620. [CrossRef] [PubMed]
69. AFNOR NF V03-402. Épices et Aromates—Détermination de la Teneur en Eau—Méthode par Entraînement. Available online: https://www.boutique.afnor.org/fr-fr/norme/nf-v03402/epices-et-aromates-determination-de-la-teneur-en-eau-methode-par-entraineme/fa032462/325 (accessed on 4 October 2021).
70. *Ph. Eur. 11.0, 0125 (04/2023)*; 2022 Animal Feeding Stuffs—Determination of Crude Ash. ISO: Geneva, Switzerland, 2022.
71. Skujins, S. *Handbook for ICP-AES (Varian-Vista): A Short Guide to Vista Series ICP-AES Operation*; Varian Int. AG: Zug, Switzerland, 1998; p. 1.
72. Dohou, N.; Yamni, K.; Tahrouch, S.; Idrissi Hassani, L.M.; Badoc, A.; Gmira, N. Screening Phytochimique d'une Endémique Ibéro-Marocaine, Thymelaea Lythroides. *Bull. Société Pharm. Bordx.* **2003**, *142*, 61–78.
73. Mezzoug, N.; Elhadri, A.; Dallouh, A.; Amkiss, S.; Skali, N.S.; Abrini, J.; Zhiri, A.; Baudoux, D.; Diallo, B.; El Jaziri, M.; et al. Investigation of the Mutagenic and Antimutagenic Effects of Origanum Compactum Essential Oil and Some of Its Constituents. *Mutat. Res./Genet. Toxicol. Environ. Mutagen.* **2007**, *629*, 100–110. [CrossRef] [PubMed]
74. Mogode, D.J. Etude Phytochimique et Pharmacologique de Cassia Nigricans Vahl (Caesalpiniaceae) Utilisé Dans Le Traitement Des Dermatoses Au Tchad. Ph.D. Thesis, Université de N'Djaména, Abidjan, Chad, 2005.
75. Bruneton, J. *Pharmacognosie, Phytochimie, Plantes Medicinales*, 4th ed.; LAVOISIER: Paris, France, 2009; ISBN 2743019042.
76. Bekro, Y.-A.; Mamyrbekova Békro, J.A.; Boua, B.B.; Fézan, H.T.B.; Ehile, E.E. Étude Ethnobotanique et Screening Phytochimique de *Caesalpinia benthamiana* (Baill.) Herend. et Zarucchi (Caesalpiniaceae). *Sci. Nat.* **2007**, *4*, 217–225. [CrossRef]

77. N'Guessan, K.; Kadja, B.; Zirihi, G.; Traoré, D.; Aké-Assi, L. Screening phytochimique de quelques plantes médicinales ivoiriennes utilisées en pays Krobou (Agboville, Côte-d'Ivoire). *Sci. Nat.* **2009**, *6*, 1–15. [CrossRef]
78. Akrout, A.; Chemli, R.; Chref, I.; Hammami, M. Analysis of the Essential Oil of *Artemisia campestris*, L. *Flavour Fragr. J.* **2001**, *16*, 337–339. [CrossRef]
79. Adams, R.P. *Identification of Essential Oil Components by Gas Chromatography/Mass Spectrometry*; Allured Publishing Corporation: Carol Stream, IL, USA, 2007; Volume 456.
80. Babushok, V.I.; Linstrom, P.J.; Zenkevich, I.G. Retention Indices for Frequently Reported Compounds of Plant Essential Oils. *J. Phys. Chem. Ref. Data* **2011**, *40*, 043101. [CrossRef]
81. Kovats, E.S. Gas Chromatographic Characterization of Organic Substances in the Retention Index System. *Adv. Chromatogr.* **1965**, *1*, 229–247.
82. Singleton, V.L.; Rossi, J.A. Colorimetry of Total Phenolics with Phosphomolybdic-Phosphotungstic Acid Reagents. *Am. J. Enol. Vitic.* **1965**, *16*, 144–158. [CrossRef]
83. Djeridane, A.; Yousfi, M.; Nadjemi, B.; Boutassouna, D.; Stocker, P.; Vidal, N. Antioxidant Activity of Some Algerian Medicinal Plants Extracts Containing Phenolic Compounds. *Food Chem.* **2006**, *97*, 654–660. [CrossRef]
84. Price, M.L.; Scoyoc, S.V.; Butler, L.G. A Critical Evaluation of the Vanillin Reaction as an Assay for Tannin in Sorghum Grain. *J. Agric. Food Chem.* **1978**, *26*, 1214–1218. [CrossRef]
85. Liu, M.H.; Otsuka, N.; Noyori, K.; Shiota, S.; Ogawa, W.; Kuroda, T.; Hatano, T.; Tsuchiya, T. Synergistic Effect of Kaempferol Glycosides Purified from Laurus Nobilis and Fluoroquinolones on Methicillin-Resistant Staphylococcus Aureus. *Biol. Pharm. Bull.* **2009**, *32*, 489–492. [CrossRef] [PubMed]
86. Oyaizu, M. Studies on Products of Browning Reaction. Antioxidative Activities of Products of Browning Reaction Prepared from Glucosamine. *Jpn. J. Nutr. Diet.* **1986**, *44*, 307–315. [CrossRef]
87. Khiya, Z.; Oualcadi, Y.; Gamar, A.; Berrekhis, F.; Zair, T.; Hilali, F.E.L. Correlation of Total Polyphenolic Content with Antioxidant Activity of Hydromethanolic Extract and Their Fractions of the Salvia Officinalis Leaves from Different Regions of Morocco. *J. Chem.* **2021**, *2021*, 8585313. [CrossRef]
88. Drioiche, A.; Baammi, S.; Zibouh, K.; Al Kamaly, O.; Alnakhli, A.M.; Remok, F.; Saidi, S.; Amaiach, R.; El Makhoukhi, F.; Elomri, A. A Study of the Synergistic Effects of Essential Oils from Origanum Compactum and Origanum Elongatum with Commercial Antibiotics against Highly Prioritized Multidrug-Resistant Bacteria for the World Health Organization. *Metabolites* **2024**, *14*, 210. [CrossRef]
89. Alam, A.; Jawaid, T.; Alam, P. In Vitro Antioxidant and Anti-Inflammatory Activities of Green Cardamom Essential Oil and in Silico Molecular Docking of Its Major Bioactives. *J. Taibah Univ. Sci.* **2021**, *15*, 757–768. [CrossRef]
90. Banerjee, P.; Eckert, A.O.; Schrey, A.K.; Preissner, R. ProTox-II: A Webserver for the Prediction of Toxicity of Chemicals. *Nucleic Acids Res.* **2018**, *46*, W257–W263. [CrossRef]
91. Van Der Spoel, D.; Lindahl, E.; Hess, B.; Groenhof, G.; Mark, A.E.; Berendsen, H.J.C. GROMACS: Fast, Flexible, and Free. *J. Comput. Chem.* **2005**, *26*, 1701–1718. [CrossRef] [PubMed]

pharmaceuticals

Article

Czech Honeydew Honeys—A Potential Source of Local Medical Honey with Strong Antimicrobial Activity

Ludovit Pudelka [1], Radek Sleha [2,*], Sylva Janovska [2], Vera Radochova [3] and Pavel Bostik [2,4]

[1] Department of Emergency Medicine and Military General Medicine, Military Faculty of Medicine, University of Defence, 500 01 Hradec Kralove, Czech Republic; ludovit.pudelka@unob.cz
[2] Department of Epidemiology, Military Faculty of Medicine, University of Defence, 500 01 Hradec Kralove, Czech Republic; sylva.janovska@unob.cz (S.J.); pavel.bostik@unob.cz (P.B.)
[3] Animal Laboratory, Military Faculty of Medicine, University of Defence, 500 01 Hradec Kralove, Czech Republic; vera.radochova@unob.cz
[4] Department of Medical Microbiology, University Hospital in Hradec Kralove, 500 01 Hradec Kralove, Czech Republic
* Correspondence: radek.sleha@unob.cz

Abstract: An increasing resistance of microbes to antibiotics, the emergence of multidrug-resistant and extremely resistant strains, and the long time needed to develop new antibiotics are driving the search for additional sources of antibacterial agents. The aim of the study was to compare the efficacy of Czech honeys with already available pharmaceutical agents containing medicinal honey, and to perform basic biochemical analysis of Czech samples, including detection of undesirable chemical substances. The results showed strong antibacterial activity of Czech honeydew honeys compared to the control group, especially against G+ pathogens, with an average MIC of 9.44% compared to 17.54%, and comparable activity against G− of 16.48% versus 16.66%. In addition to the strong antibacterial activity, this study confirmed the safety and quality of Czech honeys and helped to select the character of a possible source for in vivo testing and subsequent clinical trials.

Keywords: honeydew; antibacterial effect; hydrogen peroxide; polyphenolic compounds

1. Introduction

Natural products have been used by mankind since time immemorial. Among these products, bee honey has an irreplaceable value. Probably the first written document that mentions the use of honey in wound healing is a papyrus by Edwin Smith, which may have been a war surgeon's manual, which describes the use of honey in the prevention and treatment of wound infections in ancient Egypt [1]. The antimicrobial activity of honey was first observed in 1892 [2]. In the 20th century, interest in honey and other natural products gave way to the importance of newly discovered antibiotics in developed countries. However, with the emergence of resistant and extremely resistant bacterial species, the use and research of medicinal honey, as with other bee or natural products, is again gaining momentum.

The essence of "liquid gold", as honey is sometimes called, combines a number (180–200) of different compounds (water, sugars, minerals, vitamins, proteins, phytochemicals, and polyphenolic compounds) with antibacterial properties [3,4]. This composition depends mainly on the bee pasture, and its unique combination may be the reason why the adaptation of microorganisms to honey (e.g., by mutation of genes involved in methylglyoxal detoxification) is very slow or would lead to cross-resistance to antibiotics [5]. Basic factors include the following: (1) Low water activity, which is a scaleless quantity between 0 and 1 that expresses the amount of free, unbound water. It is the free water that microorganisms can use for their growth. Simply stated, the greater the amount of free water, the better the conditions for microbial growth and vice versa. The water activity is usually 0.6, which is sufficient to inhibit osmotolerant yeasts [6–9]. (2) The presence of polyphenolic compounds, including flavonoids and phenolic acids (nonflavonoids), which are secondary metabolites of flowers and enter honey due to their presence in nectar collected by bees from plants, contributes to the antibacterial effect of honey (nonenzymatic H_2O_2 production) [10]. Therefore, bee grazing, which is itself influenced by both the geographical location and season, can significantly affect the phytochemical spectrum and, consequently, the actual antimicrobial effect [10–14]. (3) Hydrogen peroxide is probably one of the main antibacterial factors, which is produced by the aforementioned nonenzymatic route (polyphenolic compounds) or enzymatically via the enzyme glucose oxidase (GOX), which bees add to nectar. Some studies report its production by plants, honey fungi, yeasts, and bacteria. GOX is naturally present in an inactive form and its activity increases with honey dilution, reaching a maximum in honey solutions with a concentration between 30 and 50% [15–21]. (4) Acidity—the low pH of honey is another factor that contributes to an environment unsuitable for the growth of microorganisms. A large number of microorganisms need a neutral pH for their growth, but this is not present in honey due to the presence of acids, particularly organic gluconic acid, which is produced by the activity of the enzyme GOX. According to various sources, the average pH of undiluted honey ranges from 3.2 to 4.5 [22]. (5) Honey also contains a large number of proteins, which themselves have antimicrobial activity or at least contribute to the overall antimicrobial activity of honey. One of these is defensin-1, which is found in the hemolymph of bees as part of their immune system. It is also secreted by the hypopharyngeal glands of bees, from where it enters the honey [23]. Studies have shown that defensin-1 is mainly effective against Gram-positive bacteria, but a significant potential against Gram-negative bacteria has been demonstrated as well [24]. In addition to its own antimicrobial effect, it plays an important role in wound healing by stimulating the secretion of matrix metalloproteinase-9 (MMP-9) by keratinocytes [25]. (6) 1,2-dicarbonyls: nonenzymatic reactions between glucose and free amino acid groups can occur in carbohydrate-rich foods when heated or stored for long periods of time. These processes (caramelization, Maillard reaction) can produce the highly reactive compounds mentioned above. The resulting products of these reactions are methylglyoxal and glyoxal, which are essential for the antimicrobial activity of some honeys. Methylglyoxal is a substance that is formed during honey storage by the conversion of dihydroxyacetone in the presence of arginine and lysine, which is abundantly present in the nectar of *Leptospermum* sp. Due to the presence of methylglyoxal, honey retains its antibacterial activity despite inactivation of H_2O_2 by catalase, thus demonstrating the nonperoxidase antibacterial activity of honey [26–33]. Today, there are many honeys that have found their way into human medicine. However, their price and quantity are considerable in relation to the need, for example, for the treatment of burns or chronic wounds. Along with environmental and fiscal policies, there is, therefore, an effort to find primarily local sources of honey that could be used as medical-grade honey (MGH). There is no definition of what MGH is, but based on the work of Hermann et al., MGH should meet the following criteria: natural origin, purity, absence of toxic substances and contaminants, sterilization by gamma radiation in accordance with standardized protocols to exclude pathogenic microorganisms, applicability in treatment, fulfilment of physicochemical criteria necessary for use in wound care, and compliance with standardized production and storage methods and all safety regulations [34].

However, it is not only the antibacterial properties of honey that are currently the subject of intense research. Thanks to its composition and, in particular, the presence of substances derived from nectar or honeydew, especially from the group of polyphenolic compounds, honey has a number of other properties. Recently, the results of a study have been published describing the inhibition of breast cancer cell migration by honeydew from a conifer-rich area [35], with minimal effect on the function of fibroblasts. On the other hand, honeydew from an oak-rich area showed an inhibitory effect on gastric adenocarcinoma cells, even at low concentrations [36]. The neuroprotective effect of flavonoids in honey has also been demonstrated by reducing neuroinflammation with a reduction in the production of proinflammatory cytokines and ROS [37–39]. The use of honey in the treatment of burns, which are characterized by increased ROS production leading to lipid peroxidation and subsequent scarring and contractures, has the same basis as noted [40].

In general, all honeys can be expected to possess antibacterial activity, but there is an effort to select those that have the highest potency. Based on this, we decided to analyze Czech honeys that would meet the same criteria as MGHs and at the same time show maximum antibacterial activity compared to the already available MGHs. Since previous studies [3,41,42] have shown honeydew honeys to be at least as effective as MGH control samples, we decided to focus on honeydew honeys, their qualities, antibacterial activity, and mechanism of action.

2. Results

2.1. Characteristics of Honeys

2.1.1. Physicochemical Analysis

Conductivity was measured to determine the origin of the honeys. In 30 out of 49 samples, a conductivity higher than 80 mS/cm was observed, which, in terms of origin [43], represents honeydew honeys, which are generated by the conversion of honeydew produced by hemipteran phloem-feeding insects such as aphids, mealybugs, whitefly, and psyllids, while the remaining 19 samples showed conductivities lower than 0.8 mS/cm and are therefore nomenclaturally blossom honeys produced by collecting nectar from plants and subsequently converting it into honey.

To exclude the influence of honey quality on the main parameters under investigation, hydroxymethylfurfural (HMF) level, water percentage, pH, diastase level, and free acidity were subsequently determined. These results, together with the conductivity results, are presented in Figure 1.

According to the European directive (110/2001 as amended) [44], the level of HMF must not exceed 40 mg/kg, with exceptions for honey coming from countries or regions with tropical temperatures or honeys with low enzymatic levels. This value was exceeded twice in both groups—honeydew and blossom honeys. These results may be due to poor storage or overheating of the honey during liquefaction. The average value of HMF for the blossom honeys was 25.87 mg/kg, and for the honeydew honeys, 8.28 mg/kg. The average value obtained for the blossom honeys in particular is strongly influenced by the excess level for sample H, which showed the highest value of 232.8 mg/kg among all the samples. This likely indicates a significant heating of the honey during its liquefaction.

With regards to the water content, the European directive (110/2001 as amended) [44] allows a maximum of 20%, while the Czech directive [45] allows only 18%. This is again an important criterion for the quality of honey shelf life, as the low water content guarantees the stability of the honey and reduces the risk of spoilage mainly due to fermentation processes. All our tested honeys clearly met the European honey quality criteria. Two blossom honeys (18.1–18.7%) and three honeydew honeys (18.5–18.6%) failed to meet the national (Czech) criteria [45], but only by a very narrow margin.

Although the exact recommended pH value of honey has not yet been determined by the Regulatory Committees, the literature generally indicates the pH range of honey as 3.2 to 4.5, and in some sources 3.52 to 5.13 [46]. This low pH prevents bacterial growth and reduces the risk of spoilage. The pH value of all our samples did not exceed 4.9, with a range of 3.9 to 4.9.

Free acidity/content of free acids is another parameter, values of which can indicate honey deterioration, similarly to higher pH or water content. The value depends mainly on the quantity of organic acids and inorganic ions such as phosphates, sulphates, and chlorides. European guidelines (EU Directive 110/2001 as amended) [44] allow for a maximum value of 50 mmol/kg [47]. The free acid values for our honeydew honeys ranged from 23 to 50 mmol/kg (mean 35.93 mmol/kg) and 18 to 46 mmol/kg (mean 32.19 mmol/kg) for blossom honeys.

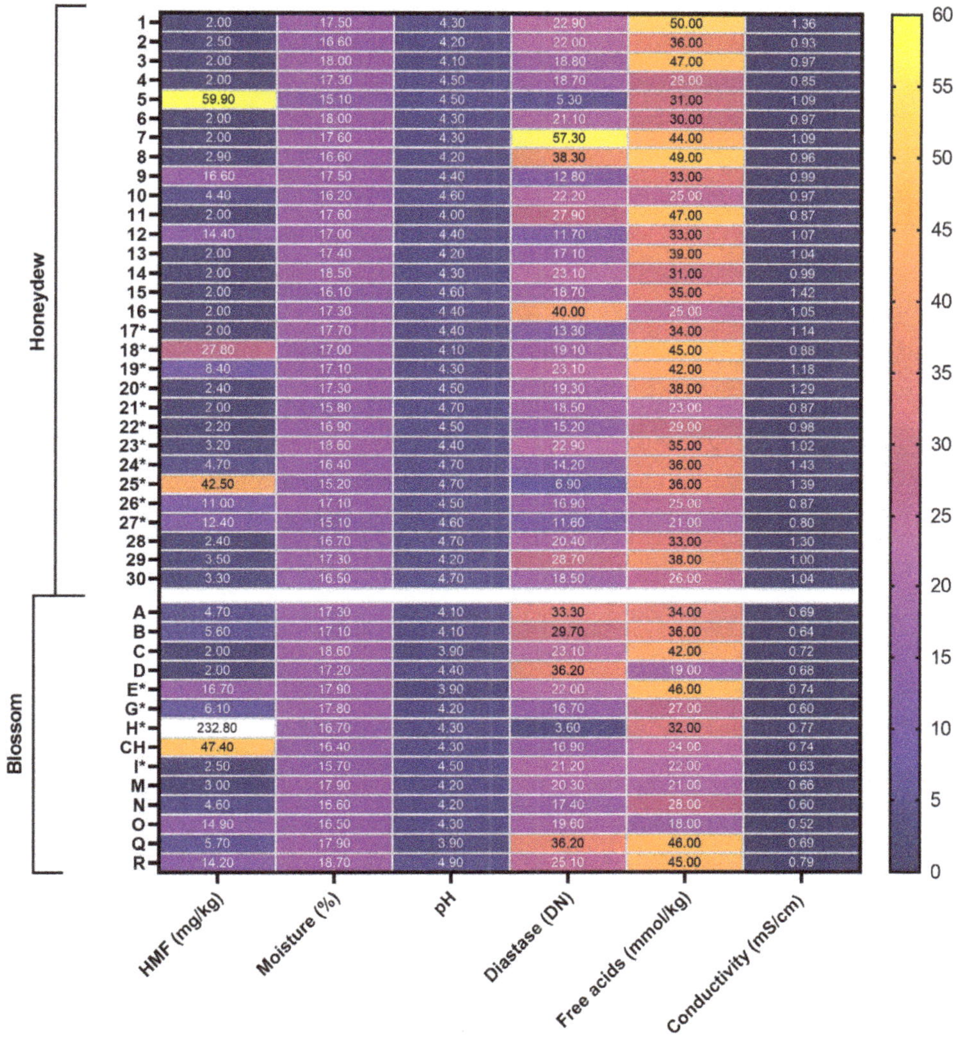

Figure 1. Results of basic physicochemical analysis including determination of HMF (5-hydroxymethylfurfural) mg/kg, moisture—water content g/100 g, pH, diastase activity (Phadebas method) DN, free acids—free acidity mmol/kg, conductivity mS/cm. Samples marked with * come from 2019.

The diastase activity value, which is given as the diastase number (DN) or Schade or Gothe unit, represents the amount of enzyme that will convert 0.01 g of starch to the prescribed endpoint in one hour at 40 °C under the test conditions, and is set at a minimum value of 8 DN under European legislation (EU Directive 110/2001, as amended) [44]. This value is mainly used on the European market as a parameter of the age/quality of the honey, since its value decreases with age or improper handling of the honey (heating). This is consistent with our results, where the measured value of diastase activity was below the required limit in only three samples (5, 25, H). At the same time, in all these samples, as well as in the CH sample, an above-limit value of 5-hydroxymethylfurfural (HMF) was found, indicating improper storage or processing (overheating) of the honey. Overall, diastase values for honeydew honeys in our samples were in the range of 5.3 to 57.3 °DN (mean 22.5 °DN) and for blossom honeys from 3.6 to 36.2 °DN (mean 21.32 °DN).

2.1.2. Melissopalynological Analysis

The most frequently represented pollen families in the honeydew honeys were Brassicaceae—present in 93% of the samples, Asteraceae 77%, Salicaceae 67%, Fabaceae 57%, Sapindaceae/Hippocastanoideae 43%, Malvaceae 40%, Boraginaceae 37%, Apiaceae 33%, Rosaceae 33%, Cornaceae 10%, and Polygonaceae 6%. The families Fagaceae and Rhamnaceae were equally represented in 3% of the samples. For blossom honeys, the families were represented in the samples as follows: Brassicaceae in 93% of the samples, Salicaceae in 73%, Fabaceae in 60%, Sapindaceae/Hippocastanoideae and Asteraceae equally in 53%, Boraginaceae in 40%, Malvaceae in 27%, Apiaceae and Rosaceae equally in 20%, and the families Polygonaceae, Balsaminaceae, and Fagaceae were similarly represented in 6% of the samples.

In terms of the number of pollen grains identified in the samples studied, the Brassicaceae family was dominant. With the exception of one sample (No. 20) out of the 44 samples examined, where more than 46% of pollen grains of a particular family were found (Nos. 2, 7, 14, 16, 17, 18, 21, 24, 26, 28, 27, B, D, E, F, G, K), it was the *Brassicaceae* family that was identified. The average percentage of pollen grains of this family in the above samples was 61%, with values ranging from 46 to 87% (see Figure 2).

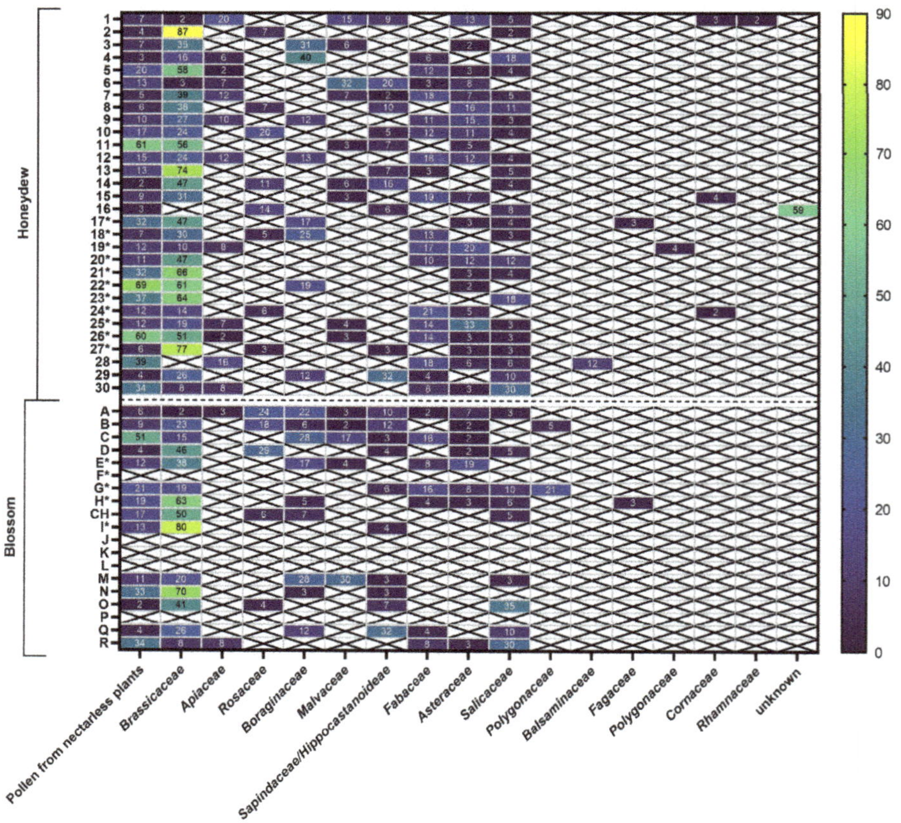

Figure 2. Pollen analysis of honey samples with relative frequency of pollen grains of different plant families (>46% very frequent pollen; 45–16% frequent pollen; 15–3% single pollen; >3% isolated pollen). Samples marked with * come from 2019.

2.1.3. Presence of Chemical Substances

In view of the possible future use of honey for medical purposes as medical-grade honey, the samples were also analyzed for the presence of undesirable substances (especially pesticides; the presence of antibiotics was not examined due to their banned use for the treatment of bee colonies in the Czech Republic). Out of all 44 samples, undesirable substances were detected in 9 honeydew samples. In 7 of these samples, substances from the acaricide group were detected (4× Acetamiprid in the range 0.012 to 0.038 mg/kg and 3× Thiacloprid, 0.01–0.072 mg/kg). For the two remaining samples, the fungicide carbendazim was present at a concentration of 0.003 mg/kg. A mixture of three substances was found in one sample—benzyldimethyloctadecylammonium BAC C18 (0.028 mg/kg), benzalkonium chloride (0.067 mg/kg), and cetalkonium chloride (0.039 mg/kg).

Carbendazim (methyl benzimidazol-2-ylcarbamate) metabolized to the bioactive substance benomyl is a broad-spectrum fungicide used worldwide to treat fungal diseases primarily of agricultural crops. However, carbendazim is no longer registered in the EU. The current European maximum residue level (MRL) for carbendazim in honey is 0.05 mg/kg.

Acetamiprid (a neonicotinoid insecticide), used mainly for the protection of agricultural crops such as oilseed rape (vs. *Meligenthes aeneus*), has its MRL set at 0.05 mg/kg in the EU. The same group also includes Thiacloprid, banned on the European market in 2020, whose MRL is 0.2 mg/kg for honey, and which was also used for the protection of agricultural crops such as oilseed rape.

Benzyldimethyloctadecylammonium BAC C18, benzalkonium chloride, and cetalkonium chloride belong to the group of quaternary ammonium compounds, which are mainly used in pharmaceutical and medical applications, as part of preservatives and disinfectants. Their European MRL is 0.1 mg/kg [48].

The analysis for the presence of undesirable chemicals was performed by an accredited laboratory as a paid-for service, and its subcontractors are listed in the Materials and Methods section.

2.2. *Antibacterial Activity of Honey Samples*

The minimum inhibitory concentrations (MICs) of the honey samples were tested against two bacterial strains representing both G+ and G- bacteria (Figure 3). In addition to the original 44 samples sent abroad for analysis, the MIC test included a further 5 samples that were received later. As controls, medical products purchased from pharmacies with medical-grade honeys (Activon®, Vivamel®, Revamil®) and a sample of manuka honey were included in the study. The MICs of the samples against *S. aureus* (SA) ranged from 5.55% to 22.22% (honey concentration in solution) for the honeydew honeys and 5.55% to 38.88% for the blossom honeys. For the control samples, the range measured was from 11.11% to 22.22%. Thus, the average MIC value for the honeydew honeys was lower, at 9.44%, compared to the average values of 17.83% for the blossom honeys and 17.54% for the control group. Fifteen honeydew samples (1, 2, 5, 8, 11, 13, 15, 17, 19, 22, 24, 26, 28, 29, 30) and four blossom samples (B, G, N, Q) were found to be more effective (5.55%) against *S. aureus* compared to control samples (11.11–22.22%). For the *P. aeruginosa* strain (PSAE), the average MIC values of the samples were very similar. The mean MICs were 16.48% (11.11–27.77%), 17.54% (11.11–33.33%), and 16.66% (11.11–22.22%) for honeydew, blossom, and control samples, respectively. The best MIC value of the control samples was 11.11% (Vivamel®). The best honeydew (10 out of 30) and blossom (8 out of 15) samples achieved the same value.

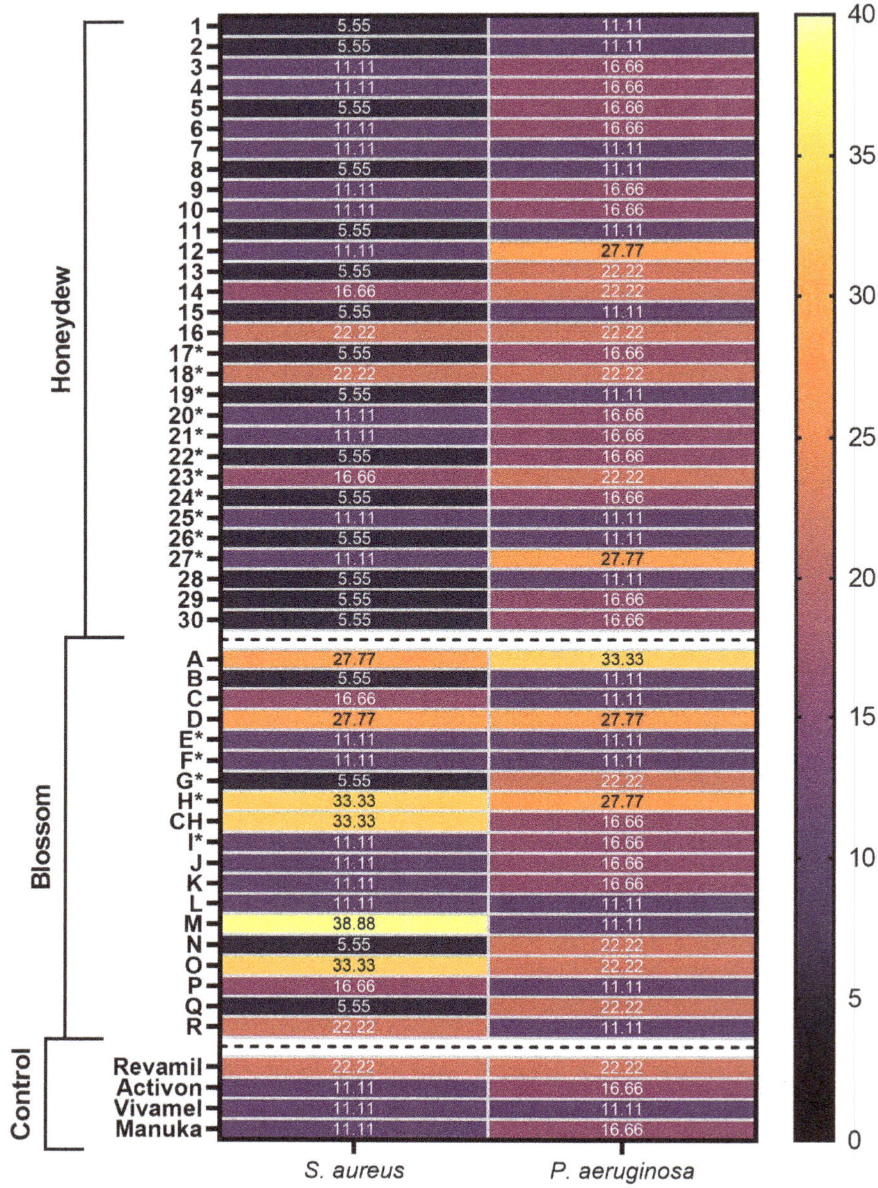

Figure 3. Antibacterial activity of honeydew, blossom, and control samples against bacterial strains of *S. aureus* and *P. aeruginosa*. Antibacterial activity was determined as minimum inhibitory concentration (MIC). MIC was defined as the lowest concentration of honey solution (%) that can inhibit bacterial growth. Samples marked with * come from 2019.

2.3. H_2O_2 and Total Polyphenolic Compound Contents in Honey Samples

Hydrogen peroxide is one of the most important antibacterial components of honey. It is known to be produced not only by the activity of the enzyme glucose oxidase (GOX) but also nonenzymatically by the contribution of polyphenolic compounds contained in the nectar of plants. In order to assess the importance of the amount of hydrogen peroxide on the overall antibacterial activity, the hydrogen peroxide content of all samples was determined in a 40% honey solution at pH 7.0 immediately after this solution reached homogeneity (Figure 4). The mean H_2O_2 value measured was 12.92 μg/g honey. The average value for the control samples was 3.67 (with a range of 1.08–3.89 μg/g honey). The lowest value was measured for the Revamil® sample and the highest value was observed for the Activon® sample. Compared to the control samples, the average level measured for both groups was higher, with 9.84 μg/g honey for the blossom samples and 16.10 μg/g honey for the honeydew samples. The highest value was measured in honey sample number 1 (34.38 μg/g honey), while the lowest value was measured in the control sample Revamil® (1.08 μg/g honey).

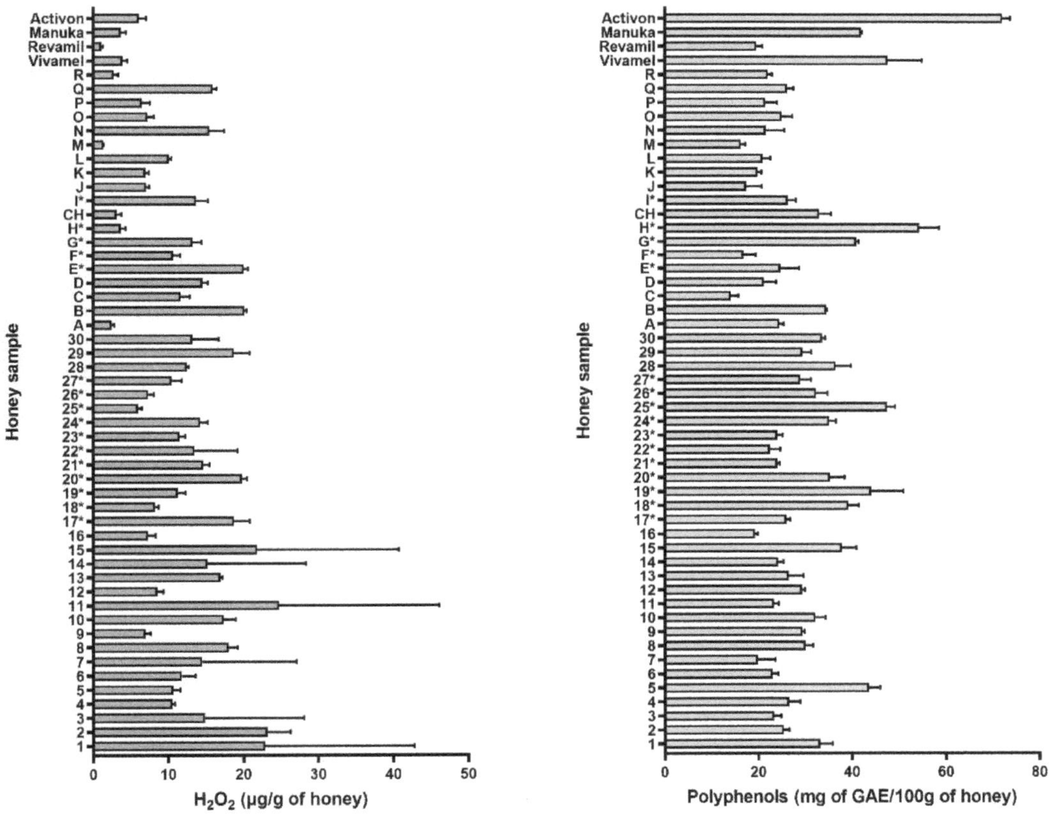

Figure 4. Hydrogen peroxide (H_2O_2) and total polyphenolic compounds (TP) in honeydew and blossom honeys. H_2O_2 content was measured in honey solution (40% *w*/*w*), immediately after the homogeneity of this solution was reached, without prior incubation. Gallic acid (GAE) was used as TP reference standard compound and results are expressed as GAE equivalents (mg GAE/100 g of honey). Data represent mean values with standard deviation. Samples marked with * come from 2019.

The polyphenol content of all 53 samples was also determined (Figure 4). As mentioned above, polyphenolic compounds may be involved in the formation of H_2O_2 and thus contribute to the production of one of the major antibacterial agents. In addition, polyphenolic compounds (phenolic acids and flavonoids) have also been shown to possess intrinsic antimicrobial activity with a broad mechanism of action (inhibition of DNA gyrase, induction of topoisomerase IV-mediated DNA cleavage, cell wall damage with pore formation, etc.) [3,10,41,49–53]. The average content in our honey samples was 28.333 mg GAE/100 g honey. In the control group, the mean was 45.348 mg GAE/100 g honey. The mean value for honeydew honeys was 30.212 mg GAE/100 g honey (range 19.332 to 47.539 mg GAE/100 g honey) and for blossom honeys 25.366 mg GAE/100 g honey (range 34.533 to 14.174 mg GAE/100 g honey). Overall, the highest value was measured for the Activon® sample from the control group (73.289 mg GAE/100 g honey).

2.4. Correlations of Parameters

As stated in the beginning, most of the honeys were subjected to a very detailed physicochemical analysis, mainly to exclude the potential influence of these parameters, in many cases used to assess the quality of honey, on the antibacterial activity of these samples. To identify possible correlations, Sperman's rho test was used, the results of which are presented graphically in Figure 5. We investigated the possible correlation between conductivity, which depends mainly on the content of mineral salts and organic acids [54,55], and the amount of free acids and MIC for both strains (SA, PSAE). The data showed a positive correlation between conductivity and the quantity of free acids, but only for blossom honey samples (r = 0.5740, p = 0.0343), and not for honeydew honey samples (r = 0.2950, p = 0.1135). Furthermore, a Spearman correlation analysis was performed to investigate the relationship between MIC and conductivity, whose value is influenced by minerals and free acids, which may also contribute to the antimicrobial activity of honey through the Fenton reaction or nonenzymatic production of hydrogen peroxide. However, no statistically significant dependence of MIC on the conductivity value for either the honeydew samples (PSAE r = −0.2115, p = 0.2619; SA r = −0.2401, p = 0.2013) or the blossom samples (PSAE r = −0.1852, p = 0.5210; SA r = 0.2840, p = 0.3207) was found. To further investigate the importance of polyphenolic compounds in honey and their influence on its antibacterial properties, correlations of factors whose levels could be influenced by the quantity of polyphenolic compounds (conductivity, pH, free acids, and MIC) were subsequently analyzed. However, no statistically significant correlation with MIC for honeydew honeys (SA r = −0.3052, p = 0.1010; PSAE r = −0.2786, p = 0.1361), or for blossom honeys (SA r = −0.1902, p = 0.5111; PSAE r = 0.2257, p = 0.4340), was observed. Similarly, no correlation with conductivity was found for blossom honeys (r = −0.0331, p = 0.9123). However, a statistically significant moderate correlation was detected for honeydew honeys (r = 0.4339, p = 0.0166). No statistically significant correlation was observed between the amount of hydrogen peroxide and polyphenolic compounds, nor in honeydew honey samples (r = −0.2232, p = 0.2359), nor in blossom honey samples (r = 0.2, p = 0.4924). No correlation between polyphenolic compounds and pH was shown for the blossom honeys (r = 0.1182, p = 0.6885), while the value for the honeydew honeys was at the borderline of statistical significance with a weak correlation (r = 0.3569, p = 0.0534). The correlation between polyphenolic compounds and free acids was not conclusive for either blossom (r = 0.0286, p = 0.9242) or honeydew (r = 0.1553, p = 0.4124) samples. The last value that the correlation analysis focused on was the amount of hydrogen peroxide, as one of the two key substances in honey reported so far, which, together with methylglyoxal, is involved in the antibacterial effect. Thus, comparisons of the MIC values against the H_2O_2 levels in both honey types for both bacterial strains were calculated. Interestingly, a statistically significant negative correlation between H_2O_2 level and MIC in blossom honeys for *S. aureus* (r = −0.7742, p = 0.0019), but not for *P. aeruginosa* (r = −0.1003, p = 0.7315), was found. For honeydew honeys, the correlations were weak, and on the borderline of statistical significance (*S. aureus* r = −0.3515, p = 0.0553, *P. aeruginosa* r = −0.3382, p = 0.0676).

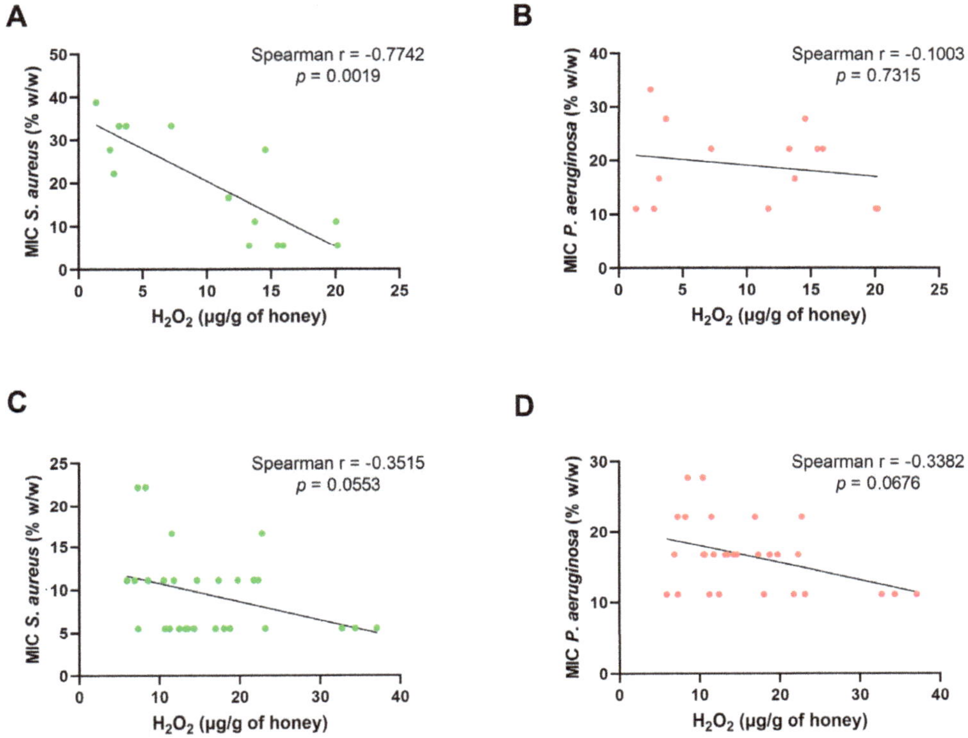

Figure 5. Graphical expression of the relationship between the amount of hydrogen peroxide and the total antibacterial activity (MIC) against both bacterial species *S. aureus* (**A**,**C**) and *P. aeruginosa* (**B**,**D**) in honeydew (**A**,**B**) and blossom (**C**,**D**) honey samples using the nonparametric Spearman's rank correlation coefficient test with a 95% confidence interval.

3. Discussion

The healing properties of honey have been known for thousands of years. Increased antibiotic resistance, the emergence of multidrug-resistant strains, and the search for possible solutions have led to a renaissance of interest in this natural product. Nowadays, there are a number of products that make use of the capabilities of honey (MGHs—medical-grade honeys) and which are used especially in the healing of chronic wounds or, for example, burns. Wider use, particularly in the area of burns, is partly hampered by the price, a significant part of which is transport. This, together with the question of the possible mechanism of action, led us to a study testing Czech honeys. On the basis of previous studies that have shown equal or higher antibacterial potential of honeydew honeys [41,42], we decided to focus on these.

3.1. Quality Parameters

We demonstrated quality and safety of Czech honeys from local producers. Of the 44 samples tested, only 4 exceeded the permitted levels of HMF, and of these 4, the majority were only slightly above the limits. For sample H in particular, it is reasonable to speculate on its liquefaction and subsequent heat damage. This would be consistent with the high HMF and high MIC values for both bacterial strains. However, this expected pattern did not occur for the remaining samples, probably due to a slightly higher HMF value. Sample 5 showed the expected decrease in diastase levels, but its MIC values were among the best. Sample 25 had borderline diastase levels but maintained average MIC values. Sample CH had a normal diastase level, but its MIC values were among the worst, especially for the

S. aureus strain. The same can be seen from another point of view in samples M, O, 16, and 18, with low HMF values, acceptable diastase values, but below average MIC values.

Moreover, the average HMF value of our blossom samples would be higher than that of the honeydew samples, which is not in agreement with a number of studies dealing with this issue [52–54]. On the other hand, the values are more in line with the general assumption that blossom honeys relatively contain a higher proportion of glucose and therefore crystallize faster, depending on the nectar source, leading to more frequent liquefaction during processing, which certainly has an effect on the HMF value of these samples.

Moisture content was exceeded only slightly in samples C, R, 14, and 23, and only when compared to Czech standards. According to the European legislation, even these samples would have easily met the required value of 20%.

3.2. *Undesirable Substances—Chemical Compounds*

In eight of the samples tested (8, 12, 14, 17, 20, 21, 22, 30), chemicals were detected that should not be present in honey. These were mainly chemical compounds from the group of fungicides and insecticides used mainly in industrial agriculture to protect crops. Paradoxically, however, one sample out of two containing a fungicide (carbendazim) did not come from an apiary that was within the range of bee grazing associated with industrial agriculture. It was, however, in the vicinity of a golf course that uses the fungicide in the protection of golf course turf against earthworms. The insecticides (neonicotinoids) acetamiprid and thiacloprid are both mainly used to protect agricultural crops such as oilseed rape. The use of thiacloprid has been banned in the EU since 2020. However, due to the honey harvesting of our samples that took place in 2020 and 2019, its presence is possible. All the samples in which the insecticide acetamiprid was detected also had a high proportion of pollen grains of Brassicaceae, the family to which oilseed rape belongs, in the range of 47 to 61% of pollen grains per sample. It can therefore be assumed that the contamination of the honey samples came from bees grazing on industrially grown plants such as oilseed rape, the cultivation of which is very intensive in terms of the use of chemicals to protect it. However, it should be noted that all the measured concepts are far below the European limits for the substances in question or their standard detection limits. Nevertheless, it appears that rigorous control of honeys that could be used as medical-grade honeys is essential, as is the choice of the locations of bees whose honey should be collected for these purposes.

3.3. *Antibacterial Activity of Samples*

As in other studies [42,56,57], our analysis confirmed the effectiveness of local—Czech—honeydew honeys compared to already available medical honeys. The average MIC against *S. aureus* was almost 32% lower in Czech honeydew honeys than in the control group containing MGHs. The situation was less pronounced for *P. aeruginosa*, where the results were almost comparable—the average MIC of the Czech honeydew honeys was 16.48, while that of the control group was 16.66.

3.4. *Relationships between Parameters*

Subsequent correlation analysis of the results showed no statistically significant relationship between diastase and MIC for either honey type or either bacterial strain. Therefore, it can be assumed that a slight exceedance of the diastase level may not affect the antibacterial capacity, depending on the type of honey.

We demonstrated a statistically significant correlation between conductivity and the quantity of polyphenolic compounds in honeydew honeys ($r = 0.4339$, $p = 0.0166$), which is consistent with the above text and demonstrates the possible influence on the resulting conductivity of the presence of organic acids belonging to the group of polyphenolic compounds. This correlation was not proven in the case of blossom honeys. On the other hand, in contrast to honeydew samples, we found a positive correlation between free acidity and conductivity values for blossom honeys ($r = 0.5740$, $r = 0.0343$), as did

Balos et al. for meadow and polyfloral honeys [58]. In contrast, for pH, the correlation with phenolic compounds is weaker and also on the borderline of statistical significance ($r = 0.3569$, $p = 0.0534$). This is again consistent with the mechanism described above and the more significant influence of mineral compounds on the resultant value. For the blossom honeys, as for the previous value, this correlation was not observed.

3.5. Mechanism of Antibacterial Activity of Honey

Another question we were attempting to answer was the possible mechanism of action of Czech honeys. A number of previous studies suggest that the unique antibacterial properties of honey are the result of the interplay of a number of factors (pH, low water activity, high sugar content, presence of proteins, H_2O_2 formation, and a number of other compounds such as methylglyoxal and polyphenolic compounds). This is also documented by a number of studies showing that the activity of one factor alone is not sufficient to achieve antibacterial capabilities and that it is, as mentioned above, a complex effect of several factors on the bacterial cell [3,59,60].

Leaving aside the antibacterial effect of honeys based on the presence of methylglyoxal, which, according to some studies, can probably inhibit other antibacterial mechanisms (low levels of GOX in manuka honeys) [28], the antibacterial activity is based on H_2O_2. Considering the results of analyses of honeys from neighboring countries, it is very difficult to assume that single-species honeys containing a unique substance similar to methylglyoxal are present in the Czech Republic and, as in other countries, their activity will be mainly the result of the cooperation of H_2O_2 and polyphenolic compounds. We based our hypothesis on this assumption and focused on these two factors.

It is known that the formation of hydrogen peroxide in honey takes place, among other mechanisms, by an enzymatic reaction mediated by the enzyme GOX. On the other hand, no correlation was found between the amount of GOX and H_2O_2 [3,41]. Interestingly, the level of this enzyme produced in the pharyngeal glands of the honey bee is controlled/dependent not only on the age of the bee and its roles in the community [61], but probably also on the composition of the honey bee forage [60] and the genetic diversity of the honey bee [62]. In the interspecies comparison of honeys, honeydew honeys produced higher amounts of H_2O_2 than blossom honeys, which was confirmed in our study, where the mean H_2O_2 value of blossom honeys was lower than that of honeydew honeys (10.40 μg/g honey vs. 16.10 μg/g honey, respectively), which is probably related to the presence of polyphenolic compounds in honeydew honeys [41,42,60,62]. Another explanation may lie in the presence of the enzyme catalase. Catalase is abundant mainly in flower pollen, and much less in nectar. Nevertheless, it can be considered that in certain situations, such as the availability of intensive monofloral bee pasture, the type of which (pollen, nectar) contains high levels of catalase, the resulting production and, hence, the overall antibacterial activity may be more significantly affected. This is particularly the case if the flower constancy aspect is also taken into account. This hypothesis is also supported by the knowledge of the origin of honeydew honey, the source of which is predominantly not nectar but honeydew, as we wrote earlier [63,64].

In our study we showed a statistically significant negative correlation ($r = -0.7742$, $p = 0.0019$) between the amount of hydrogen peroxide and MIC in blossom honeys for G+ (*S. aureus*) bacteria, similarly to other authors [3]. For honeydew honeys, the correlation was weaker and, moreover, at the borderline of statistical significance ($r = -0.3515$, $p = 0.0553$). For G− bacteria, represented by *P. aeruginosa*, we did not demonstrate the above-described correlation for either type of honey.

The second option of hydrogen peroxide formation is the nonenzymatic pathway, in which polyphenolic compounds play an important role due to their oxidation–reduction potential. An example is the flavonoid quercetin, which, according to various studies, is one of the most common in honeys, as are chrysin, pinocembrin, galangin from propolis [65], or ferulic acid and kaempherol [41,66,67]. The oxidation of quercetin to quinone (an oxidized derivative of aromatic compounds) produces, among other things, H_2O_2 [68].

The relationship between MIC for *S. aureus*/*P. aeruginosa* and the content of polyphenolic compounds that has been shown in blossom honeys [3] was not confirmed in our sample of honeydew or blossom honeys. Thus, the resulting effects of the two main factors can be expected to be much more complex. Honeydew honeys are known to contain higher mineral content than blossom honeys, the amount and type of which depend mainly on the type of bee foraging, its geographical location, and possible secondary environmental contamination [69]. In relation to the previous text, this is mainly due to the presence of elements with oxidation–reduction potential such as Fe and Cu. It is in the presence of these elements that the abovementioned reactions of polyphenolic compounds take place. Analysis of Polish blossom honeys (acacia, buckwheat, linden, oilseed rape, raspberry, mixed) showed the highest abundance of Fe together with Mn and Zn in buckwheat honeys and a negative correlation between copper and, on the other hand, sodium and calcium [69]. A Swiss study showed a high Fe and Cu content in honeydew honey (electrical conductivity 97 mS/cm), probably with a predominant pollen content of fir (designated as fir in the study) [70]. A final clue is the formation of reactive oxygen species in the Fenton reaction requiring the presence of elements with high redox potential such as the elements iron and copper. It is in the presence of these elements and hydrogen peroxide that superoxide and hydroxyl radicals are formed [71]. The interdependence was presented in a study by Rane (2021) [72], where inactivation of hydrogen peroxide by catalase led to inhibition of polyphenol autooxidation. At the same time, it confirmed the assumption that it is the combination of these two factors that is responsible for DNA degradation, as opposed to H_2O_2 alone [72]. Indeed, as Brudzynski et al. report in their article, H_2O_2 is a substrate for hydroxyl radical formation [73]. The above assumption is then indirectly confirmed by the results of our study and the study of Bucekova et al., where honey samples with the highest H_2O_2 values do not automatically have the lowest MIC values [74].

3.6. Holy Grail

Based both on the data presented above and previous studies, it can thus be assumed that the imaginary holy grail should be honey with a high content of polyphenolic compounds and sufficient minerals. The data in this study show that such criteria are best fulfilled by honeydew honeys. This hypothesis is supported by studies showing a correlation between honey color and mineral and polyphenol content [21,75,76]. Thus, these honeys should likely originate in areas with honeydew sources and plants that are rich in polyphenolic compounds contained in nectar/pollen (heather, chestnut, buckwheat, fir). However, at present, the authors are not aware of any study that answers the above hypothesis of the complex relationship between the amount and nature of minerals, honey color, quantity of phenolic compounds, pollen analysis, and H_2O_2 content in relation to overall antibacterial activity.

4. Material and Methods

4.1. Honey Samples

A total of 49 honey samples from local producers (33 from 2020 and 16 marked with * in the graphs from 2019) were included in the study. The control group consisted of 3 commercial products containing medical-grade honey (MGH) purchased on the market: Revamil® (Rhenen, The Netherlands), Activon® (Nottingham, UK), Vivamel® (Domžale, The Republic of Slovenia), and 1 package of Manuka Honey MGO 550+ (Manuka Health NZ Ltd., JMH12560, produced 13 August 2019 (Auckland, New Zealand)).

4.2. Physical and Biochemical Analysis of Honeys

Forty-four samples were sent for complex analysis to the Eurofins Food Integrity Control Services GmbH laboratory (Ritterhude, Germany) to determine the quality and origin of individual honey samples and their possible comparison or the influence of these factors on the main parameter under investigation—antimicrobial efficacy. The analysis included microscopic analysis (microscopic examination of pollen—500 pollen grains counted, 30 species identified, starch and yeast content, number of honeydew particles, pollen from nectarless plants, percentage of individual pollen grains: >46%, 45–16%, 15%–3%, >3%), physicochemical analysis (electrical conductivity at 20 °C, free acids, diastase activity, pH value, moisture, 5-hydroxymethylfurfural), analysis of undesirable chemical substances—reporting limit in mg/kg (acaricides 0.2–0.002, organophosphorus pesticides 0.01–0.05, organochlorine pesticides, pyrethroids 0.001–0.05). According to the protocol, the analysis consisted of the following methods: gas chromatography with conventional (flame photometric detector—FDP and electron capture detector—ECD) and mass-selective detectors (mass detector—MS), and tandem mass spectrometry—MS/MS. MS/MS was used to detect acaricide residues. GC-ECD was used to detect organochlorine pesticides and pyrethroids, and GC-FDP to detect organophosphorus pesticides. Pesticide screening was then carried out using a multimethod approach for the determination of pesticide residues using GC and liquid chromatography-based analysis after acetonitrile extraction/partitioning and clean-up by dispersive SPE—modular QuEChERS method. QuEChERS is an acronym for quick, easy, cheap, effective, rugged, and safe.

4.3. Bacterial Strains and Culture Conditions

The bacterial strains of *Staphylococcus aureus* (CCM 4223) and *Pseudomonas aeruginosa* (CCM 1960) were obtained from the Czech collection of microorganisms. Strains were cultured on Nutrient agar (Merck, Czech Republic). Bacterial stocks for cryopreservation were prepared on porous beads (ITEST, Hradec Kralove, Czech Republic). For each experiment, fresh bacterial culture was prepared as follows. The porous bead with appropriate bacteria was inoculated onto the agar plate. Culture was performed under aerobic conditions at 37 °C for 24 h.

4.4. Determination of H_2O_2 Content

The content of H_2O_2 in honey samples was determined using a modified protocol by Megazyme GOX assay kit (Megazyme International Ireland, Wicklow, Ireland) as published [3]. Briefly, the dilution range of 9.8 to 312.5 μM of H_2O_2 was prepared as calibration standard. Then, 40% (*w*/*w*) honey solutions were prepared in 0.1 M potassium phosphate buffer (pH 7.0) and immediately measured. For the blank control, the sample or H_2O_2 standard was substituted with distilled water. Each sample was tested at least in three replicates. The absorbance was then measured at 510 nm using a Synergy H1 microplate reader, and data were analyzed using Gene5 (version 3.05.11, Biotek, Winooski, VT, USA) software.

4.5. Determination of Polyphenolic Content

The content of polyphenolic compounds was determined from 20% (*w*/*v*) honey samples using Folin–Ciocalteau Phenolic Content Quantification Assay Kit (BioQuochem, Oviedo, Spain) according to the manufacturer's instructions. The absorbance was measured at 700 nm using a Synergy H1 (Biotek, Winooski, VT, USA) microplate reader, and the polyphenolic content was calculated using Gene5 (version 3.05.11, Biotek Winooski, VT, USA) software.

4.6. In Vitro Antimicrobial Testing of Honey Samples

The evaluation of antimicrobial activities of tested honey samples was performed using a microdilution broth method. Briefly, dilutions of each honey were prepared with a Mueller–Hinton broth resulting in final percentage concentrations of 50, 44, 38, 33, 27, 22, 16, 11, 5.5, 2.75, 1.38, and 0 (*w*/*w*). Subsequently, the bacterial inoculum was prepared from overnight bacterial culture in a saline solution to a final concentration of 10^6 colony forming units/mL. Afterward, 90 μL of each diluted honey sample was applied into the wells and inoculated with 10 μL of bacterial suspension. A positive growth control consisting of tested bacteria in broth and a negative sterility control consisting of sterile broth were included for each assay. Each testing was performed at least in three replicates. The minimal inhibitory concentration (MIC) was determined after incubation at 37 °C for 24 h. The MIC was defined as the lowest concentration of honey sample in which no visible bacterial growth was detected.

4.7. Data Analysis

GraphPad Prism 9 software (version 9.40, GraphPad Software Inc., San Diego, CA, USA) was utilized for graphical outputs and basic statistical evaluation. Normality evaluation was performed using the Anderson–Darling test and Shapiro–Wilk test. For the correlation analyses, the nonparametric Spearman's rank correlation coefficient test with a 95% confidence interval was used.

5. Conclusions

In this study, we compared the antibacterial efficacy of Czech honeys with three representatives of commercially available products containing medicinal honey (Revamil®, Activon®, Vivamel®) and with Manuka Honey MGO 550+ pack (Manuka Health NZ Ltd.). We demonstrated their safety, quality, and efficacy against both G+ and G− pathogens and, based on the results and comparison with published sources, we defined the type of honey that should meet our requirements for a local source of medical-grade honey. However, a series of further analyses are needed to confirm our hypothesis and the possibility of testing this source in vivo and in subsequent clinical trials.

Author Contributions: Conceptualization, L.P.; Methodology, L.P., R.S. and S.J.; Formal analysis, R.S., V.R. and P.B.; Investigation, L.P. and R.S.; Writing—original draft, L.P.; Supervision, P.B. All authors have read and agreed to the published version of the manuscript.

Funding: This research was funded by the Specific University Research provided by Ministry of Education Youth and Sports (SV/FVZ202009), the Ministry of Defence of the Czech Republic (long-term organization development plan), and by the MH-CZ DRO (UHHK, 00179906).

Institutional Review Board Statement: Not applicable.

Informed Consent Statement: Not applicable.

Data Availability Statement: The original contributions presented in the study are included in the article, further inquiries can be directed to the corresponding author.

Acknowledgments: The authors are grateful to Ian McColl for his assistance with the manuscript.

Conflicts of Interest: The authors do not have any commercial or other associations or interests that might pose a conflict of interest with the work presented in this manuscript.

References

1. van Middendorp, J.J.; Sanchez, G.M.; Burridge, A.L. The Edwin Smith Papyrus: A Clinical Reappraisal of the Oldest Known Document on Spinal Injuries. *Eur. Spine J.* **2010**, *19*, 1815–1823. [CrossRef] [PubMed]
2. Dustmann, J.H. Antibacterial Effect of Honey. *Apiacta* **1979**, *14*, 7–11.
3. Bucekova, M.; Jardekova, L.; Juricova, V.; Bugarova, V.; Di Marco, G.; Gismondi, A.; Leonardi, D.; Farkasovska, J.; Godocikova, J.; Laho, M.; et al. Antibacterial Activity of Different Blossom Honeys: New Findings. *Molecules* **2019**, *24*, 1573. [CrossRef] [PubMed]
4. El Sohaimy, S.A.; Masry, S.H.D.; Shehata, M.G. Physicochemical Characteristics of Honey from Different Origins. *Ann. Agric. Sci.* **2015**, *60*, 279–287. [CrossRef]
5. Bischofberger, A.M.; Pfrunder Cardozo, K.R.; Baumgartner, M.; Hall, A.R. Evolution of Honey Resistance in Experimental Populations of Bacteria Depends on the Type of Honey and Has No Major Side Effects for Antibiotic Susceptibility. *Evol. Appl.* **2021**, *14*, 1314–1327. [CrossRef] [PubMed]
6. Troller, J.; Christian, J.H.B. *Water Activity and Food*; Elsevier Science: Amsterdam, The Netherlands, 1978; ISBN 978-0-12-700650-5.
7. Chirife, J.; Zamora, M.; Motto, A. The Correlation between Water Activity and % Moisture in Honey: Fundamental Aspects and Application to Argentine Honeys. *J. Food Eng.* **2006**, *72*, 287–292. [CrossRef]
8. Beckh, G.; Wessel, P.; Lüllmann, C. Natürliche Bestandteile des Honigs: Hefen und deren Stoffwechselprodukte–Teil 2: Der Wassergehalt und die Wasseraktivität als Qualitätsparameter mit Bezug zum Hefewachstum. *Dtsch. Lebensm. -Rundsch.* **2004**, *100*, 14–17.

9. The Water Activity of Honey and Related Sugar Solutions. Available online: https://ira.agroscope.ch/en-US/Page/Publikation?einzelpublikationId=12356&parentUrl=/de-CH/Page/Publikationsliste?guid=85894ecf-e9e1-4c3f-8499-314daea7244c&page=1693 (accessed on 20 April 2024).
10. Cianciosi, D.; Forbes-Hernández, T.Y.; Afrin, S.; Gasparrini, M.; Reboredo-Rodriguez, P.; Manna, P.P.; Zhang, J.; Bravo Lamas, L.; Martínez Flórez, S.; Agudo Toyos, P.; et al. Phenolic Compounds in Honey and Their Associated Health Benefits: A Review. *Molecules* **2018**, *23*, 2322. [CrossRef] [PubMed]
11. Sherlock, O.; Dolan, A.; Athman, R.; Power, A.; Gethin, G.; Cowman, S.; Humphreys, H. Comparison of the Antimicrobial Activity of Ulmo Honey from Chile and Manuka Honey against Methicillin-Resistant *Staphylococcus aureus*, *Escherichia coli* and *Pseudomonas aeruginosa*. *BMC Complement. Altern. Med.* **2010**, *10*, 47. [CrossRef] [PubMed]
12. Vasić, V.; Đurđić, S.; Tosti, T.; Radoičić, A.; Lušić, D.; Milojković-Opsenica, D.; Tešić, Ž.; Trifković, J. Two Aspects of Honeydew Honey Authenticity: Application of Advance Analytical Methods and Chemometrics. *Food Chem.* **2020**, *305*, 125457. [CrossRef]
13. Lachman, J.; Orsák, M.; Hejtmánková, A.; Kovářová, E. Evaluation of Antioxidant Activity and Total Phenolics of Selected Czech Honeys. *LWT—Food Sci. Technol.* **2010**, *43*, 52–58. [CrossRef]
14. Alaerjani, W.M.A.; Abu-Melha, S.; Alshareef, R.M.H.; Al-Farhan, B.S.; Ghramh, H.A.; Al-Shehri, B.M.A.; Bajaber, M.A.; Khan, K.A.; Alrooqi, M.M.; Modawe, G.A.; et al. Biochemical Reactions and Their Biological Contributions in Honey. *Molecules* **2022**, *27*, 4719. [CrossRef] [PubMed]
15. Brudzynski, K. A Current Perspective on Hydrogen Peroxide Production in Honey. A Review. *Food Chem.* **2020**, *332*, 127229. [CrossRef] [PubMed]
16. Grzesik, M.; Bartosz, G.; Stefaniuk, I.; Pichla, M.; Namieśnik, J.; Sadowska-Bartosz, I. Dietary Antioxidants as a Source of Hydrogen Peroxide. *Food Chem.* **2019**, *278*, 692–699. [CrossRef] [PubMed]
17. Da Silva, P.M.; Gauche, C.; Gonzaga, L.V.; Costa, A.C.O.; Fett, R. Honey: Chemical Composition, Stability and Authenticity. *Food Chem.* **2016**, *196*, 309–323. [CrossRef] [PubMed]
18. Endo, A.; Salminen, S. Honeybees and Beehives Are Rich Sources for Fructophilic Lactic Acid Bacteria. *Syst. Appl. Microbiol.* **2013**, *36*, 444–448. [CrossRef] [PubMed]
19. Carter, C.; Thornburg, R.W. Tobacco Nectarin I. Purification and Characterization as a Germin-like, Manganese Superoxide Dismutase Implicated in the defensE of Floral Reproductive Tissues. *J. Biol. Chem.* **2000**, *275*, 36726–36733. [CrossRef] [PubMed]
20. Carter, C.J.; Thornburg, R.W. Tobacco Nectarin V Is a Flavin-Containing Berberine Bridge Enzyme-like Protein with Glucose Oxidase Activity. *Plant Physiol.* **2004**, *134*, 460–469. [CrossRef] [PubMed]
21. Brudzynski, K. Unexpected Value of Honey Color for Prediction of a Non-Enzymatic H_2O_2 Production and Honey Antibacterial Activity: A Perspective. *Metabolites* **2023**, *13*, 526. [CrossRef]
22. Almasaudi, S. The Antibacterial Activities of Honey. *Saudi J. Biol. Sci.* **2021**, *28*, 2188–2196. [CrossRef]
23. McLoone, P.; Warnock, M.; Fyfe, L. Honey: A Realistic Antimicrobial for Disorders of the Skin. *J. Microbiol. Immunol. Infect.* **2016**, *49*, 161–167. [CrossRef] [PubMed]
24. Tseng, J.-M.; Huang, J.-R.; Huang, H.-C.; Tzen, J.T.C.; Chou, W.-M.; Peng, C.-C. Facilitative Production of an Antimicrobial Peptide Royalisin and Its Antibody via an Artificial Oil-Body System. *Biotechnol. Prog.* **2011**, *27*, 153–161. [CrossRef] [PubMed]
25. Bucekova, M.; Sojka, M.; Valachova, I.; Martinotti, S.; Ranzato, E.; Szep, Z.; Majtan, V.; Klaudiny, J.; Majtan, J. Bee-Derived Antibacterial Peptide, Defensin-1, Promotes Wound Re-Epithelialisation in Vitro and in Vivo. *Sci. Rep.* **2017**, *7*, 7340. [CrossRef] [PubMed]
26. Nolan, V.C.; Harrison, J.; Cox, J.A.G. Dissecting the Antimicrobial Composition of Honey. *Antibiotics* **2019**, *8*, 251. [CrossRef]
27. Grainger, M.N.C.; Manley-Harris, M.; Lane, J.R.; Field, R.J. Kinetics of the Conversion of Dihydroxyacetone to Methylglyoxal in New Zealand Mānuka Honey: Part II--Model Systems. *Food Chem.* **2016**, *202*, 492–499. [CrossRef] [PubMed]
28. Majtan, J.; Klaudiny, J.; Bohova, J.; Kohutova, L.; Dzurova, M.; Sediva, M.; Bartosova, M.; Majtan, V. Methylglyoxal-Induced Modifications of Significant Honeybee Proteinous Components in Manuka Honey: Possible Therapeutic Implications. *Fitoterapia* **2012**, *83*, 671–677. [CrossRef] [PubMed]
29. Adams, C.J.; Manley-Harris, M.; Molan, P.C. The Origin of Methylglyoxal in New Zealand Manuka (*Leptospermum scoparium*) Honey. *Carbohydr. Res.* **2009**, *344*, 1050–1053. [CrossRef] [PubMed]
30. Roberts, A.E.L.; Brown, H.L.; Jenkins, R.E. On the Antibacterial Effects of Manuka Honey: Mechanistic Insights. *RRB* **2015**, *6*, 215–224. [CrossRef]
31. Arena, E.; Ballistreri, G.; Tomaselli, F.; Fallico, B. Survey of 1,2-Dicarbonyl Compounds in Commercial Honey of Different Floral Origin. *J. Food Sci.* **2011**, *76*, C1203–C1210. [CrossRef]
32. Degen, J.; Hellwig, M.; Henle, T. 1,2-Dicarbonyl Compounds in Commonly Consumed Foods. *J. Agric. Food Chem.* **2012**, *60*, 7071–7079. [CrossRef]
33. Laallam, H.; Boughediri, L.; Bissati, S.; Menasria, T.; Mouzaoui, M.S.; Hadjadj, S.; Hammoudi, R.; Chenchouni, H. Modeling the Synergistic Antibacterial Effects of Honey Characteristics of Different Botanical Origins from the Sahara Desert of Algeria. *Front. Microbiol.* **2015**, *6*, 01239. [CrossRef] [PubMed]
34. Hermanns, R.; Mateescu, C.; Thrasyvoulou, A.; Tananaki, C.; Wagener, F.A.D.T.G.; Cremers, N.A.J. Defining the Standards for Medical Grade Honey. *J. Apic. Res.* **2020**, *59*, 125–135. [CrossRef]
35. Dzugan, M.; Ciszkowicz, E.; Tomczyk, M.; Miłek, M.; Lecka-Szlachta, K. Coniferous Honeydew Honey: Antibacterial Activity and Anti-Migration Properties against Breast Cancer Cell Line (MCF-7). *Appl. Sci.* **2024**, *14*, 710. [CrossRef]

36. Kocyigit, A.; Aydogdu, G.; Balkan, E.; Yenigun, V.B.; Guler, E.M.; Bulut, H.; Koktasoglu, F.; Gören, A.C.; Atayoglu, A.T. Quercus Pyrenaica Honeydew Honey With High Phenolic Contents Cause DNA Damage, Apoptosis, and Cell Death Through Generation of Reactive Oxygen Species in Gastric Adenocarcinoma Cells. *Integr. Cancer Ther.* **2019**, *18*, 1534735419876334. [CrossRef] [PubMed]
37. Zulkifli, N.A.; Hassan, Z.; Mustafa, M.Z.; Azman, W.N.W.; Hadie, S.N.H.; Ghani, N.; Mat Zin, A.A. The Potential Neuroprotective Effects of Stingless Bee Honey. *Front. Aging Neurosci.* **2023**, *14*, 1048028. [CrossRef] [PubMed]
38. Fadzil, M.A.M.; Mustar, S.; Rashed, A.A. The Potential Use of Honey as a Neuroprotective Agent for the Management of Neurodegenerative Diseases. *Nutrients* **2023**, *15*, 1558. [CrossRef] [PubMed]
39. Che Mohd Nassir, C.M.N.; Abdul Hamid, H.; Hambali, A.; Abd Manan, N.; Mehat, M.Z.; Ismail, N.I.; Mustapha, M. Neuroprotective Potentials of Honey for Cerebral Small Vessel Disease. *OBM Neurobiol.* **2022**, *6*, 144. [CrossRef]
40. Nweze, J.A.A.; Nweze, E.I.; Olovo, C.V.; Obi, O.J.; Chidebelu, P. *Therapeutic Properties of Honey;* IntechOpen: London, UK, 2019.
41. Bucekova, M.; Buriova, M.; Pekarik, L.; Majtan, V.; Majtan, J. Phytochemicals-Mediated Production of Hydrogen Peroxide Is Crucial for High Antibacterial Activity of Honeydew Honey. *Sci. Rep.* **2018**, *8*, 9061. [CrossRef] [PubMed]
42. Tsavea, E.; Vardaka, F.-P.; Savvidaki, E.; Kellil, A.; Kanelis, D.; Bucekova, M.; Grigorakis, S.; Godocikova, J.; Gotsiou, P.; Dimou, M.; et al. Physicochemical Characterization and Biological Properties of Pine Honey Produced across Greece. *Foods* **2022**, *11*, 943. [CrossRef] [PubMed]
43. FAO; WHO. Search Results. CODEXALIMENTARIUS. Available online: https://www.fao.org/fao-who-codexalimentarius/search/en/?cx=018170620143701104933:qq82jsfba7w&q=honey&cof=FORID:9 (accessed on 8 May 2024).
44. European Parliament. *Council Directive 2001/110/EC of 20 December 2001 Relating to Honey;* European Parliament: Strasbourg, France, 2001; Volume 10.
45. Vyhláška 76/2003 Sb., Kterou se Stanoví Požadavky pro Přírodní Sladidla, Med, Cukrovinky, Kakaový Prášek a Směsi. Available online: https://www.zakonyprolidi.cz/cs/2003-76 (accessed on 24 April 2024).
46. Chakir, A.; Romane, A.; Marcazzan, G.L.; Ferrazzi, P. Physicochemical Properties of Some Honeys Produced from Different Plants in Morocco. *Arab. J. Chem.* **2016**, *9*, S946–S954. [CrossRef]
47. Kirs, E.; Pall, R.; Martverk, K.; Laos, K. Physicochemical and Melissopalynological Characterization of Estonian Summer Honeys. *Procedia Food Sci.* **2011**, *1*, 616–624. [CrossRef]
48. EU Pesticides Database-MRLs. Available online: https://ec.europa.eu/food/plant/pesticides/eu-pesticides-database/start/screen/mrls (accessed on 11 May 2024).
49. Gunes, E.; Şahin, S.; Demir, C.; Borum, E.; Bilisik Tosunoglu, A. Determination of Phenolic Compounds Profile in Chestnut and Floral Honeys and Their Antioxidant and Antimicrobial Activities: Güneş et Al. *J. Food Biochem.* **2016**, *41*, e12345. [CrossRef]
50. Jibril, F.; Abu Bakar, M.H.; Manivannan, L. Isolation and Characterization of Polyphenols in Natural Honey for the Treatment of Human Diseases. *Bull. Natl. Res. Cent.* **2019**, *43*, 4. [CrossRef]
51. Estevinho, L.; Pereira, A.P.; Moreira, L.; Dias, L.G.; Pereira, E. Antioxidant and Antimicrobial Effects of Phenolic Compounds Extracts of Northeast Portugal Honey. *Food Chem. Toxicol.* **2008**, *46*, 3774–3779. [CrossRef] [PubMed]
52. Lou, Z.; Wang, H.; Zhu, S.; Ma, C.; Wang, Z. Antibacterial Activity and Mechanism of Action of Chlorogenic Acid. *J. Food Sci.* **2011**, *76*, M398–M403. [CrossRef] [PubMed]
53. Eumkeb, G.; Siriwong, S.; Phitaktim, S.; Rojtinnakorn, N.; Sakdarat, S. Synergistic Activity and Mode of Action of Flavonoids Isolated from Smaller Galangal and Amoxicillin Combinations against Amoxicillin-Resistant *Escherichia coli*. *J. Appl. Microbiol.* **2012**, *112*, 55–64. [CrossRef] [PubMed]
54. Grigoryan, K. Chapter 12-Safety of Honey. In *Regulating Safety of Traditional and Ethnic Foods;* Prakash, V., Martín-Belloso, O., Keener, L., Astley, S., Braun, S., McMahon, H., Lelieveld, H., Eds.; Academic Press: San Diego, CA, USA, 2016; pp. 217–246, ISBN 978-0-12-800605-4.
55. Habib, H.M.; Al Meqbali, F.T.; Kamal, H.; Souka, U.D.; Ibrahim, W.H. Physicochemical and Biochemical Properties of Honeys from Arid Regions. *Food Chem.* **2014**, *153*, 35–43. [CrossRef] [PubMed]
56. Bucekova, M.; Bugarova, V.; Godocikova, J.; Majtan, J. Demanding New Honey Qualitative Standard Based on Antibacterial Activity. *Foods* **2020**, *9*, 1263. [CrossRef] [PubMed]
57. Ng, W.-J.; Sit, N.-W.; Ooi, P.A.-C.; Ee, K.-Y.; Lim, T.-M. The Antibacterial Potential of Honeydew Honey Produced by Stingless Bee (*Heterotrigona itama*) against Antibiotic Resistant Bacteria. *Antibiotics* **2020**, *9*, 871. [CrossRef] [PubMed]
58. Baloš, M.; Popov, N.; Vidakovic Knezevic, S.; Ljubojević Pelić, D.; Pelić, M.; Mihaljev, Ž.; Jakšić, S. Electrical Conductivity and Acidity of Honey. *Arch. Vet. Med.* **2018**, *11*, 91–101. [CrossRef]
59. Masoura, M.; Passaretti, P.; Overton, T.W.; Lund, P.A.; Gkatzionis, K. Use of a Model to Understand the Synergies Underlying the Antibacterial Mechanism of H_2O_2-Producing Honeys. *Sci. Rep.* **2020**, *10*, 17692. [CrossRef] [PubMed]
60. Bugarova, V.; Godocikova, J.; Bucekova, M.; Brodschneider, R.; Majtan, J. Effects of the Carbohydrate Sources Nectar, Sucrose and Invert Sugar on Antibacterial Activity of Honey and Bee-Processed Syrups. *Antibiotics* **2021**, *10*, 985. [CrossRef] [PubMed]
61. Kubo, T.; Sasaki, M.; Nakamura, J.; Sasagawa, H.; Ohashi, K.; Takeuchi, H.; Natori, S. Change in the Expression of Hypopharyngeal-Gland Proteins of the Worker Honeybees (*Apis mellifera* L.) with Age and/or Role. *J. Biochem.* **1996**, *119*, 291–295. [CrossRef] [PubMed]

62. Bucekova, M.; Valachova, I.; Kohutova, L.; Prochazka, E.; Klaudiny, J.; Majtan, J. Honeybee Glucose Oxidase--Its Expression in Honeybee Workers and Comparative Analyses of Its Content and H_2O_2-Mediated Antibacterial Activity in Natural Honeys. *Naturwissenschaften* **2014**, *101*, 661–670. [CrossRef] [PubMed]
63. Weston, R.J. The Contribution of Catalase and Other Natural Products to the Antibacterial Activity of Honey: A Review. *Food Chem.* **2000**, *71*, 235–239. [CrossRef]
64. Dustmann: Über Die Katalaseaktivität in Bienenhonig-Google Scholar. Available online: https://scholar.google.com/scholar_lookup?title=%C3%9Cber%20die%20Katalaseaktivit%C3%A4t%20in%20Bienenhonig%20aus%20der%20Tracht%20der%20Heidekrautgew%C3%A4chse%20&publication_year=1971&author=J.H.%20Dustman (accessed on 11 May 2024).
65. Tomás-Barberán, F.; Martos, I.; Ferreres, F.; Radovic, B.; Anklam, E. HPLC Flavonoid Profile as Markers for the Botanical Origin of European Honey. *J. Sci. Food Agric.* **2001**, *81*, 485–496. [CrossRef]
66. Nešović, M.; Gašić, U.; Tosti, T.; Trifković, J.; Baošić, R.; Blagojević, S.; Ignjatović, L.; Tešić, Ž. Physicochemical Analysis and Phenolic Profile of Polyfloral and Honeydew Honey from Montenegro. *RSC Adv.* **2020**, *10*, 2462–2471. [CrossRef] [PubMed]
67. Kurek-Górecka, A.; Górecki, M.; Rzepecka-Stojko, A.; Balwierz, R.; Stojko, J. Bee Products in Dermatology and Skin Care. *Molecules* **2020**, *25*, 556. [CrossRef] [PubMed]
68. Bellion, P.; Olk, M.; Will, F.; Dietrich, H.; Baum, M.; Eisenbrand, G.; Janzowski, C. Formation of Hydrogen Peroxide in Cell Culture Media by Apple Polyphenols and Its Effect on Antioxidant Biomarkers in the Colon Cell Line HT-29. *Mol. Nutr. Food Res.* **2009**, *53*, 1226–1236. [CrossRef] [PubMed]
69. Kędzierska-Matysek, M.; Florek, M.; Wolanciuk, A.; Barłowska, J.; Litwińczuk, Z. Concentration of Minerals in Nectar Honeys from Direct Sale and Retail in Poland. *Biol. Trace Elem. Res.* **2018**, *186*, 579–588. [CrossRef]
70. Rt, A.; Bogdanov, S.; Haldimann, M.; Luginbühl, W.; Gallmann, P. Minerals in Honey: Environmental, Geographical and Botanical Aspects. *J. Apic. Res. Bee World* **2007**, *46*, 269–275. [CrossRef]
71. Kurek-Górecka, A.; Rzepecka-Stojko, A.; Górecki, M.; Stojko, J.; Sosada, M.; Świerczek-Zięba, G. Structure and Antioxidant Activity of Polyphenols Derived from Propolis. *Molecules* **2014**, *19*, 78–101. [CrossRef] [PubMed]
72. Rane, M.; Deshmukh, K.; Mulik, P.; Mulani, N.; Patwardhan, R. Resolving a Mechanism of Honey Antibacterial Action: Polyphenol/H_2O_2-Induced Oxidative Effect on Bacterial Cell Growth and on DNA Degradation. *Indian J. Appl. Pure Bio.* **2021**, *36*, 1–10.
73. Brudzynski, K.; Abubaker, K.; Laurent, M.; Castle, A. Re-Examining the Role of Hydrogen Peroxide in Bacteriostatic and Bactericidal Activities of Honey. *Front. Microbiol.* **2011**, *2*, 213. [CrossRef] [PubMed]
74. Bucekova, M.; Juricova, V.; Di Marco, G.; Gismondi, A.; Leonardi, D.; Canini, A.; Majtan, J. Effect of Thermal Liquefying of Crystallised Honeys on Their Antibacterial Activities. *Food Chem.* **2018**, *269*, 335–341. [CrossRef] [PubMed]
75. González-Miret, M.L.; Terrab, A.; Hernanz, D.; Fernández-Recamales, M.A.; Heredia, F.J. Multivariate Correlation between Color and Mineral Composition of Honeys and by Their Botanical Origin. *J. Agric. Food Chem.* **2005**, *53*, 2574–2580. [CrossRef]
76. Škrovánková, S.; Snopek, L.; Mlček, J.; Volaří ková, E. Bioactive Compounds Evaluation in Different Types of Czech and Slovak Honeys. *Potr. S. J. F. Sci.* **2019**, *13*, 94–99. [CrossRef]

pharmaceuticals

MDPI

Article

Phytochemical Analysis, Biological Activities, and Molecular Docking Studies of Root Extracts from *Paeonia* Species in Serbia

Petar Batinić [1,*], Aleksandra Jovanović [2], Dejan Stojković [3], Gökhan Zengin [4], Ilija Cvijetić [5], Uroš Gašić [3], Natalija Čutović [1], Mirjana B. Pešić [6], Danijel D. Milinčić [6], Tamara Carević [3], Aleksandar Marinković [7], Branko Bugarski [7] and Tatjana Marković [1]

[1] Institute for Medicinal Plant Research "Dr Josif Pančić", Tadeuša Košćuška 1, 11000 Belgrade, Serbia; ncutovic@mocbilja.rs (N.Č.); tmarkovic@mocbilja.rs (T.M.)
[2] Institute for the Application of Nuclear Energy INEP, University of Belgrade, Banatska 31b, Zemun, 11080 Belgrade, Serbia; ajovanovic@inep.co.rs
[3] Institute for Biological Research "Siniša Stanković", National Institute of the Republic of Serbia, University of Belgrade, Bulevar Despota Stefana 142, 11060 Belgrade, Serbia; dejanbio@ibiss.bg.ac.rs (D.S.); uros.gasic@ibiss.bg.ac.rs (U.G.); tamara.carevic@ibiss.bg.ac.rs (T.C.)
[4] Science Faculty, Selcuk University, 42130 Konya, Turkey; gokhanzengin@selcuk.edu.tr
[5] Faculty of Chemistry, University of Belgrade, Students Square 10-13, 11000 Belgrade, Serbia; ilija@chem.bg.ac.rs
[6] Faculty of Agriculture, Institute of Food Technology and Biochemistry, University of Belgrade, Nemanjina 6, Zemun, 11080 Belgrade, Serbia; mpesic@agrif.bg.ac.rs (M.B.P.); danijel.milincic@agrif.bg.ac.rs (D.D.M.)
[7] Faculty of Technology and Metallurgy, University of Belgrade, Karnegijeva 4, 11000 Belgrade, Serbia; marinko@tmf.bg.ac.rs (A.M.); branko@tmf.bg.ac.rs (B.B.)
* Correspondence: pbatinic@mocbilja.rs

Abstract: Without being aware of their chemical composition, many cultures have used herbaceous peony roots for medicinal purposes. Modern phytopreparations intended for use in human therapy require specific knowledge about the chemistry of peony roots and their biological activities. In this study, ethanol–water extracts were prepared by maceration and microwave- and ultrasound-assisted extractions (MAE and UAE, respectively) in order to obtain bioactive molecules from the roots of *Paeonia tenuifolia* L., *Paeonia peregrina* Mill., and *Paeonia officinalis* L. wild growing in Serbia. Chemical characterization; polyphenol and flavonoid content; antioxidant, multianti-enzymatic, and antibacterial activities of extracts; and *in vitro* gastrointestinal digestion (GID) of hot water extracts were performed. The strongest anti-cholinesterase activity was observed in PT extracts. The highest anti-ABTS (2,2′-azino-bis(3-ethylbenzothiazoline-6-sulphonic acid) radical potential was observed in PP extracts, whereas against DPPH (2,2-diphenyl-1-picrylhydrazyl radicals), the best results were achieved with PO extracts. Regarding antibacterial activity, extracts were strongly potent against *Bacillus cereus.* A molecular docking simulation was conducted to gather insights into the binding affinity and interactions of polyphenols and other *Paeonia*-specific molecules in the active sites of tested enzymes. *In vitro* GID of *Paeonia* teas showed a different recovery and behavior of the individual bioactives, with an increased recovery of methyl gallate and digallate and a decreased recovery of paeoniflorin and its derivatives. PT (Gulenovci) and PP (Pirot) extracts obtained by UAE and M were more efficient in the majority of the bioactivity assays. This study represents an initial step toward the possible application of *Paeonia* root extracts in pharmacy, medicine, and food technologies.

Keywords: peony roots; chemical characterization; Fourier-transform infrared spectroscopy; antibacterial activity; enzyme-inhibitory activity; *in vitro* gastrointestinal digestion

1. Introduction

The genus *Paeonia* (fam. Paeoniaceae) consists of 32 species and is divided into three sections, which are well supported by morphological and molecular studies: (1)

Paeonia L., (2) *Onaepia* Lindl (a herbaceous species that is distributed around the Mediterranean region and in the countries of the Far East), and (3) *Moutan* DC (a woody species predominantly growing on the South American continent) [1]. Section *Paeonia* L., which contains 22 species, has the widest distribution among the three sections, and the distribution center is in China. Also, it is known that the herbaceous peony flowers are significant ornamentally for Chinese people, while their roots have a variety of biological activities and effects shown in alternative medicine [2,3].

In recent years, the secondary metabolites of the herbaceous peonies have been intensively studied, and over 20 active compounds have been identified [2]. Monoterpene glycosides, phenol-carboxylic acids, flavonoids, and tannins are considered major organic groups of molecules in the root extracts of herbaceous peonies. Despite the use of herbaceous peonies for medicinal purposes, there is only one report of the contemporary age on the chemical analysis of their root extracts, and it was related to peony populations widespread in China [2]. On the other hand, water or water–ethanol extracts are one of the forms that make the use of herbal drugs, that is, bioactive molecules from medicinal plants, more suitable in conventional pharmacotherapy [4,5]. The researchers are looking for the most efficient extraction protocol that captures and preserves all of the bio-constituents while retaining their healthy and nutritional properties. Regarding that, the extraction protocols, which include liquid and solid phases, are rudely divided into traditional and novel (eco-friendly) methods, referring to Soxhlet, maceration (M), CO_2-extraction, heat- and microwave-assisted extraction (MAE), and ultrasound-assisted extraction (UAE) [6–8]. Some of these procedures require a high consumption of toxic extraction medium and prolonged extraction time, making them non-economic and harmful to the environment. Therefore, recent investigations favor the use of MAE and UAE in the extraction of active molecules from herbal material [9]. In addition, there is a theory that high temperature and pressure guarantee high extractability of bioactive compounds from herbal material with a short extraction time and a satisfactory degree of preservation of active molecules responsible for various biological and pharmacological activities [10].

As species of the *Paeonia* genus have become more favored for their edible, medicinal, and ornamental properties, in the first 20 years of the 21st century, large-scale chemical investigations and biological and medicinal tests have been performed, focusing especially on their generative organs (e.g., flowers, leaves, and stems) used to treat various diseases, including female sterility, neurological and urogenital disorders, and trauma [11]. The roots of *Paeonia officinalis* (PO) have been used in the therapy of sluggish liver, hepatomegaly, and chronic hepatitis [12]. On the other hand, in Chinese, Indian, and Perso-Arabic ethnomedicine, the root of PO was used as an ingredient in different antioxidant (i.e., natural) concoctions [11]. From the toxicological point of view, the root and root bark of PO were safe for administration up to a dose of 0.2 g/kg body weight/per day [13]. The root of *Paeonia peregrina* (PP) was a source of specific "cage-like" monoterpene glucosides, condensed tannins, and mono(di)-saccharides (e.g., aldoses) [14]. Even though the biological activity of PP is still very poorly investigated and refers only to the chemistry and biological potential of roots, flowers, and petals [15,16], its use for the treatment of epilepsy, spasms, and hemorrhage is documented [14,15]. Regarding the roots of *Paeonia tenuifolia* (PT), in the available literature, there is no published data about their biological activity.

Numerous studies have been carried out utilizing different methods to evaluate the antioxidant, antibacterial, and enzyme-inhibitory properties of medicinal plants of importance with regard to food and functional food products and human health [16,17]. For this purpose, the most common methods for *in vitro* determination of the antioxidant, antibacterial, and enzyme-inhibitory activities of peony root extract were employed [18]. The antioxidant activity suggests that extracts could be used to alleviate the effects of oxidative stress caused by factors from the external environment (free radicals, pollution, ultraviolet radiation, etc.), which can lead to hindrance of a variety of diseases [16,17].

The extract's antibacterial activity demonstrates its capacity to prevent the growth of pathogen bacteria that are already present in the human gastrointestinal tract (GIT), as evidenced by its ability to reduce the presence of these bacteria in people with impaired immune systems or digestive disorders [17,18]. The theory of enzymatic inhibition uses a bulk-based, deterministic approach to quantitatively evaluate how inhibitors influence the progression of enzyme action. However, single-enzyme catalysis is intrinsically stochastic, which may result in significant discrepancies from traditional requirements [18]. Cholinesterase inhibitors serve as a strategy for the treatment of neurological disorders (Alzheimer's and Parkinson's diseases, AD and PD, respectively); amylase and glucosidase inhibitors act as anti-diabetes mellitus factors, while tyrosinase inhibitors can be useful for dermatological disorders linked to excessive amounts of melanin, which can lead to skin cancer [19].

Up until today, there have been no comprehensive reports on the composition and content of secondary metabolites in the roots of any wild herbaceous peony species distributed in Serbia. For that reason, this study aimed to obtain root extracts of PT, PP, and PO using M, UAE, and MAE and to investigate their phytochemical composition by employing Ultra High Performance Liquid Chromatography (UHPLC-LTQ-OrbiTrap MS), UV-Visible (UV-Vis), and Fourier-transform infrared (FTIR) analyses. Also, this study aimed to systematically evaluate their biological potential through antioxidant, antibacterial, and enzyme inhibitory assays. A molecular docking simulation was conducted to gather valuable insights into the binding affinity and interactions of polyphenols and other *Paeonia*-specific molecules in the active sites of tested enzymes (acetylcholinesterase (AChE), butyrylcholinesterase (BuChE), human pancreatic α-amylase (HPA), human intestinal α-glucosidase (HIG), and tyrosinase). Additionally, the aim was to evaluate the bioaccessibility of the bioactive compounds in hot water extracts (teas) and estimate their potential for use in the food industry. As a result of the overall research, the goal of this study was also to recommend the best plant resources for further cultivation that would enable the continuous supply of interested industries with herbal raw materials (herbaceous peony roots) of standardized quality.

2. Results and Discussion

In the present study, PT, PP, and PO root extracts were prepared using M, UAE, and MAE. The obtained extracts were characterized via identification and determination of bioactives, *in vitro* estimation of biological activities, and *in vitro* release of biologically active compounds in simulated gastrointestinal fluids.

2.1. Chemical Characterization

The chemical characterization of the roots of the wild peonies that grow in Serbia is summarized in Table 1. The extracts of roots PT, PP, and PO are a rich source of phenolic compounds, and four groups of polyphenols were identified: (1) gallic acid derivatives (compounds **1–7**), (2) flavan-3-ols (compounds **8–13**), (3) *Paeonia* terpenes (compounds **14–26**), and (4) other metabolites (compounds **27–33**). From the full-scan MS spectra, molecular formulas of the compounds were obtained using isotopic exact masses, while the exact structure was suggested by further study of the MS^{2-4} spectra. The chemical structures of major active compounds identified in PT, PP, and PO obtained by microwave-assisted extraction (MAE) are presented in Figure 1. All listed compounds in Table 1 have been previously isolated or identified in *Paeonia* taxa.

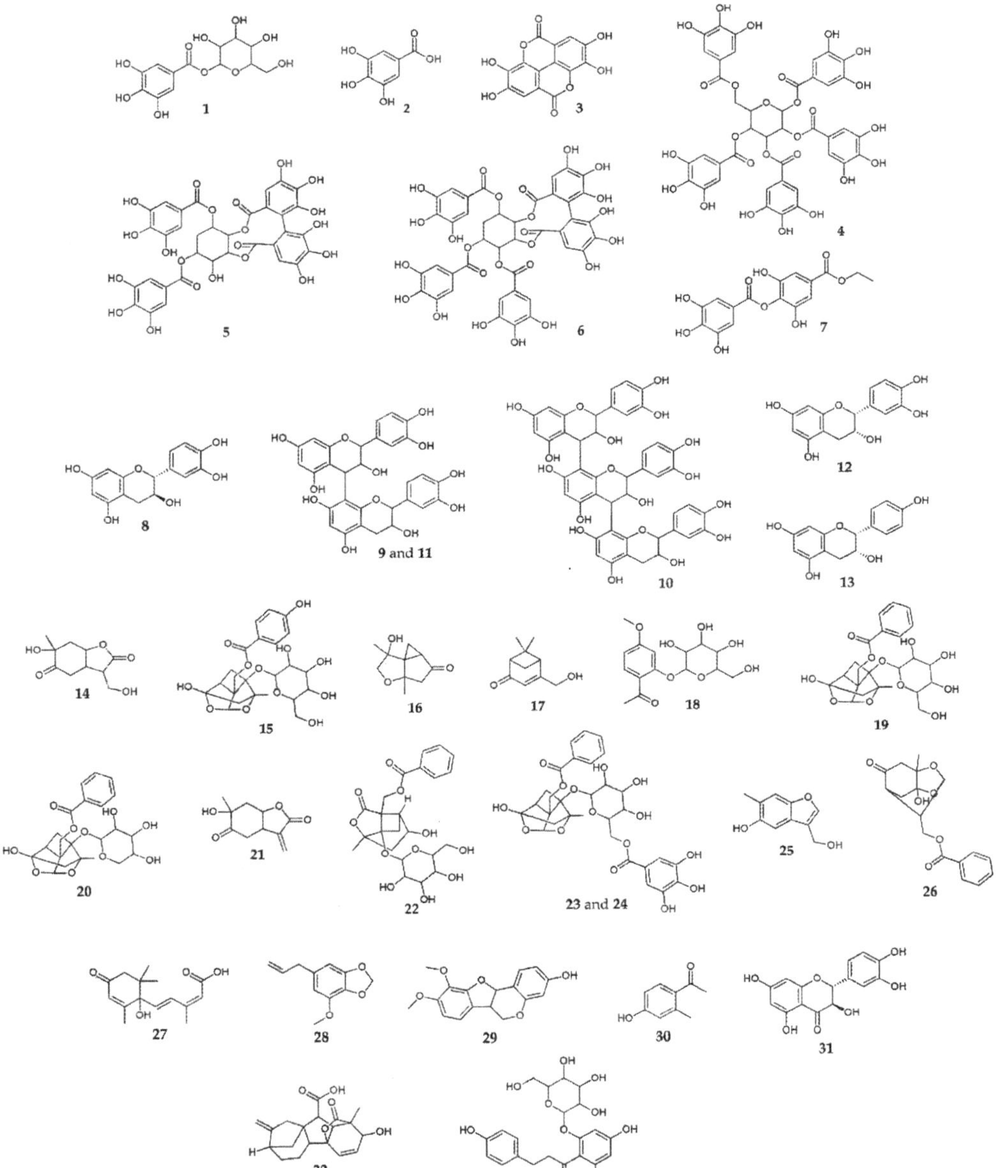

Figure 1. Chemical structures of major active compounds identified in the root extracts of *Paeonia tenuifolia* L., *Paeonia peregrina* Mill., and *Paeonia officinalis* L.

Gallic acid derivatives. This group of molecules presents the major peony antioxidants. The MS data of compounds **1, 2, 3,** and **7** matched with galloyl-hexose, gallic acid, ellagic acid, and ethyl-digallate, respectively [20–23]. Compound **4** eluted at 5.00 min showed a molecular ion at 939 *m*/*z*, and from its exact mass, the chemical formula was calculated–$C_{41}H_{31}O_{26}^-$. The MS^2 base peak, formed by the neutral loss of one gallic acid molecule (170 Da), was found at 769 *m*/*z*. MS^3 and MS^4 base peaks were formed by subsequent loss of 152 Da, respectively, and fragments at 617 and 465 *m*/*z* were obtained.

Finally, with all the abovementioned facts, this compound was identified as pentagalloyl-hexose, and its fragmentation agrees with the available literature [18]. Also, it is reported that pentagalloyl-hexose (**4**) is exclusively based on 1,2,3,4,6-pentagalloylglucose core, so that the depside of the galloyl group is mainly connected at the C-3 and C-4 positions of the glucose group through *m*- and *p*-deleterious linkages [24–26]. On the other hand, compounds **5** and **6**, derivatives of protoquercitol, have not been previously found in the chemical composition of the roots of plants belonging to the *Paeonia* taxa. Compounds **1, 2, 3, 4,** and **7** have previously been found to be the main constituents of the chemical composition of the plant species belonging to the *Paeonia* taxa [16,17].

Flavon-3-ols. Compounds **8, 12,** and **13** were identified as flavan-3-ol monomers (catechin, epicatechin, and epiafzelechin, respectively) by comparing their fragment ions with the reference standards in the online database [27–29]. The characteristic MS fragmentation pattern of catechin and epicatechin was previously described by Xu et al. [27]. Compound **12** was detected at 4.23 min with a molecular ion at 291 m/z. Its MS^2 base peak found at 139 m/z was formed by characteristic retro-Diels-Alder (RDA) fragmentation and the loss of 152 Da—1,3 + RDA fragment [30]. The MS^3 base peak was at 111 m/z (generated by a loss of CO—28 Da), while its MS^4 base peak (83 m/z) was generated by a further loss of CO (28 Da). Compounds **9, 10,** and **11** showed molecular ions of 579, 867, and 579 m/z, respectively. These compounds could be tentatively identified as B-type procyanidin dimers 1 and 2 (compounds **9** and **11**) and B-type procyanidin trimer (compound **10**).

Paeonia terpenes. This group of compounds was the main chemical constituent of the extracts of PT, PP, and PO. Therefore, **12** compounds from this class were detected, and all of them were previously reported as characteristic of the *Paeonia* taxa [16]. Compounds **15** (t_R = 3.28 min) and **22** (t_R = 4.91 min), as well as their isomers (compounds **23**, t_R = 5.02) and **24**, t_R = 5.32) were identified as oxypaeoniflorin, albiflorin, galloyl-paeonoflorin (631 m/z), and galloyl-paeoniflorin isomer, respectively [31]. The typical paeoniflorin derivatives had the characteristic fragment ion $[M-H_2O-H]^-$, and for the pinane skeleton of a molecule of paeniflorin, it was easy to lose the neutral H−COH (30 Da), mainly due to the instability of the hemiketal group [27]. Oxypaeoniflorin had a negative molecular ion $[M-H]^-$ of 495 m/z, and a prominent MS^2 base peak fragment ion of 465 m/z. Also, several organic molecules identified in this study were previously reported in other herbaceous and tree peonies: compound **16** with molecular ion at 183 m/z was found in the cortex of a mountain peony (*Paeonia suffruticosa*) [32]; compound **17** with molecular ion at 167 m/z was found in the root of herbaceous *Paeonia lactiflora* [31]; and compound **18** (paenol glycoside) with molecular ion at 327 m/z was found both in the roots of *P. suffruticosa* and *P. lactiflora* [1]. Furthermore, the identification of compound **25**, precisely paeoveitol D, with a molecular ion at 179 m/z, was achieved by its characteristic MS fragmentations. Compound **26** (paeoniflorigenone), a new monoterpene that modulates the neuromuscular junction in mouse-isolated phrenic nerve-diagram preparation, was previously isolated from the roots of *Paeonia albiflora* Pall. [33] and from the root bark of *P. suffriticosa* [34].

Other metabolites. In this group, several specific organic compounds were identified, and some of them are strong repellents and plant hormones that regulate numerous aspects of plant growth, development, and stress responses. Abscisic acid (**27**) with a molecular ion at 265 m/z was first found in the leaves of *P. lactiflora* Pall., and it was responsible for the positive impact of leaf senescence [34]. Myristicin (**28**), with a molecular ion at 193 m/z, was a strong acaricide that inhibits monoamine oxidase responsible for the promotion of angiogenesis [34], and it was previously found in the essential oil of *Paeonia mascula* [35–37]. Compound **29** was previously detected in the dried root of *P. lactiflora* Pall. [38] and *Paeonia veitchii* Lynch, while compound **30** was found in the root-bark of *Paeonia ostii* [39]. Taxifolin (**31**) is a natural antioxidant that belongs to the subclass of flavanonols in the flavonoids, and it was found in the fruit extracts of the tree *Paeonia rockii* [40]. Compounds **32** and **33** (gibberellin and phloridzin) were found in the trees *P. ostii, P. rockii,* and *P. suffruticosa* [38–40].

Table 1. HRMS and MS^4 data for secondary plant metabolites identified in the root extracts of *Paeonia tenuifolia* L. (PT), *Paeonia peregrina* Mill. (PP), and *Paeonia officinalis* L. (PO).

No	Compound Name	t_R, min	Molecular Formula, $[M \pm H]^{\pm}$	Calculated Mass, *m/z*	Exact Mass, *m/z*	Δ ppm	MS^2 Fragments, (% Base Peak)	MS^3 Fragments, (% Base Peak)	MS^4 Fragments, (% Base Peak)	PT	PP	PO	Refs.
						Gallic acid derivatives							
1	Galloyl-hexose	0.59	$C_{13}H_{15}O_{10}^-$	331.06707	331.06588	3.61	125 (19), **169** (100), 193 (10), 211 (24), 271 (50)	**125** (100)	67 (58), 73 (59), **107** (100)	+	−	+	[19]
2	Gallic acid	0.91	$C_7H_5O_5^-$	169.01425	169.01355	4.14	**125** (100)	53 (57), 63 (50), **97** (100)	NA	+	+	+	[20]
3	Ellagic acid	4.62	$C_{14}H_5O_8^-$	300.99899	300.99744	5.16	185 (45), 201 (25), **229** (100), 257 (77), 284 (44)	129 (28), 157 (34), 173 (44), 185 (84), **201** (100)	NA	+	+	+	[15]
4	Pentagalloyl-hexose	5.00	$C_{41}H_{31}O_{26}^-$	939.11091	939.10833	2.74	617 (6), **769** (100), 787 (9)	429 (16), 447 (29), 599 (34), 601 (22), **617** (100)	193 (10), 313 (15), 429 (9), 447 (40), **465** (100)	+	−	+	[25]
5	Digalloyl-HHDP-protoquercitol	5.23	$C_{34}H_{27}O_{21}^+$	771.10394	771.10271	1.59	233 (29), 261 (75), 279 (50), **305** (100), 413 (14), 431 (60)	**153** (100)	**125** (100), 143 (25)	+	+	+	[24]
6	Trigalloyl-HHDP-protoquercitol	5.57	$C_{41}H_{31}O_{25}^+$	923.11489	923.11375	1.23	**305** (100), 431 (53), 457 (30), 601 (22), 771 (42)	**153** (100)	**125** (100), 143 (26)	+	+	+	[41]
7	Ethyl-digallate	5.93	$C_{16}H_{13}O_9^-$	349.05651	349.05455	5.61	**197** (100)	**125** (14), 169 (100)	**125** (100)	+	−	+	[21]
						Flavan-3-ols							
8	Catechin	3.47	$C_{15}H_{15}O_6^+$	291.08632	291.08529	3.52	**123** (100), 139 (97), 147 (8), 151 (21), 165 (43), 273 (15)	67 (73), 77 (53), 95 (55), **105** (100), 199 (12)	NA	+	+	+	[25]
9	B-type procyanidin dimer 1	3.53	$C_{30}H_{27}O_{12}^+$	579.14970	579.14788	3.14	247 (28), 289 (33), 291 (66), 301 (20), 409 (60), **427** (100)	247 (14), 275 (62), 287 (18), 301 (69), **409** (100)	257 (20), **287** (100), 299 (10), 391 (11)	+	+	+	[42,43]
10	B-type procyanidin trimer	3.79	$C_{45}H_{39}O_{18}^+$	867.21309	867.2118	1.48	425 (19), 559 (20), 577 (88), **579** (100), 715 (19)	289 (23), 291 (48), 301 (27), 409 (75), **427** (100)	247 (23), 275 (43), 287 (8), 301 (43), **409** (100)	+	−	+	[42,43]
11	B-type procyanidin dimer 2	4.02	$C_{30}H_{27}O_{12}^+$	579.14970	579.14836	2.32	247 (23), 289 (38), 291 (71), 301 (17), 409 (37), **427** (100)	247 (19), 275 (67), 287 (14), 301 (68), **409** (100)	257 (19), **287** (100), 299 (7), 391 (11)	+	+	+	[42,43]
12	Epicatechin	4.23	$C_{15}H_{15}O_6^+$	291.08632	291.08547	2.9	123 (98), **139** (100), 147 (8), 151 (21), 165 (42), 273 (10)	67 (19), 83 (13), 93 (14), **111** (100)	65 (26), 69 (70), **83** (100), 93 (73), 111 (24)	+	+	+	[25]
13	Epiafzelechin	5.92	$C_{15}H_{15}O_5^+$	275.09140	275.09057	3.03	**107** (100), 127 (15), 149 (22), 169 (33)	53 (80), 77 (46), **79** (100), 93 (33), 99 (36)	NA	+	+	+	[26]

Table 1. *Cont.*

No	Compound Name	t_R, min	Molecular Formula, $[M \pm H]^{\pm}$	Calculated Mass, *m*/*z*	Exact Mass, *m*/*z*	Δ ppm	MS² Fragments, (% Base Peak)	MS³ Fragments, (% Base Peak)	MS⁴ Fragments, (% Base Peak)	PT	PP	PO	Refs.
							Paeonia terpenes						
14	9-Hydroxypaeonilactone A	2.42	$C_{10}H_{15}O_5{}^+$	215.09140	215.09072	3.16	**155** (100), 158 (26), 169 (19), 173 (14), 197 (81)	95 (26), 109 (42), 113 (26), 127 (28), **137** (100)	69 (47), 81 (25), 95 (39), 106 (7), **109** (100)	+	+	−	[29]
15	Oxypaeoniflorin	3.28	$C_{23}H_{27}O_{12}{}^-$	495.15080	495.14796	5.74	331 (20), 333 (22), 427 (32), 449 (27), **465** (100)	NA	NA	+	−	+	[44]
16	Paeonisothujone	3.71	$C_{10}H_{15}O_3{}^+$	183.10157	183.10085	3.96	137 (14), 147 (69), **165** (100)	123 (18), 137 (24), **147** (100)	**119** (100), 129 (20)	+	+	−	[30]
17	Paeonisuffrone C	3.94	$C_{10}H_{15}O_2{}^+$	167.10666	167.10622	2.63	109 (22), 121 (27), 125 (17), **149** (100)	93 (11), 107 (24), 109 (8), **121** (100), 131 (81)	64 (14), 77 (15), 91 (40), **93** (100), 105 (30)	+	+	+	[29]
18	Paeonoside	4.28	$C_{15}H_{19}O_8{}^-$	327.10854	327.10743	3.39	123 (14), **165** (100), 309 (12)	95 (29), 121 (19), **123** (100)	NA	+	−	−	[22]
19	Paeoniflorin + FA	4.39	$C_{24}H_{29}O_{13}{}^-$	525.16137	525.15874	5.00	**449** (100), 479 (33)	165 (42), 309 (8), **327** (100)	123 (10), **165** (100), 309 (16)	+	+	+	[44]
20	Paeoniflorigenin 1-O-pentoside	4.40	$C_{22}H_{25}O_{10}{}^-$	449.14532	449.14346	4.13	165 (25), 309 (3), **327** (100)	123 (15), **165** (100), 309 (28)	**123** (100), 147 (21), 150 (14)	+	+	+	[45]
21	Paeonilactone B	4.53	$C_{10}H_{13}O_4{}^+$	197.08084	197.07993	4.57	125 (41), **138** (100), 179 (20)	69 (13), 83 (7), **110** (100)	69 (94), **83** (100), 94 (30)	+	+	+	[25]
22	Albiflorin + FA	4.91	$C_{24}H_{29}O_{13}{}^-$	525.16137	525.15859	5.29	**449** (100), 479 (41)	165 (38), 309 (7), **327** (100)	123 (11), **165** (100), 309 (11)	+	−	+	[44,45]
23	Galloyl-paeoniflorin	5.02	$C_{30}H_{31}O_{15}{}^-$	631.16684	631.16434	3.96	271 (20), 313 (10), 399 (10), 479 (12), 491 (23), **613** (100)	**271** (100), 313 (33), 375 (16), 399 (27), 491 (67)	169 (8), 210 (7), **211** (100)	+	−	+	[44,45]
24	Galloyl-paeoniflorin isomer	5.32	$C_{30}H_{31}O_{15}{}^-$	631.16684	631.16451	3.70	**313** (100), 463 (9), 481 (25), 483 (6), 509 (12)	125 (37), 151 (31), **169** (100), 209 (11), 223 (12)	**125** (100)	+	−	+	[44,45]
25	Paeoveitol D	5.38	$C_{10}H_{11}O_3{}^+$	179.07027	179.06977	2.82	93 (21), 107 (32), 135 (97), **151** (100), 161 (14)	95 (21), 105 (19), **109** (100), 123 (80), 133 (31)	65 (3), 69 (10), 79 (6), **81** (100), 91 (14)	+	+	+	[46]
26	Paeoniflorigenone	8.13	$C_{17}H_{19}O_6{}^+$	319.11762	319.11663	3.07	179 (15), **197** (100), 259 (8), 273 (10), 301 (8)	119 (21), 137 (33), 155 (59), 161 (14), **179** (100)	85 (13), 133 (21), **137** (100), 151 (10), 161 (24)	+	+	+	[32]

Table 1. *Cont.*

No	Compound Name	t_R, min	Molecular Formula, $[M \pm H]^{\pm}$	Calculated Mass, *m/z*	Exact Mass, *m/z*	Δ ppm	MS^2 Fragments, (% Base Peak)	MS^3 Fragments, (% Base Peak)	MS^4 Fragments, (% Base Peak)	PT	PP	PO	Refs.
Other metabolites													
27	Abscisic acid	3.80	$C_{15}H_{21}O_4^+$	265.14344	265.14258	3.22	175 (13), 203 (17), 229 (12), 235 (8), **247** (100)	157 (52), 187 (36), 201 (48), 217 (56), **229** (100)	159 (27), 173 (21), 187 (40), **201** (100), 211 (68)	–	+	+	[33]
28	Myristicin	3.96	$C_{11}H_{13}O_3^+$	193.08592	193.08535	2.98	138 (18), **161** (100), 166 (14)	105 (22), **133** (100)	**105** (100)	+	+	+	[35]
29	3-Hydroxy-9,10-dimethoxypterocarpan	4.53	$C_{17}H_{17}O_5^+$	301.10705	301.10602	3.40	187 (18), 243 (40), **283** (100), 285 (16)	211 (31), 235 (19), **239** (100), 247 (24), 265 (23)	**211** (100), 213 (3)	+	+	+	[36]
30	4-Hydroxy-2-methylacetophenone	4.58	$C_9H_{11}O_2^+$	151.07536	151.07499	2.40	95 (30), 105 (25), **109** (100), 123 (93), 133 (38)	69 (8), 79 (8), **81** (100), 91 (12)	NA	+	+	+	[37]
31	Taxifolin	4.80	$C_{15}H_{13}O_7^+$	305.06558	305.06445	3.69	153 (99), 195 (35), 259 (87), **287** (100)	105 (9), **259** (100), 269 (3)	149 (76), **231** (100), 241 (10)	+	+	+	[40]
32	Gibberellin A7	5.06	$C_{19}H_{23}O_5^+$	331.15400	331.15286	3.45	151 (35), 189 (18), 285 (13), 287 (47), **313** (100)	137 (8), **151** (100), 189 (76), 249 (10), 281 (28)	91 (40), 95 (20), **119** (100), 123 (4), 136 (8)	+	+	+	[39]
33	Phloridzin	5.66	$C_{21}H_{23}O_{10}^-$	435.12967	435.12705	6.03	205 (4), 271 (5), **273** (100), 293 (5), 399 (5)	123 (15), **167** (100)	**123** (100)	+	–	+	[47]

The **bold** numbers indicate 100% of the base peak, as well as which peaks were further fragmented in the MS^3 and MS^4 experiments; NA indicates not available. FA: formic acid; + stands for detected and – stands for not detected compounds; refs: the literature that indicates that the given compound was identified in *Paeonia*.

2.2. FTIR Study

Structural characterization via FTIR with the attenuated total reflectance (ATR) technique was used to identify characteristic functional groups presented in the extracts of PT, PP, and PO. As shown in Figure 2, the *Paeonia* root extracts (obtained by MAE) exhibited characteristic peaks that can be attributed to stretching and bending vibrations in different areas, as follows: O–H stretching (a broad band of a hydroxyl group bonded directly to the aromatic (phenol) hydrocarbon group at 3385 cm^{-1} and C–O stretching at 1274 cm^{-1}); C–H asymmetric and symmetric stretching (–CH_3 group at 2925 cm^{-1}; –CH_2/methoxy/–CH_3 at 2897 cm^{-1}); C=O stretching: from the aromatic organic molecules in flavonols (ester functionalities) at 1630 cm^{-1}; –CH_3 bending (the bands at 1440 and 1340 cm^{-1}); C–O–C stretching that can be attributed to the carbohydrate residues (strong bands in the region between 1150 and 1000 cm^{-1} that is characteristic for the C–O stretching of –C–O–C– glycosidic linkages), and –CH bending (from an aromatic compound, band at 864 cm^{-1}) [48,49].

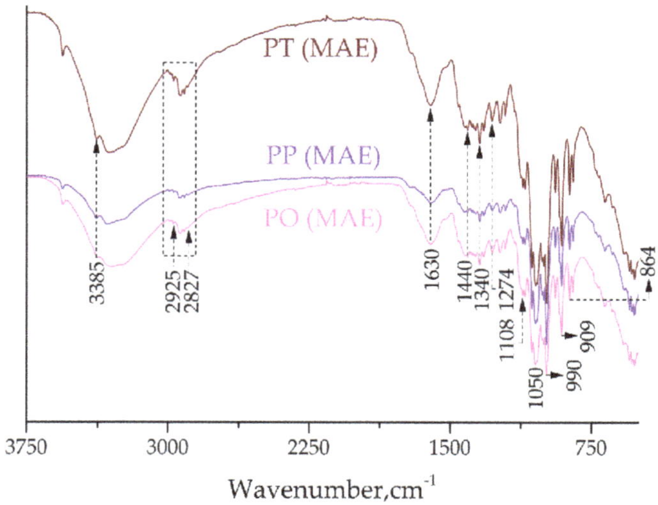

Figure 2. ATR-FTIR spectra of the root extracts of *Paeonia tenuifolia* L. (PT), *Paeonia peregrina* Mill. (PP), and *Paeonia officinalis* L. (PO). MAE: microwave-assisted extraction.

The results of the FTIR study are in accordance with others reported earlier [4,5]. The weak absorption bands in the region of 1000–860 cm^{-1} can be assigned to the $\alpha-$ and $\beta-$glycosidic linkages [48,49]. The FTIR spectra of PT, PP, and PO obtained by UAE and M were provided in the Supplementary Materials (Figures S1 and S2).

2.3. Optimization of the Polyphenol Extraction Process from Paeonia Roots

The values of the polyphenol yield of all prepared *Paeonia* root extracts are shown in Table 2. The total phenol content (TPC) values in PT extracts were in the range of 31.14 to 99.64 mg GAE (gallic acid equivalents)/g, depending on the employed extraction procedure and locality. Furthermore, the polyphenol concentration was between 32.39 and 161.2 mg GAE/g in the PP samples, while the TPC of the PO extracts varied from 35.01 to 165.6 mg GAE/g.

Preliminary screening of factor levels. The influence of all levels of each factor (locality and extraction method) on the TPC was examined. The results are presented in the Supplementary Materials (Figure S3). Statistical significance among all factor levels was estimated on triplicate values through a one-way ANOVA and Duncan's post hoc test

($p < 0.05$). Selected two levels of each factor with the highest polyphenol yield were further included in the experimental design (Table 3).

Table 2. Total polyphenol content (TPC) of the root extracts of *Paeonia tenuifolia* L., *Paeonia peregrina* Mill., and *Paeonia officinalis* L.

Plant Species (Root Extract)	Locality	Extraction Method	TPC [mg GAE/g]
PT	Gulenovci	MAE	77.20 ± 2.56
	Deliblato sand		67.64 ± 0.75
	Bogovo gumno		31.14 ± 1.38
	Gulenovci	UAE	87.89 ± 1.38
	Deliblato sand		99.64 ± 0.25
	Bogovo gumno		36.45 ± 3.94
	Gulenovci	M	53.70 ± 2.94
	Deliblato sand		47.76 ± 1.00
	Bogovo gumno		72.58 ± 2.56
PP	Pirot	MAE	161.2 ± 2.19
	Južni Kučaj		110.7 ± 4.63
	Golina		82.20 ± 3.94
	Bogovo gumno		72.45 ± 0.94
	Krivi vir		48.20 ± 0.81
	Pančevo		91.14 ± 4.63
	Pirot	UAE	93.58 ± 0.56
	Južni Kučaj		32.39 ± 0.13
	Golina		57.01 ± 6.63
	Bogovo gumno		43.20 ± 4.19
	Krivi vir		69.01 ± 0.63
	Pančevo		143.7 ± 2.56
	Pirot	M	105.9 ± 15.8
	Južni Kučaj		81.01 ± 5.63
	Golina		83.89 ± 6.13
	Bogovo gumno		54.26 ± 0.00
	Krivi vir		95.08 ± 1.06
	Pančevo		109.3 ± 3.06
PO	Rujevica	MAE	35.01 ± 2.50
	Božurna		82.58 ± 8.56
	Rujevica	UAE	49.26 ± 2.63
	Božurna		77.58 ± 3.44
	Rujevica	M	165.6 ± 5.00
	Božurna		101.2 ± 3.81

MAE: microwave-assisted extraction; UAE: ultrasound-assisted extraction; M: maceration; PT: *Paeonia tenuifolia* L.; PP: *Paeonia peregrina* Mill.; PO: *Paeonia officinalis* L.; GAE: gallic acid equivalents.

Table 3. Statistical analysis of optimization of polyphenol extraction of roots from three *Paeonia* species (*Paeonia tenuifolia* L., *Paeonia peregrina* Mill., and *Paeonia officinalis* L.) collected in different localities and employing maceration and microwave- and ultrasound-assisted extractions.

	TPC [mg GAE/g]	Effect.	Std. Err.	Effect Estimates	Coeff.	Std. Err. Coeff.	*p*
PT	Constant				82.910	0.449	0.000
	Locality (1)	1.267	0.898	1.410	0.633	0.449	0.196
	Extraction procedure (2)	−21.527	0.898	−23.965	−10.763	0.449	0.000
	1 by 2	−10.573	0.898	−11.771	−5.287	0.449	0.000

Table 3. *Cont.*

	TPC [mg GAE/g]	Effect.	Std. Err.	Effect Estimates	Coeff.	Std. Err. Coeff.	*p*
PP	Constant				123.727	1.530	0.000
	Locality (1)	13.342	3.061	4.358	6.671	1.530	0.002
	Extraction procedure (2)	56.908	3.061	18.591	28.454	1.530	0.000
	1 by 2	4.555	3.061	1.488	2.277	1.530	0.175
PO	Constant				71.032	0.417	0.000
	Locality (1)	41.532	0.835	49.731	20.766	0.417	0.000
	Extraction procedure (2)	24.535	0.835	29.379	12.267	0.417	0.000
	1 by 2	−5.998	0.835	−7.182	−2.999	0.417	0.000

TPC: total polyphenol content; PT: *Paeonia tenuifolia* L.; PP: *Paeonia peregrina* Mill.; PO: *Paeonia officinalis* L.; GAE: gallic acid equivalents.

Locality represents an important parameter that significantly influenced the TPC in all tested roots of *Paeonia* species (Figure S3). Namely, the effect of the locality of PT follows the trend: Gulenovci and Deliblato sand > Bogovo gumno (Figure S3). In the case of PP: Pirot and Pančevo > Južni kučaj ≥ Krivi vir and Golina ≥ Bogovo gumno (Figure S3), whereas in PO: Božurna ≥ Rujevica (Figure S3). Namely, the chemical composition and quantity of the target compounds in the harvested plant matrix are significantly affected by the geographic location, climate, soil, seasonal variations, and altitude [16]. It can be an explanation for the presence of a significant difference between the TPC values of the extracts prepared using roots from various localities. Therefore, Gulenovci and Deliblato sand (for PT), Pirot and Pančevo (for PP), and Božurna and Rujevica (for PO) were included in further experimental design. As can be seen in Figure S3, UAE provided the PT extracts with the highest TPC values; however, there were no statistically significant differences between UAE and MAE. Additionally, the extracts prepared using M method possessed the lowest TPC, but there were no statistically significant differences between the M method and MAE. According to the literature data, UAE represents a good alternative extraction procedure in comparison to traditional techniques due to its high efficiency, lower price, simplicity, reduced extraction time and solvent consumption, and employment of a wide range of extraction solvents. Namely, ultrasound waves in the extraction solvent induce mechanical, thermal, and cavitation reactions causing the degradation of cell structures without significant changes in the structural and functional characteristics of most target compounds [50]. Higher contents of polyphenol components in extracts obtained in the UAE, apart from reduced extraction time in comparison to traditional extraction procedures, were shown in several publications [51–53]. MAE also provides numerous benefits, including a shorter extraction time, a reduced amount of extraction medium, and higher extraction efficiency due to the high vapor pressure of free water molecules in the plant cells and the breaking of the cell walls that provide a higher release of the compounds in the surrounding medium [8]. On the other hand, the M method as a traditional procedure possesses several disadvantages, such as low extraction yield and prolonged extraction time [8]. According to the literature, the high power of microwaves can ensure the degradation of cell walls and better diffusion of polyphenols into extraction surroundings in shorter extraction periods. However, prolonged extraction time and a higher yield of MAE do not mean a large quantity of target components, such as polyphenols, because microwaves cause the release of a large amount of ballast compounds, including lipids, proteins, and sugars [8]. MAE is a widely and successfully applied procedure for preparing polyphenol-rich extracts from different plant materials [54]. In the case of PT, the results showed that the M method provided significantly lower values of polyphenol yield in comparison to MAE (Figure S3), therefore, it was excluded for further experimental design. Regarding the TPC of PP extracts, the impact of the extraction procedure follows the trend: MAE > UAE and M methods (Figure S3). Since there was no statistically significant difference in the TPC between UAE and M method and the M method does not require an expensive device, UAE was excluded from further experimental design related to the PT samples. In the PO extracts, there was no statistically significant difference between all employed extraction procedures (Figure S3), thus MAE and M method were included in future experimental design (MAE due to very short extraction time, while M method due to simple operation). According to the results of one-way ANOVA and Duncan's post hoc test and the highest TPC values, the following two levels of two parameters (locality and extraction method) were included in the experimental design (Table 3): for PP—Gulenovci and Deliblato (among localities), and UAE and MAE (among extraction methods); for PT—Pirot and Pančevo, and M method and MAE; and for PO—Rujevica and Božurna, and MAE and M methods.

Experimental design. The influence of two factors (locality and extraction techniques) with two selected levels on the polyphenol yield was observed through the effects and corresponding regression coefficients of parameters and parameter interactions, as presented in Table 3.

In the PT samples, the extraction technique (variable number 2, UAE and MAE) and interaction among locality and extraction technique have a significant effect on the TPC, while locality (variable number 1, Gulenovci and Deliblato sand) did not show statistically significant influence (Table 3). Among all the variables mentioned, the extraction technique had the most significant impact on the dependent variable (TPC). In the PP samples, both variables (locality—Pirot and Pančevo, and extraction technique—MAE and M methods) possessed a significant impact on the polyphenol yield, whereas interaction did not have a significant effect (Table 3). The extraction method had the most significant effect on the polyphenol yield, followed by locality. On the other hand, in PO, both variables (locality–Božurna and Rujevica and extraction technique–MAE and M) and their interaction showed a significant influence on the TPC, and significance followed the trend: locality > extraction technique > interaction (Table 3). The significant influence of the interaction between parameters indicated that the effect of one parameter was not the same at all levels of another parameter. Specifically, the influence of locality differed when different extraction techniques were employed. Hence, every herbal material requires the examination of the appropriate extraction procedures that will provide the highest polyphenol content in the samples. Measured and predicted values for the TPC (as the dependent variable) of the selected extracts are presented in Table S1.

According to the results of the experimental design (the measured and predicted values of the polyphenol yield in root extracts listed in Table S1), it can be seen that the highest measured polyphenol concentration was achieved under the following factors: PP (species), Pirot (locality), and MAE (extraction method), and it was 161.2 $\pm$ 2.2 mg GAE/g. The model has predicted the maximal polyphenol yield under the same parameters, PP (species), Pirot (locality), and MAE (extraction method), to be 161.1 $\pm$ 3.5 mg GAE/g. Among PT extracts, the highest TPC was reached under the following factors: Deliblato sand (locality) and UAE (extraction method), and it was 99.6 $\pm$ 0.2 mg GAE/g. The model has predicted the highest TPC under the same factors, Deliblato sand (locality) and UAE (extraction method), to be 99.6 $\pm$ 1.9 mg GAE/g. Among PO samples, the highest polyphenol yield was obtained using the following factors: Božurna (locality) and MAE (extraction method), and it was 101.2 $\pm$ 2.8 mg GAE/g. The model has predicted the highest TPC under the same factors, Božurna (locality) and MAE (extraction method), to be 101.1 $\pm$ 1.8 mg GAE/g. Since the differences between predicted and observed values (Table S1) were all less than 1%, a full factorial design may be recommended as an appropriate model for optimizing polyphenol extraction from *Paeonia* roots.

2.4. Total Flavonoid Content (TFC) of Root Extracts

TFC values of all prepared *Paeonia* root extracts were also determined, and the results are displayed in Table 4. Following the PT extracts, the roots from Deliblato sand were found to have the highest TFC after UAE, followed by the extracts prepared using Gulenovci roots and UAE and MAE methods and Bogovo gumno and M method (Table 4). The lowest TFC of PT extracts was detected in the samples obtained using Deliblato sand and MAE, and Bogovo gumno and the M method. TFC values in all PT extracts ranged from 0.94 to 3.27 mg catechin equivalents (CE)/g. In the case of PP extracts, the highest flavonoid yield was measured in the sample prepared using roots from Pirot and MAE and from Pančevo and UAE, followed by Južni Kučaj and MAE, while the lowest flavonoid yield was detected in the extracts prepared using roots from Bogovo gumno and UAE (Table 4). The flavonoid yield of all PP samples varied from 0.74 to 5.75 mg CE/g. The root from Rujevica was found to have the highest flavonoid concentration after the M method, followed by Božurna and the M method. The lowest TFC was measured in the samples obtained by Rujevica root and MAE or UAE (Table 4). The TFC of PO extracts was from 1.01 to 5.92 mg CE/g. The explanation for why the flavonoid yield did not follow the trend of polyphenol concentration at all examined levels can be found in the fact that the chemical composition of the herbal matrix is greatly influenced by the harvested region [16]. Additionally, it can be seen that the flavonoid yield was significantly lower in comparison to the polyphenol content in all prepared *Paeonia* root extracts, which is in agreement with the literature data. Namely, Sut et al.'s [19] study has shown that there were significant differences between the TPC and TFC of root extracts in comparison to the aerial parts of the plant.

Table 4. Total flavonoid content of the root extracts of *Paeonia tenuifolia* L., *Paeonia peregrina* Mill., and *Paeonia officinalis* L.

Plant Species (Root Extract)	Locality	Extraction Method	TFC [mg CE/g]
PT	Gulenovci	MAE	2.30 ± 0.38^{d}
	Deliblato sand		1.84 ± 0.28^{de}
	Bogovo gumno		0.94 ± 0.45^{fg}
	Gulenovci	UAE	2.97 ± 0.85^{d}
	Deliblato sand		3.27 ± 0.55^{cd}
	Bogovo gumno		1.09 ± 0.27^{f}
	Gulenovci	M	1.29 ± 0.23^{f}
	Deliblato sand		0.99 ± 0.50^{fg}
	Bogovo gumno		2.24 ± 0.12^{d}
PP	Pirot	MAE	5.75 ± 0.37^{ab}
	Južni Kučaj		4.10 ± 0.35^{c}
	Golina		2.34 ± 0.28^{d}
	Bogovo gumno		2.14 ± 0.22^{d}
	Krivi vir		1.10 ± 0.17^{fg}
	Pančevo		2.99 ± 0.42^{d}
	Pirot	UAE	3.03 ± 0.65^{d}
	Južni Kučaj		0.99 ± 0.15^{gh}
	Golina		1.53 ± 0.10^{ef}
	Bogovo gumno		0.74 ± 0.15^{h}
	Krivi vir		1.93 ± 0.30^{e}
	Pančevo		5.35 ± 0.03^{b}
	Pirot	M	3.99 ± 0.53^{cd}
	Južni Kučaj		2.14 ± 0.85^{d}
	Golina		2.32 ± 0.13^{d}
	Bogovo gumno		1.37 ± 0.18^{f}
	Krivi vir		3.14 ± 0.65^{cd}
	Pančevo		4.00 ± 0.92^{c}

Table 4. *Cont.*

Plant Species (Root Extract)	Locality	Extraction Method	TFC [mg CE/g]
PO	Rujevica Božurna	MAE	1.01 ± 0.10 [g] 2.39 ± 0.15 [d]
	Rujevica Božurna	UAE	1.01 ± 0.06 [g] 2.39 ± 0.07 [d]
	Rujevica Božurna	M	5.92 ± 0.33 [a] 3.72 ± 0.23 [cd]

MAE: microwave-assisted extraction; UAE: ultrasound-assisted extraction; M: maceration; CE: catechin equivalents; PT: *Paeonia tenuifolia* L.; PP: *Paeonia peregrina* Mill.; PO: *Paeonia officinalis* L.; TFC: total flavonoid content; values with the same letter in the column showed no statistically significant difference ($p > 0.05$; $n = 3$, one-way ANOVA, analysis of variance, Duncan's post hoc test).

2.5. Antioxidant Activity of Root Extracts

The antioxidant capacity of all prepared *Paeonia* root extracts was examined employing two antioxidant assays: ABTS (2,2′-azino-bis(3-ethylbenzothiazoline-6-sulphonic acid) and DPPH (2,2-diphenyl-1-picrylhydrazyl radicals). The obtained results are displayed in Table 5.

Table 5. Antioxidant activity of root extracts of *Paeonia tenuifolia* L., *Paeonia peregrina* Mill., and *Paeonia officinalis* L. obtained by different extraction methods.

Plant Species (Root Extract)	Locality	Extraction Method	Antioxidant Activity	
			ABTS [μg TE/mL]	DPPH [IC_{50}, mg/mL]
PT	Gulenovci Deliblato sand Bogovo gumno	MAE	15.0 ± 0.5 [e] 8.0 ± 0.2 [j] 15.0 ± 0.2 [e]	0.207 ± 0.054 [ab] 0.203 ± 0.022 [b] 0.250 ± 0.000 [c]
	Gulenovci Deliblato sand Bogovo gumno	UAE	19.5 ± 0.5 [bc] 12.0 ± 1.0 [fg] 8.0 ± 0.5 [ij]	0.179 ± 0.052 [ab] 0.168 ± 0.056 [ab] 0.199 ± 0.048 [ab]
	Gulenovci Deliblato sand Bogovo gumno	M	28.5 ± 1.8 [a] 10.5 ± 0.8 [gh] 13.0 ± 0.9 [f]	0.190 ± 0.0843 [ab] 0.188 ± 0.055 [ab] 0.184 ± 0.034 [ab]
PP	Pirot Južni Kučaj Golina Bogovo gumno Krivi vir Pančevo	MAE	8.5 ± 0.5 [ij] 10.5 ± 0. 5 [gh] 6.0 ± 0.5 [k] 9.0 ± 0.5 [i] 18.0 ± 1.5 [bc] 30.0 ± 1.0 [a]	0.221 ± 0.014 [b] 0.188 ± 0.039 [ab] 0.244 ± 0.068 [bc] 0.235 ± 0.037 [bc] 0.266 ± 0.047 [bc] 0.196 ± 0.037 [ab]
	Pirot Južni Kučaj Golina Bogovo gumno Krivi vir Pančevo	UAE	12.0 ± 0.5 [g] 8.5 ± 0.5 [ij] 16.5 ± 0.5 [cd] 14.0 ± 1.0 [ef] 15.0 ± 1.0 [de] 11.5 ± 0.5 [g]	0.186 ± 0.056 [ab] 0.190 ± 0.019 [ab] 0.269 ± 0.048 [bc] 0.235 ± 0.034 [bc] 0.224 ± 0.014 [bc] 0.186 ± 0.044 [ab]
	Pirot Južni Kučaj Golina Bogovo gumno Krivi vir Pančevo	M	13.5 ± 0.5 [f] 10.5 ± 0.9 [gh] 11.0 ± 0.7 [g] 20.5 ± 0.8 [b] 16.0 ± 0.3 [d] 18.5 ± 0.9 [c]	0.191 ± 0.033 [ab] 0.187 ± 0.057 [ab] 0.233 ± 0.039 [bc] 0.171 ± 0.058 [ab] 0.199 ± 0.059 [ab] 0.165 ± 0.055 [ab]

Table 5. *Cont.*

Plant Species (Root Extract)	Locality	Extraction Method	Antioxidant Activity	
			ABTS [μg TE/mL]	DPPH [IC_{50}, mg/mL]
PO	Rujevica	MAE	13.0 ± 0.5 [c]	0.170 ± 0.039 [ab]
	Božurna		10.5 ± 0. 5 [gh]	0.207 ± 0.015 [b]
	Rujevica	UAE	10.5 ± 0.7 [gh]	0.190 ± 0.032 [ab]
	Božurna		20.0 ± 1.0 [bc]	0.213 ± 0.021 [b]
	Rujevica	M	19.5 ± 0.8 [bc]	0.168 ± 0.054 [ab]
	Božurna		12.0 ± 0.8 [g]	0.145 ± 0.0350 [a]

MAE: microwave-assisted extraction; UAE: ultrasound-assisted extraction; M: maceration; PT: *Paeonia tenuifolia* L.; PP: *Paeonia peregrina* Mill.; PO: *Paeonia officinalis* L.; ABTS: 2,2′-azino-bis(3-ethylbenzothiazoline-6-sulfonic acid); DPPH: 2,2-diphenyl-1-picrylhydrazyl; TE: Trolox equivalent; IC_{50}: the concentration of the root extract required to neutralize 50% of DPPH• radicals; values with the same letter in each column showed no statistically significant difference ($p > 0.05$; $n = 3$, one-way ANOVA, analysis of variance, Duncan's post hoc test).

As can be seen in Table 5, in PT samples, the highest ABTS radical scavenging potential was determined in the extracts prepared from Gulenovci roots and using the M method, followed by Gulenovci and UAE, while the lowest values were obtained for the samples prepared using Deliblato sand root and MAE and Bogovo gumno root and UAE. The highest anti-ABTS activity was measured in the PT extracts obtained from Pančevo roots and MAE, followed by Bogovo gumno and the M method. On the other hand, low values were detected in the samples prepared using Golina roots and MAE (Table 5). In the case of PO, there were no differences between the extracts prepared using Božurna root and UAE, and Rujevica root and M method; thus, the mentioned extracts showed the highest ABTS radical scavenging potential. Among PO extracts, Božurna and MAE, as well as Rujevica and UAE, possessed the lowest anti-ABTS capacity (Table 5). The ABTS radical scavenging capacity did not follow the trend of polyphenol and flavonoid yields at all tested levels, which can be explained by the fact that numerous secondary metabolites (apart from polyphenols) and their interactions can have an important role in the radical scavenging potential of the plant extracts [51].

Regarding the results of the DPPH radical scavenging capacity of the root extracts, there was no statistically significant difference between the PT samples obtained using the roots from different localities and various extraction procedures (0.168–0.207 mg/mL), except in the case of Bogovo gumno (MAE), which possessed a higher value of IC_{50} (0.250 mg/mL), implying a lower anti-DPPH potential. Further, the IC_{50} values of PP and PO extracts varied in the range of 0.165 to 0.221 mg/mL and from 0.145 to 0.213 mg/mL, respectively. Additionally, there was no statistically significant difference between the anti-DPPH activity of all PP extracts, as in the case of PO extracts (Table 5). The absence of a correlation between anti-ABTS and the anti-DPPH activities of the extracts can be attributed to in the fact that the characteristics and reactivity of free radicals, as well as the mechanism of the reactions, are different. Specifically, ABTS radicals react via electron transfer, and they are more reactive than DPPH radicals, which are involved in the transfer of hydrogen atoms [53]. Hence, higher reactivity of ABTS radicals resulted in a statistically significant difference between the extracts that could not be detected using lower reactive DPPH radicals. Thus, it is important to employ various antioxidant assays to gain a better insight into the overall antioxidant potential of *Paeonia* root extracts. Since the literature data also showed a correlation between the anti-DPPH activity of the extracts and flavonoid yield [55], it can also explain the absence of statistically significant differences among various *Paeonia* root extracts in terms of DPPH radical scavenging capacity (Table 5) due to very low TFC (Table 4).

2.6. Enzyme Inhibitory Activity of Root Extracts

AD, followed by diabetes mellitus 2 (DM 2), is a major global health problem in the 21st century. Today, the prevalence of AD is in progression and is estimated to sharply increase over the next 20 years [56].

Cholinesterases are the key enzymes in the synaptic cleft of the brain that terminate the cholinergic signal transfer and are considered key targets for the treatment of AD [56]. Normal cholinergic activity depends on the fast hydrolysis of the neurotransmitter acetylcholine (ACh) by cholinesterases. The fact that naturally occurring active molecules from medicinal and aromatic plants are considered to be new therapeutics has led to the discovery of secondary plant metabolites, extracts, and essential oils with the ability to inhibit AChE activity, which can cause a parallel increase in the level of ACh in the brain, reducing the symptoms of AD and PD. Based on their widespread use as neuroprotectants in conventional therapy, some publications suggest that *Paeonia* spp. could be used as potential cholinesterase inhibitors [17,19]. Therefore, this study evaluates different *Paeonia* root extracts as possible AChE and BuChE inhibitors. As can be seen in Table 6, for the AChE and BuChE assays, the highest anti-enzymatic activity was observed for the extracts of PT (obtained by MAE) collected from Bogovo gumno. These outcomes are similar to the antioxidant activity, indicating that the Bogovo gumno PT extract prepared using the M technique has a high potential to react with ABTS radicals and eliminate them. Similarly, the most effective AChE/BuChE inhibitor among the extracts of PP was one collected from Pirot (obtained by the M method). Its antioxidant activity against DPPH and ABTS radicals was assessed as moderate. The third group of extracts (PO) displayed moderate cholinesterase inhibitory potential when the UAE was implemented. Earlier studies on this topic have shown the positive effects of the polyphenols on inhibiting AChE activity [57]. Epicatechin, a monomeric flavanol, has been found to reduce tremors and enhance learning and memory ability in mouse models of PD [58]. Also, there is a claim that terpenoid-derived chemicals and other related compounds are the major responsible phytoconstituents for AChE inhibitory potential [59]. Besides, the paper of Ji and Zhang [56] suggests that flavonoids, as inhibitors of AChE and BuChE, might be functional in the treatment of AD. The extract with the highest inhibitory potential against AChE/BuChE was PT collected from Bogovo gumno (MAE), with values of 2.43 and 2.94 mg GALAE (galanthamine equivalents)/g, respectively, so it might be considered to have therapeutic potential.

DM 2 is a metabolic disease characterized by hyperglycemia, followed by a lack of insulin, which is considered to be one of the five leading causes of death worldwide. Also, the prevalence of DM 2 has risen dramatically on the global level, which will affect 438 million people by the end of the third decade of the 21st century [60]. HPA and HIG are the key enzymes involved in the metabolism of carbohydrates and are of crucial importance for decreasing post-prandial blood glucose levels, resulting in the normal level of insulin [59]. Recent publications on this topic have shown that polyphenolic compounds and polyphenol-rich products are beneficial for preventing DM 2 [20,61]. The benefits of polyphenolic derivatives for DM 2 can be mirrored in the protection of $\beta-$cells against the toxicity of glucose; enzyme inhibitory activity through the mechanism of the action of HPA and HIG, and thus a decrease in the digestion of starch; and inhibition of the formation and accumulation of advanced glycation end products (AGEs) [62]. On the other hand, the scientific society is still in search of effective drugs from plant resources with high absorption in the GIT, a long duration of action, low toxicity, and immunostimulant effects. Therefore, the aim of this experiment is to investigate whether PT, PP, and PO contain active substances that enhance anti-diabetic activity through the inhibition of HPA/HIG (Table 6). In HPA inhibitory activity, the extract of PP (Bogovo gumno) obtained by UAE showed the highest inhibitory activity with a value of 0.26 mmol ACAE (acarbose equivalents)/g, respectively. A similar pattern was observed for PP collected from Južni Kučaj—the most effective HPA inhibitor was the extract of PP (obtained by the M method), with a value of 0.25 mmol ACAE/g. These experimental results are supported by the findings of Sut et al. [19] who reported that isoprenoid derivatives and polyphenolic compounds present in the root extract of *Paeonia arietina* and *Paeonia kesrounansis* exhibited antidiabetic activities. In addition, it was documented that gallic acid (also present in the tested *Paeonia* extracts) can reduce HPA activity, increase glucose-induced insulin secretion and glucose uptake in peripheral blood glucose uptake *in vitro*, and increase serum insulin levels and glycogen in the liver *in vivo* [61]. On the other hand, in HIG inhibitory activity, the most prominent inhibitory potential was observed in the extract of PO (Rujevica) obtained by the M method. Considering the results by the study of Sut et al. [19], it can be seen that the ethyl acetate extracts of *P. arietina* and *P. kesrounansis* possess about 40 times higher HIG inhibitory activity compared to our outputs. The potential explanation could be that some of the polyphenol compounds that cause the enzyme inhibitory potential are more soluble in ethyl acetate than in their alcoholic counterparts (in this research, ethyl alcohol (50%, *v*/*v*) was used as a solvent). Zengin et al. [63] also reported that there is a direct correlation between the nature/polarity of the solvent (due to its ability to extract target compounds) and enzyme inhibitory activity. The nature of extract (herbaceous or tree peony) and its chemical profile (ratio and concentration between secondary plant metabolites) can affect the results of enzyme-inhibitory activity as well. According to the literature review, this is the first report concerning the enzyme-inhibitory activity of extracts of PT, PP, and PO wild-grown in Serbia. Keeping this in mind, further chemical and biological studies are needed for the identification of responsible active compounds and the evaluation of the molecular mechanism of their anti-enzymatic action.

Table 6. Enzyme-inhibitory activity of the root extracts of *Paeonia tenuifolia* L., *Paeonia peregrina* Mill., and *Paeonia officinalis* L.

Plant Species (Root Extract)	Locality	Extraction Method	Ache Inhibition	Buche Inhibition	HPA Inhibition	HIG Inhibition	Tyrosinase Inhibition
			[mg GALAE/g]		[mmol ACAE/g]		[mg KAE/g]
PT	Gulenovci	MAE	1.14 ± 0.02 ^{j}	0.90 ± 0.14 ^{cd}	0.24 ± 0.00 ^{b}	1.21 ± 0.01 ^{f}	24.02 ± 0.66 ^{e}
	Deliblato sand		1.78 ± 0.07 ^{cd}	1.41 ± 0.18 ^{b}	0.17 ± 0.01 ^{f}	1.02 ± 0.02 ^{j}	28.73 ± 2.26 ^{cd}
	Bogovo gumno		2.43 ± 0.03 ^{a}	2.94 ± 0.23 ^{a}	0.15 ± 0.01 ^{g}	1.23 ± 0.01 ^{f}	24.29 ± 0.55 ^{e}
	Gulenovci	UAE	1.35 ± 0.02 ^{h}	1.01 ± 0.19 ^{c}	0.22 ± 0.00 ^{c}	1.28 ± 0.01 ^{bc}	29.59 ± 2.36 ^{c}
	Deliblato sand		1.81 ± 0.05 ^{c}	0.78 ± 0.06 ^{de}	0.20 ± 0.00 ^{e}	1.19 ± 0.01 ^{g}	29.99 ± 1.76 ^{c}
	Bogovo gumno		1.62 ± 0.02 ^{e}	0.98 ± 0.12 ^{cd}	0.18 ± 0.00 ^{f}	1.13 ± 0.02 ^{h}	24.83 ± 1.57 ^{e}
	Gulenovci	M	1.22 ± 0.06 ^{i}	0.96 ± 0.06 ^{cd}	0.24 ± 0.00 ^{b}	1.28 ± 0.01 ^{bc}	28.63 ± 0.51 ^{d}
	Deliblato sand		1.92 ± 0.07 ^{bc}	1.09 ± 0.07 ^{c}	0.16 ± 0.00 ^{fg}	1.16 ± 0.03 ^{g}	32.68 ± 1.33 ^{b}
	Bogovo gumno		1.70 ± 0.09 ^{de}	1.14 ± 0.04 ^{c}	0.15 ± 0.01 ^{g}	1.09 ± 0.01 ^{i}	24.12 ± 1.38 ^{e}
PP	Pirot	MAE	1.63 ± 0.02 ^{e}	1.01 ± 0.04 ^{c}	0.15 ± 0.01 ^{g}	1.25 ± 0.00 ^{f}	31.05 ± 1.63 ^{bc}
	Južni Kučaj		1.69 ± 0.06 ^{de}	1.18 ± 0.28 ^{bc}	0.18 ± 0.01 ^{ef}	1.29 ± 0.00 ^{b}	32.34 ± 1.05 ^{b}
	Golina		1.25 ± 0.03 ^{i}	1.10 ± 0.08 ^{c}	0.18 ± 0.00 ^{f}	0.62 ± 0.01 ^{m}	25.37 ± 2.05 ^{de}
	Bogovo gumno		1.41 ± 0.02 ^{g}	1.05 ± 0.20 ^{c}	0.20 ± 0.01 ^{de}	1.22 ± 0.02 ^{ef}	26.07 ± 1.32 ^{de}
	Krivi vir		0.48 ± 0.08 ^{k}	1.11 ± 0.14 ^{c}	0.16 ± 0.01 ^{fg}	0.90 ± 0.04 ^{k}	22.95 ± 1.43 ^{f}
	Pančevo		1.35 ± 0.04 ^{gh}	1.14 ± 0.17 ^{c}	0.21 ± 0.00 ^{d}	1.27 ± 0.01 ^{cd}	25.68 ± 0.22 ^{e}
	Pirot	UAE	1.67 ± 0.05 ^{e}	0.68 ± 0.06 ^{e}	0.18 ± 0.00 ^{f}	1.29 ± 0.00 ^{b}	33.99 ± 0.48 ^{b}
	Južni Kučaj		1.63 ± 0.03 ^{e}	0.74 ± 0.07 ^{de}	0.25 ± 0.02 ^{a}	1.29 ± 0.00 ^{b}	35.50 ± 1.91 ^{ab}
	Golina		1.23 ± 0.02 ^{i}	0.74 ± 0.07 ^{de}	0.24 ± 0.01 ^{ab}	0.71 ± 0.06 ^{l}	22.18 ± 0.28 ^{f}
	Bogovo gumno		1.53 ± 0.04 ^{f}	0.67 ± 0.05 ^{e}	0.21 ± 0.00 ^{d}	1.24 ± 0.02 ^{ef}	25.36 ± 1.43 ^{e}
	Krivi vir		1.82 ± 0.04 ^{c}	1.03 ± 0.19 ^{c}	0.23 ± 0.01 ^{b}	1.03 ± 0.02 ^{j}	27.44 ± 0.77 ^{d}
	Pančevo		1.54 ± 0.03 ^{f}	1.26 ± 0.16 ^{bc}	0.18 ± 0.00 ^{f}	1.14 ± 0.03 ^{h}	30.22 ± 0.68 ^{c}
	Pirot	M	2.00 ± 0.01 ^{b}	1.38 ± 0.03 ^{b}	0.20 ± 0.00 ^{e}	1.28 ± 0.00 ^{c}	35.33 ± 1.71 ^{ab}
	Južni Kučaj		1.73 ± 0.02 ^{d}	1.17 ± 0.04 ^{c}	0.23 ± 0.01 ^{b}	1.29 ± 0.00 ^{b}	30.57 ± 0.60 ^{c}
	Golina		1.31 ± 0.02 ^{h}	0.81 ± 0.02 ^{d}	0.18 ± 0.00 ^{f}	0.66 ± 0.05 ^{lm}	23.28 ± 1.22 ^{ef}
	Bogovo gumno		1.40 ± 0.01 ^{g}	0.82 ± 0.05 ^{d}	0.26 ± 0.01 ^{a}	1.28 ± 0.01 ^{bc}	27.61 ± 2.67 ^{cd}
	Krivi vir		1.42 ± 0.02 ^{g}	1.10 ± 0.04 ^{c}	0.20 ± 0.01 ^{de}	1.01 ± 0.01 ^{j}	23.16 ± 1.16 ^{ef}
	Pančevo		1.46 ± 0.08 ^{fg}	1.10 ± 0.08 ^{c}	0.19 ± 0.01 ^{ef}	1.26 ± 0.00 ^{e}	27.97 ± 2.13 ^{cd}

Table 6. *Cont.*

Plant Species (Root Extract)	Locality	Extraction Method	Ache Inhibition	Buche Inhibition	HPA Inhibition	HIG Inhibition	Tyrosinase Inhibition
			[mg GALAE/g]		[mmol ACAE/g]		[mg KAE/g]
PO	Rujevica	MAE	1.69 ± 0.02 [de]	1.21 ± 0.09 [bc]	0.23 ± 0.01 [b]	1.26 ± 0.00 [e]	33.67 ± 1.19 [b]
	Božurna		1.65 ± 0.05 [de]	0.79 ± 0.06 [d]	0.21 ± 0.00 [d]	1.27 ± 0.00 [d]	30.08 ± 0.90 [c]
	Rujevica	UAE	1.85 ± 0.06 [c]	1.42 ± 0.17 [b]	0.24 ± 0.00 [b]	1.29 ± 0.00 [b]	35.96 ± 1.05 [ab]
	Božurna		1.82 ± 0.03 [c]	0.66 ± 0.04 [e]	0.21 ± 0.00 [d]	1.29 ± 0.00 [b]	30.44 ± 1.18 [c]
	Rujevica	M	1.72 ± 0.02 [d]	1.34 ± 0.07 [b]	0.24 ± 0.01 [ab]	1.30 ± 0.00 [a]	37.06 ± 1.33 [a]
	Božurna		1.62 ± 0.03 [e]	1.20 ± 0.09 [bc]	0.20 ± 0.00 [e]	1.28 ± 0.00 [c]	26.80 ± 0.63 [d]

GALAE: galanthamine equivalents; ACAE: acarbose equivalents; KAE: kojic acid equivalents; AChE: acetylcholinesterase; BuChE: butyrylcholinesterase; HPA: human pancreatic α-amylase; HIG: human intestinal α-glycosidase; PT: *Paeonia tenuifolia* L.; PP: *Paeonia peregrina* Mill.; PO: *Paeonia officinalis* L.; values with the same letter in each column showed no statistically significant difference ($p > 0.05$; $n = 3$, one-way ANOVA, analysis of variance, Duncan's post hoc test); MAE: microwave-assisted extraction; UAE: ultrasound-assisted extraction; M: maceration.

Melanin, a major pigment in the skin, is known to protect the mentioned organ against the harmful effects of ultraviolet irradiation, oxidative stress, and DNA damage [64]. The accumulation of melanin can affect health problems associated with hyperpigmentation and other related skin disorders, such as acanthosis nigricans, melasma, and skin cancer [65]. Tyrosinase is a tetramer that contains four atoms of Cu^{2+} per molecule, which catalyzes the *o*-hydroxylation of monophenols to *o*-diphenols [64,65]. Its main drawback is the acceleration of melanogenesis, which can cause, as mentioned above, skin degeneration and malignancies [65]. Thus, the identification of novel tyrosinase inhibitors was crucial to the development of new therapeutic agents that may be used to treat diseases associated with skin-pathological disorders. Many active compounds, including kojic acid, vitamin C, hydroquinone, and arbutin, are reported to exhibit inhibition of tyrosinase and are extensively used in pharmacology, clinical research, and similar fields [66]. However, due to their lack of safety, unsatisfactory efficacy, and cytotoxicity, further studies for proper use are exclusively necessary.

Regarding that, the presented findings revealed that all examined extracts of PT, PP, and PO inhibited tyrosinase (Table 6). Among all tested extracts, the extract of PO (Rujevica) obtained by the M method, followed by the extracts of PP (Južni Kučaj and Pirot) obtained by UAE and the M method, displayed the highest tyrosinase inhibition. Previous investigations showed that root extracts of *P. arietina* and *P. kesrounansis* show high tyrosinase-inhibitory activity, about four times higher compared to our results [19]. Also, in the literature, it can be found that other organs of *Paeonia* species, specifically the aerial parts of *P. mascula* ssp. *hellenica,* possess a strong potential to inhibit tyrosinase [67]. The reason for this atypical occurrence could be that the synthesis of secondary plant metabolites—tyrosinase inhibitors, such as flavonoids and galloyl derivatives—in aerial parts of peony is more intense compared to the roots, which are not directly exposed to sunlight. However, further investigations are necessary to support this claim. In addition, kaempferol-3-*O*-(6-β-*O*-galloyl-β-D-glucopyranoside) isolated from the flowers of *P. lactiflora* was found to inhibit tyrosinase, with greater effectiveness compared to reference anti-tyrosinase inhibitors (e.g., kojic acid) [19,67].

2.7. Molecular Docking

The chemical profile of the *Peaonia* root extracts was analyzed by molecular docking on five enzymes (AChE, BuChE, HPA, HIG, and tyrosinase) with the aim of highlighting individual compounds that contribute most to the observed activities of the extracts. The heatmap representation of calculated binding affinities is shown in Figure 3. The binding modes of several protein–ligand complexes are presented in Figures 4 and 5, indicating the most important interactions that stabilize these structures.

	1	2	3	4	5	7	9	11	12	13	14	15	16	17	18	19	20	21	22	23	24	25	26	27	28	29	30	31	32	33
AChE	-8	-7.5	-8.5	-6.2	-7	-9.6	-7.1	-7.6	-8.5	-7.6	-7.4	-7.2	-6.1	-6.9	-7.2	-7.5	-7.6	-7.5	-7.1	-7.4	-7.6	-7	-9	-7.3	-7.3	-6.9	-6.8	-9.2	-6.8	-7.1
BChE	-7.6	-6.4	-9.9	-11.6	-11	-8.8	-10.8	-11.6	-8.4	-8.2	-6.5	-9.7	-6.9	-6.2	-7.7	-10.1	-10.3	-6.7	-10.3	-10.8	-10.8	-6.7	-9.6	-7.8	-6.2	-8.7	-6.2	-9.5	-9.3	-9.1
Amylase	-7.4	-5.9	-8	-8	-9.6	-7.8	-9.3	-8	-8.8	-8.8	-6.5	-9.1	-6.8	-6.2	-6.8	-8.6	-7.9	-6.5	-9	-9.5	-9.4	-6.4	-8.9	-7.4	-5.9	-7.7	-6.2	-9.2	-8.6	-8.4
Glucosidase	-6.6	-5.7	-6.3	-8.4	-8.2	-7.1	-7.6	-8.3	-7	-6.5	-5.4	-7.8	-5	-4.7	-6.3	-8.2	-7.7	-4.9	-7.1	-8.5	-8.4	-5.7	-7.2	-6.7	-6	-6.6	-4.7	-6.8	-7.6	-6.8
Tyrosinase	-7.7	-6.5	-6.2	-7.5	-7.6	-7.8	-7.8	-7.7	-8.3	-7.7	-5.8	-7.8	-5.8	-5.9	-6.7	-7.8	-7.4	-6.1	-7	-8	-8	-6.2	-7.7	-6.5	-6.7	-6.9	-6.2	-8.6	-7	-7.9

Figure 3. Docking scores of 33 compounds identified in the *Paeonia* root extracts to five enzymes. The red color indicates a higher binding affinity. AChE: acetylcholinesterase; BuChE: butyrylcholinesterase.

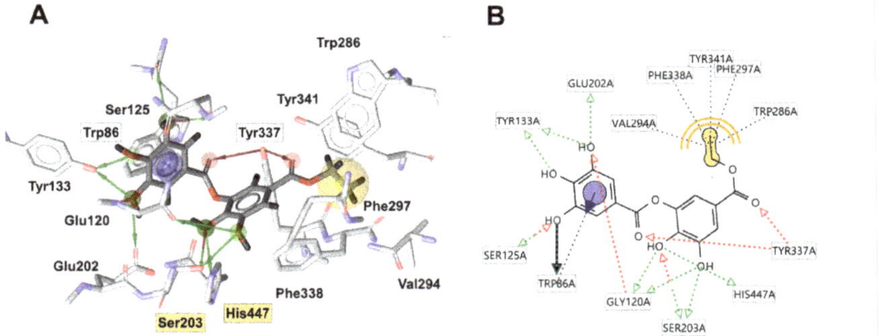

Figure 4. (**A**) Binding mode of ethyl digallate (**7**) within the acetylcholinesterase binding pocket; (**B**) 2D ligand interaction diagram for this macromolecular complex. Hydrogen bond donor, hydrogen bond acceptor, hydrophobic, and π–π stacking interactions are represented by green arrows, red arrows, yellow spheres, and blue rings, respectively.

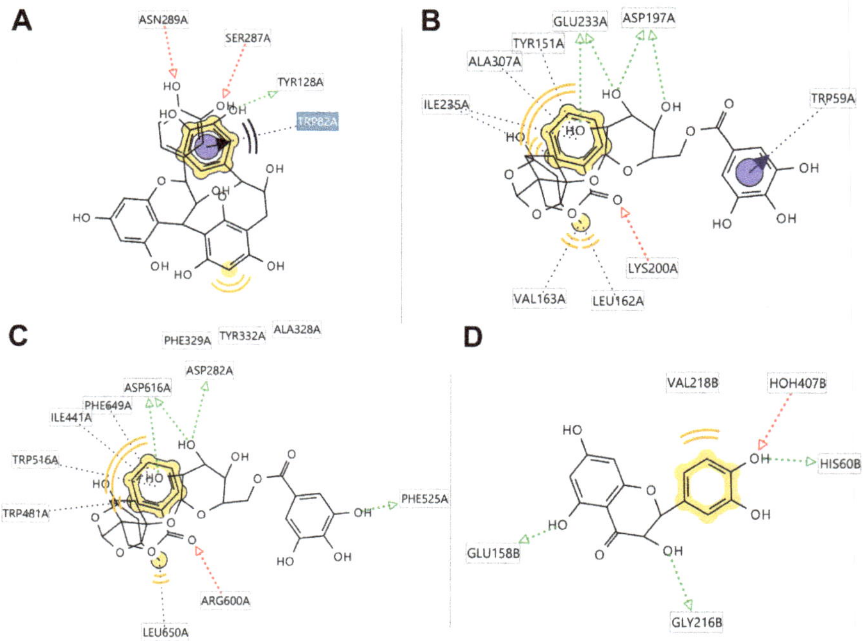

Figure 5. 2D ligand interaction diagrams showing the most important interactions that stabilize the protein–ligand complexes depicted for: (**A**) butyrylcholinesterase-B-type procyanidin dimer 2, (**B**) amylase-galloyl-paeoniflorin, (**C**) glucosidase-galloyl-paeoniflorin, and (**D**) tyrosinase-taxifolin. Hydrogen bond donor, hydrogen bond acceptor, hydrophobic, and π–π stacking interactions are represented by green arrows, red arrows, yellow spheres, and blue rings, respectively.

Ethyl gallate (**7**) and paeoniflorigenone (**26**) exhibited notable binding affinities toward AChE (−9.6 and −9.0 kcal/mol, respectively). Ethyl gallate interacts with Ser203 and His447 from the catalytic triad by serving as a hydrogen-bond donor (HBD) (Figure 4). Additionally, it binds to Trp86 from the anionic site via HBD and π–π stacking interactions and to Tyr337 from the peripheral anionic site (PAS) through hydrogen-bond acceptor (HBA) interactions involving two carbonyl oxygens. Moreover, the ethyl group establishes a rich pattern of hydrophobic interactions with Val294, Phe338, Tyr341, Phe297, and Trp286.

In addition, pentagalloyl-hexose (**4**) and B-type procyanidin dimer 2 (**11**) displayed the highest binding activities of −11.6 kcal/mol toward BuChE. The ligand-interaction diagram for the BChE-**4** complex (Figure 4A) illustrates interactions with Trp82 and Phe329 from the anionic site, as well as with Tyr332 from the PAS, which stabilize this structure. Galloyl-paeoniflorin (**23**) showed the highest binding affinities toward amylase and glucosidase (−9.5 and −8.5 kcal/mol, respectively) among all compounds identified in the chemical profile of root extracts, indicating the significant role of *Paeonia* terpenes in the overall biological activities. The most important protein–ligand interactions for binding to these two enzymes are displayed in Figures 4B and 5C. Finally, taxifolin (**31**) exhibited the highest binding affinity to tyrosinase (−8.6 kcal/mol), attributed to hydrogen-bonding interactions of the taxifolin B-ring with His60 and catalytic water 407, which bridges two cooper cations within the active site of the enzyme.

In order to fully explore the pharmaceutical potential of the high-affinity compounds identified through molecular docking, it is essential to conduct experimental validation of their binding affinity and binding kinetics. Furthermore, optimizing their pharmacokinetic properties to enhance drug-likeness is likely necessary for the development of viable drug candidates.

2.8. Antibacterial Activity of Root Extracts

In humans, *Listeria monocytogenes*, *Staphylococcus aureus*, and *Escherichia coli* are of the GIT and urogenital tract (UGT), including gastroenteritis, hemorrhagic colitis, urinary infections, and other GIT- and UGT-related disorders [68,69]. While the use of synthetic drugs has lowered the severity and spread of many infectious diseases, food toxoinfections remain the leading cause of death in both high- and low-income countries. Synthetic anti-inflammatory medications have come under investigation due to the recent advances in our comprehension of the human GIT, digestion, intestinal peristalsis, and similar.

The bacteria selected for the present study were chosen based on several factors. First, *L. monocytogenes* NCTC 7973, *S. aureus* ATCC 11632, and *Bacillus cereus* human isolate were selected due to their significance as common pathogens known to cause foodborne illnesses and infections in humans. Additionally, these bacteria represent a range of Gram-positive species, providing insight into the efficacy of the tested antimicrobial agents against this bacterial group. Furthermore, three Gram-negative bacteria species were included, namely, *Salmonella* Typhimurium ATCC 13311, *Pseudomonas aeruginosa* ATCC 27853, and *E. coli* ATCC 25922. These bacteria were chosen to broaden the scope of the study and assess the antimicrobial activity against Gram-negative pathogens, which are also prevalent causes of various infectious diseases. Finally, the selection of these bacterial strains aimed to provide a comprehensive evaluation of the antimicrobial agents under investigation across different bacterial types, encompassing both Gram-positive and Gram-negative species commonly associated with human infections and food contamination. Some literature reports suggest that polyphenols (phenolic acids, flavonoids, anthocyanins, condensed tannins, etc.) are the main class of active compounds in medicinal plants associated with antibacterial activity [70,71]. Also, the antibacterial activity can be attributed to the number and position of hydroxyl and carboxylic groups in the benzoic ring of phenol-carboxylic acids [16,70]. Much effort has been focused on plant medicinal formulations and their bioconstituents as potential sources of valuable antibacterial agents for the prevention or eradication of *Salmonella*, *E. coli*, and other pathogens. In particular, it was reported that some *Paeonia* species had growth-inhibitory activity toward human GIT pathogens [72].

Herein, water–ethanolic extracts of PT, PP, and PO were analyzed as a potential source of antibacterial agents intended for use in the therapeutic treatment of the disease of human GIT.

The results of the antibacterial activity tested by the broth microdilution method are summarized in Table 7. The antimicrobial assay showed that extracts of PT, PP, and PO can inhibit the growth of the tested bacterial strains. Minimal inhibitory concentration (MIC) values range from 0.125 to 4.0 mg/mL, and minimal bactericidal concentration (MBC) values range from 0.25 to 8.0 mg/mL. The PP extract (Južni Kučaj) obtained by the M method had the highest antibacterial activity against *B. cereus* (Gram-negative), followed by roots from Golina and Bogovo gumno (both prepared by M method). Further, the PO extract (Rujevica) obtained by the M method shows a lower ability to inhibit bacterial growth, being the most effective against *L. monocytogenes* (Gram-positive) and *P. aeruginosa* (Gram-negative). Similarly, the extract of PT shows slightly poorer antimicrobial activity compared to PP and PO, except for roots originating from Bogovo gumno (obtained by UAE and M).

Table 7. Antibacterial activity of the root extracts of *Paeonia tenuifolia* L., *Paeonia peregrina* Mill., and *Paeonia officinalis* L. expressed as MIC and MBC (mg/mL).

Plant Species (Root Extract)	Locality	Extraction Method	*Salmonella* Typhimurium		*Listeria monocytogenes*		*Bacillus cereus*		*Pseudomonas aeruginosa*		*Staphylococcus aureus*		*Escherichia coli*	
			MIC	MBC	MIC	MBC	MIC	MBC	MIC	MBC	MIC	MBC	MIC	MBC
PT	Gulenovci	MAE	2.0	4.0	4.0	8.0	2.0	4.0	4.0	8.0	4.0	8.0	2.0	4.0
	Deliblato sand		1.0	2.0	2.0	4.0	2.0	4.0	2.0	4.0	2.0	4.0	2.0	4.0
	Bogovo gumno		4.0	8.0	4.0	8.0	4.0	8.0	4.0	8.0	4.0	8.0	2.0	4.0
	Gulenovci	UAE	1.0	2.0	1.0	2.0	0.5	1.0	1.0	2.0	2.0	4.0	1.0	2.0
	Deliblato sand		2.0	4.0	1.0	2.0	1.0	2.0	2.0	4.0	2.0	4.0	1.0	2.0
	Bogovo gumno		0.5	1.0	1.0	2.0	1.0	2.0	0.5	1.0	2.0	4.0	1.0	2.0
	Gulenovci	M	1.0	2.0	2.0	4.0	1.0	2.0	1.0	2.0	1.0	2.0	1.0	2.0
	Deliblato sand		1.0	2.0	1.0	2.0	1.0	2.0	1.0	2.0	2.0	4.0	1.0	2.0
	Bogovo gumno		2.0	4.0	1.0	2.0	1.0	2.0	1.0	2.0	2.0	4.0	0.5	1.0
PP	Pirot	MAE	4.0	8.0	4.0	8.0	4.0	8.0	4.0	8.0	4.0	8.0	4.0	8.0
	Južni Kučaj		2.0	4.0	2.0	4.0	1.0	2.0	2.0	4.0	2.0	4.0	1.0	2.0
	Golina		2.0	4.0	2.0	4.0	1.0	2.0	1.0	2.0	2.0	4.0	1.0	2.0
	Bogovo gumno		4.0	8.0	4.0	8.0	2.0	4.0	4.0	8.0	2.0	4.0	2.0	4.0
	Krivi vir		2.0	4.0	2.0	4.0	2.0	4.0	1.0	2.0	2.0	4.0	2.0	4.0
	Pančevo		4.0	8.0	2.0	4.0	1.0	2.0	2.0	4.0	2.0	4.0	0.5	1.0
	Pirot	UAE	2.0	4.0	1.0	2.0	1.0	2.0	2.0	4.0	2.0	4.0	1.0	2.0
	Južni Kučaj		1.0	2.0	1.0	2.0	1.0	2.0	1.0	2.0	1.0	2.0	2.0	4.0
	Golina		4.0	8.0	2.0	4.0	1.0	2.0	2.0	4.0	2.0	4.0	1.0	2.0
	Bogovo gumno		1.0	2.0	1.0	2.0	1.0	2.0	1.0	2.0	2.0	4.0	1.0	2.0
	Krivi vir		4.0	8.0	1.0	2.0	1.0	2.0	2.0	4.0	4.0	8.0	1.0	2.0
	Pančevo		1.0	2.0	1.0	2.0	2.0	4.0	0.5	1.0	2.0	4.0	2.0	4.0
	Pirot	M	1.0	2.0	0.5	1.0	0.5	1.0	1.0	2.0	1.0	2.0	1.0	2.0
	Južni Kučaj		1.0	2.0	1.0	2.0	0.125	0.25	1.0	2.0	1.0	2.0	0.5	1.0
	Golina		1.0	2.0	1.0	2.0	0.25	0.5	1.0	2.0	1.0	2.0	0.5	1.0
	Bogovo gumno		1.0	2.0	0.5	1.0	1.0	2.0	0.5	1.0	2.0	4.0	1.0	2.0
	Krivi vir		0.5	1.0	1.0	2.0	0.25	0.5	0.5	1.0	0.5	1.0	0.5	1.0
	Pančevo		1.0	2.0	2.0	4.0	1.0	2.0	1.0	2.0	2.0	4.0	0.5	1.0
PO	Rujevica	MAE	2.0	4.0	2.0	4.0	2.0	4.0	2.0	4.0	2.0	4.0	2.0	4.0
	Božurna		2.0	4.0	1.0	2.0	0.5	1.0	2.0	4.0	2.0	4.0	0.5	1.0
	Rujevica	UAE	2.0	4.0	1.0	2.0	0.5	1.0	0.5	1.0	2.0	4.0	1.0	2.0
	Božurna		1.0	2.0	1.0	2.0	0.5	1.0	0.5	1.0	2.0	4.0	1.0	2.0
	Rujevica	M	1.0	2.0	0.25	0.5	0.5	1.0	0.25	0.5	1.0	2.0	0.5	1.0
	Božurna		1.0	2.0	1.0	2.0	0.5	1.0	0.5	1.0	1.0	2.0	0.5	1.0

MAE: microwave-assisted extraction; UAE: ultrasound-assisted extraction; M: maceration; MIC: minimal inhibitory concentration; MBC: minimal bactericidal concentration; GALAE: galanthamine equivalents; ACAE: acarbose equivalents; KAE: kojic acid equivalents; AChE: acetylcholinesterase; BuChE: butyrylcholinesterase; PT: *Paeonia tenuifolia* L.; PP: *Paeonia peregrina* Mill.; PO: *Paeonia officinalis* L. The antibacterial study was repeated three times (n = 3); the highest values obtained in the test were used as MIC and MBC (like with most antimicrobial tests, the "stricter criteria" rule was applied).

The extraction method proven to produce the most effective antibacterial agents is the M method, due to the fact that the M method is a cold extraction method, without an aggressive regime of extraction, so the high ratio of preservation of polyphenols, the carriers of antimicrobial activity, is completely enabled.

On the other hand, the results of phytochemical screening suggest that the obtained macerates of PT, PP, and PO abound in the content of phenolic acid, flavonoids, and other phenol-core-related substances. To date, the exact mode of action of polyphenols or other bioactive molecules found in the different herbaceous *Paeonia* root extracts on bacteria has not been well documented. Namely, there are several hypotheses suggesting that polyphenols from plant sources can disrupt the bacterial cell wall and cytoplasmic membrane, which leads to the dissolution of the protein fraction and the leaching out of essential ions/biomolecules (K^+, PO_4^{3-}, nucleic acids, etc.), reducing the cellular activity of bacteria [73–75]. Flavonoids can inhibit cell membrane functions, energy metabolism, and the synthesis of DNA and RNA material through the mechanism of linkage with the soluble protein fractions located outside the cell walls of bacteria, or nucleic material might be broken down into small pieces after the flavonoids enter the cell [76,77].

Based on the results of our experiment, it is evident that the tested extracts of PP and PO exhibit potent antibacterial activity and contribute to significantly lower survival of bacteria, which are the most common mediators of health problems in human GIT. According to Aligiannis et al. [78], extracts with MIC values up to 0.5 mg/mL can be classified as strong inhibitors of bacteria and can be useful for therapeutic applications.

Furthermore, a correlation between the achieved antibacterial activity of the tested root extracts and their chemical assembly insinuates that the observed activity can be attributed to the high presence of the major extract phytoconstituents (e.g., gallic acid, catechin, myristicin, and taxifolin). Since the extracts of PT, PP, and PO are complex and impure mixtures, their antibacterial activities vary in accordance with the biological molecules that they include. Moreover, strong antibacterial activity can be a result of the synergistic effect that is formed by the active molecules coming together. There is also an assumption that some differences in antibacterial activity observed for three *Paeonia* root samples might be attributed to environmental factors and/or possible plant infection that might interfere during the synthesis of antibacterial active compounds [74].

Finally, the comparison of all determined antibacterial effects indicated that the general susceptibility of the pathogens in the tested extracts of PT, PP, and PO could be given in the following order: the most sensitive were isolates of *B. cereus*, followed by *P. aeruginosa*, *E. coli*, and *L. monocytogenes*. As mentioned, it seems that the M method had a superior effect on the preservation of polyphenols compared to the other two extraction techniques, enabling the best impact on the antibacterial activity of root extracts.

2.9. Simulated In Vitro GID and Bioaccessibility

A total of 58 bioactive compounds (BCs) were identified in various water extracts—tea samples before and after *in vitro* gastrointestinal digestion (GID). All identified BCs were categorized into different classes and subclasses: (1) phenolic acids and derivatives (primarily gallic acid, ellagic acid, and their derivatives); (2) flavonoid and derivatives (primarily flavan-3-ols and procyanidins); and (3) terpenoids of *Paeonia* root. The relative content of total identified terpenoids was similar in all control tea samples (30.53–34.66%), mainly due to the high relative content of paeoniflorin (Table 8). On the other hand, the relative contents of total phenolic acids and flavonoid derivatives in control tea samples were different and strongly depended on the peony root species (Table 8). Thus, flavan-3-ols and procyanidins (catechin, chalcan flavan-3-ol dimer isomer I, and B-type procyanidin dimer and trimer isomers) predominated in the PTc (control (initial) PT tea) and PPc (control (initial) PP tea samples) (46.39–49.82%), while gallic acid derivatives (33.59%) and ellagic acid (4.18%) were the most abundant in POc (control (initial) PO tea) (Table 8). The PTc control tea had the highest total relative content of identified BCs, while their relative content was lower at 7.63% and 21% in the PPc and POc control tea samples, respectively.

Table 8. Relative content of identified bioactive compounds (%) in tea samples before and after GID using UHPLC Q-ToF MS.

No.	Compound Name	Relative Content (%) *					
		PTc	DPT	PPc	DPP	POc	DPO
	Phenolic acids and derivatives						
	Gallic acid and derivatives						
1	Gallic acid	0.69	0.27	1.10	0.19	2.24	0.38
2	Methyl gallate	0.09	7.14	0.18	3.80	2.34	21.30
3	Gallic acid derivative	0.79	0.14	0.14	0.03	1.05	0.08
4	Digallic acid isomer I	0.21	0.05	-	-	1.00	-
5	Digallic acid isomer II	0.52	0.09	0.19	-	1.58	0.05
6	Gallic acid hexoside	1.21	0.62	1.62	0.62	1.54	0.41
7	Methyl digallate	0.22	1.21	-	0.11	0.03	1.70
8	Methyl gallic acid hexoside	0.06	-	0.34	0.06	0.05	-
9	Galloyl-vanilloyl-rhamoside	0.31	0.11	0.06	-	2.82	1.57
10	Gallic acid dihexoside	7.98	2.44	4.26	1.21	13.70	5.01
11	Galloyl-HHDP-hexose isomer II	0.97	0.11	0.44	0.04	1.58	0.15
12	Galloyl-HHDP-hexose isomer I	0.78	0.10	0.50	-	1.21	0.08
13	Trigalloyl-hexoside	0.33	0.08	0.26	0.09	-	-
14	Digalloyl-HHDP-protoquercitol	0.14	-	0.20	0.12	0.75	0.53
15	Tetragalloyl-hexoside	0.17	0.12	0.35	0.19	1.31	0.61
16	Pentagalloyl-hexoside	0.39	0.33	0.43	0.30	2.40	1.50
	∑	14.66	12.83	10.07	6.64	33.59	33.38
	Ellagic acid and derivatives						
17	Ellagic acid	0.83	0.29	2.37	0.73	4.18	1.53
18	Methyl ellagic acid	0.41	0.19	0.80	0.28	1.25	0.43
19	Dimethyl ellagic acid	0.13	0.04	0.20	0.19	1.19	1.49
20	Trimethyl ellagic acid	-	-	1.48	1.12	0.06	0.07
21	Ellagic acid hexoside	0.35	0.03	0.45	0.06	0.82	0.11
22	Methyl ellagic acid hexoside	0.46	0.18	0.28	0.12	0.52	0.22
	∑	2.18	0.73	5.58	2.50	8.03	3.86
	Other phenolic acids and their glycosides						
23	Hydroxybenzoic acid	1.26	0.84	1.46	1.10	1.98	1.33
24	Dihydroxybenzoic acid isomer I	0.38	-	0.50	-	0.29	-
25	Dihydroxybenzoic acid isomer II	0.15	0.0.04	-	-	0.45	0.25
26	Dihydroxybenzoic acid hexoside	0.23	0.18	0.45	0.27	0.77	0.25
27	Vanillic acid hexoside	0.39	0.10	1.12	0.33	0.16	-
	∑	2.42	1.16	3.53	1.70	3.64	1.83
	∑RC of total phenolic acid	19.26	14.71	19.18	10.84	45.26	39.06
	Flavonoids and derivatives						
	Flavan-3-ols and procyanidins						
28	Catechin	13.86	12.97	16.28	12.58	5.08	2.57
29	Epicatechin	1.10	0.74	2.57	1.74	0.65	0.27
30	Methyl epigallocatechin	0.14	0.02	0.13	-	0.12	-
31	Epicatechin-gallate	0.27	0.21	0.16	-	0.04	-
32	Catechin hexoside	0.81	0.56	3.92	3.66	4.35	3.00
33	Epicatechin-hexoside	0.38	0.22	0.55	0.41	0.21	-
34	B-type procyanidin dimer isomer I	22.20	18.55	8.88	1.94	6.02	2.35
35	B-type procyanidin dimer isomer II	1.12	0.82	2.58	2.35	0.67	0.43
36	Chalcan flavan-3-ols dimer isomer II	0.20	0.16	0.87	0.50	-	-
37	Chalcan flavan-3-ol dimer isomer I	6.41	6.08	7.11	4.88	0.71	0.23
38	Methyl B-type prodelphinidin	0.27	-	0.26	-	0.21	-
39	Procyanidin trimer B-type isomer I	2.48	1.85	2.72	2.39	0.50	0.38
40	Procyanidin trimer B-type isomer II	0.58	0.18	0.37	-	0.08	-
	∑	49.82	42.35	46.39	42.02	18.65	9.24

Table 8. *Cont.*

No.	Compound Name	Relative Content (%) *					
		PTc	DPT	PPc	DPP	POc	DPO
				Other detected flavonoids			
41	Kaempferol	0.06	-	0.08	0.04	0.04	0.02
42	Naringenin	0.07	0.07	0.12	0.12	0.14	0.17
43	Phloridzin	0.26	0.33	0.36	0.45	1.25	1.22
	∑	0.39	0.40	0.56	0.61	1.43	1.41
	∑RC of total flavonoids	50.21	42.75	46.94	31.06	20.07	10.65
				Peonia root terpenoids			
44	Nor-paeonilactone	-	-	0.08	0.03	0.18	-
45	Paeoveitol D	0.91	0.58	0.71	-	0.64	-
46	Paeonisothujone	0.57	0.03	0.44	-	1.44	-
47	Paeonilactone B	0.34	0.09	0.46	0.21	0.93	0.23
48	Paeonilactone A	-	-	0.39	0.22	1.73	-
49	9-Hydroxypaeonilactone A	0.09	-	2.55	0.67	1.07	-
50	Paeoniflorigenone	0.31	0.18	4.22	7.18	2.66	1.96
51	Oxypaeoniflorin	6.18	5.53	4.81	4.14	5.02	4.66
52	Mudanpioside D	-	-	0.23	0.22	-	-
53	Paeoniflorin + HCOOH	12.91	8.61	14.17	13.28	15.72	10.24
54	Albiflorin + HCOOH	3.64	4.36	3.29	3.40	1.96	2.19
55	Galloyl desbenzoyl paeoniflorin	0.82	0.39	0.84	0.26	-	-
56	Benzoyl paeoniflorin	-	-	-	-	0.21	0.11
57	Mudanpioside J	1.03	1.10	0.26	0.24	1.39	1.30
58	Galloyl-paeoniflorin	3.74	3.58	1.44	0.73	1.72	1.32
	∑RC of total terpenoids	30.53	24.45	33.88	30.58	34.66	22.03
		100	-	100	-	100	-
	**	100	-	92.37	-	79.00	-

GID: digestion in the gastrointestinal tract; * The relative content (%) of bioactive compounds in each sample (before and after gastrointestinal digestion) (share of total area is defined as 100% for each sample). ** Comparison of the share of total identified bioactive compounds among tea samples. "-" nonidentified compounds. DPT: digested of *Paeonia tenuifolia* tea; PTc: control (initial) *Paeonia tenuifolia* tea; DPP: digested of *Paeonia peregrina* tea; PPc: control (initial) *Paeonia peregrina* tea; DPO: digested of *Paeonia officinalis* tea; POc: control (initial) *Paeonia officinalis* tea.

The recovery of total and individual BCs of the tea samples after *in vitro* gastrointestinal digestion is shown in Table 9. As can be seen, a total recovery of all identified BCs was reduced and similar for all digested tea samples (DPT–digested of PT tea, DPP–digested of PP tea, and DPO–digested of PO tea) and ranged from 71.75 to 81.91%. These results are higher or similar to those reported by Qin et al. [79] and Koláčková et al. [80] for the recovery of total phenolic compounds of green tea infusion after GID (68.71% and 62–84%, respectively), but they are significantly higher than the recovery of total phenolic compounds of teas prepared from the flowers of *P. lactiflora* (21.25%) [81] and *P. suffruticosa* (12.63%) [82]. On the other hand, an increase in the total amount of total phenolic compounds was found for Guayusa after an *in vitro* GID of 3% [83]. However, the recovery for each identified compound was different and was highly dependent on their structure, their tendency to react with digestive enzymes, solubilization in the digestive cocktail, and their presence in the initial sample [84–86]. The majority of the identified phenolic acid derivatives showed reduced recovery, with the exception of methyl gallate and methyl digallate, whose relative content (Table 8) and recovery (Table 9) increased significantly after *in vitro* GID. It is known that peony root is a rich source of various galloylated macromolecules (tannins or some carbohydrates) from which the methyl gallate derivatives were probably released. This is also confirmed by the significantly lower recovery of all identified high-molecular-weight galloyl derivatives (compounds **8–16**, Table 9). In addition, some high-molecular-weight galloyl derivatives were digested but not detected in the initial tea samples, as they were probably removed by filtration prior to chromatographic analysis. The high percentage of released methyl gallate in the digested tea samples was due to the high recovery of total phenolic acid derivatives (56.53–86.30%). A high recovery of phenolic acid derivatives after GID was also observed by Kelebek et al. [83] for Guayusa tea. These results may contribute significantly to the future evaluation of the biological activity of peony root tea, as methyl gallate has been shown to have a variety of biological functions [87]. Ellagic acid and its derivatives exhibited lower recovery after *in vitro* GID (Table 9), except for the recovery of dimethyl and trimethyl ellagic acid (DPP and DPO). However, their relative contents in the initial PPc and POc were low (about 1%, Table 8), so they have no significant effect on the overall recovery of total phenolic acid derivatives. As expected, the flavan-3-ols and procyanidins showed lower recovery, as these molecules have a high tendency to react with enzymes and compounds of the digestive cocktail [86,88]. Other authors also reported a low recovery of flavan-3-ols from green tea flowers [80,89] and *P. lactiflora* Pall. flower tea [81]. Other detected flavonoids were present in trace amounts, so their recovery has a negligible effect on the recovery of total flavonoid derivatives. The majority of the detected monoterpenoids (compounds **44–49**, Table 9) and galloyl/benzoyl paeoniflorin derivatives (compounds **55**, **56**, and **58**, Table 9), showed low recovery or were not found in digested tea samples. However, the predominantly found paeoniflorin and its derivatives (oxypaeoniflorin, paeoniflorigenone, with the exception of DPP, and the selectively detected mudanpioside) showed a reduced recovery after *in vitro* GID. Albiflorin, on the other hand, showed an increased recovery, as it was probably released during digestion.

It is worth mentioning that in vivo studies have reported low bioavailability of paeoniflorin, only 2.3% [90], which is due to poor permeation and its hydrolysis by the gut mircrobiota to various metabolites such as benzoic acid, paeoniflorgenin, 7S- or 7R-paeonimetabolin I, paeonimetabolin II, and sinomenine [91].

Table 9. Recovery of total and individual bioactive compounds detected in the selected *Paeonia* root teas after *in vitro* GID using UHPLC Q-ToF MS. The expected retention time (RT), molecular formula, and exact *m*/*z* mass of the confirmed compounds are presented in Table 1.

No	RT	Compound Name	Formula	*m/z* Exact Mass	Recovery after In Vitro GID (%) DPT	DPP	DPO	Recovery Range (%)
			Phenolic acids and derivatives					
			Gallic acid and derivatives					
1	1.14	Gallic acid	$C_7H_5O_5^-$	169.01443	39.18	17.11	17.02	17.02–39.18
2	4.24	Methyl gallate	$C_8H_7O_5^-$	183.02825	7538.45	2060.68	910.95	910.95–7538.45
3	1.75	Gallic acid derivative	$C_{10}H_{11}O_7^-$	243.05244	17.62	20.88	7.57	7.57–20.88
4	3.77	Digallic acid isomer I	$C_{14}H_9O_9^-$	321.02654	23.72	-	0	0–23.72
5	5.59	Digallic acid isomer II	$C_{14}H_9O_9^-$	321.02743	17.21	0	3.11	3.11–17.21
6	0.90	Gallic acid hexoside	$C_{13}H_{15}O_{10}^-$	331.06817	50.75	38.39	26.64	26.64–50.75
7	8.02	Methyl digallate	$C_{15}H_{11}O_9^-$	335.04267	5484	**	5686.48	>5484
8	1.75	Methyl gallic acid hexoside	$C_{14}H_{17}O_{10}^-$	345.08617	0	16.97	0	0–16.97
9	7.34	Galloyl-vanilloyl-rhamoside	$C_{21}H_{21}O_{12}^-$	465.10780	35.54	0	55.84	0–55.84
10	1.00	Gallic acid dihexoside	$C_{19}H_{25}O_{15}^-$	493.12260	30.64	28.33	36.54	28.33–36.54
11	5.93	Galloyl-HHDP-hexose isomer II	$C_{27}H_{21}O_{18}^-$	633.07382	11.28	9.49	9.24	9.24–11.28
12	2.89	Galloyl-HHDP-hexose isomer I	$C_{27}H_{21}O_{18}^-$	633.07577	13.45	0	6.82	0–13.45
13	6.80	Trigalloyl-hexoside	$C_{27}H_{23}O_{18}^-$	635.09260	25.11	34.26	-	25.11–34.26
14	8.15	Digalloyl-HHDP-protoquercitol	$C_{34}H_{27}O_{21}^+$	771.10856	0	60.06	70.22	0–70.22
15	7.55	Tetragalloyl-hexoside	$C_{34}H_{27}O_{22}^-$	787.10066	70.80	54.59	46.96	46.96–70.80
16	7.95	Pentagalloyl-hexoside	$C_{41}H_{31}O_{26}^-$	939.11237	85.75	69.30	62.73	62.73–85.75
		Σ			87.49	65.93	99.37	65.93–99.37

Table 9. *Cont.*

No	RT	Compound Name	Formula	*m/z* Exact Mass	Recovery after In Vitro GID (%) DPT	DPP	DPO	Recovery Range (%)
		Ellagic acid and derivatives						
17	7.68	Ellagic acid	$C_{14}H_5O_8^-$	301.00097	34.42	31.04	36.58	31.04–36.58
18	8.42	Methyl ellagic acid	$C_{15}H_7O_8^-$	315.01710	46.31	35.33	34.48	34.48–46.31
19	9.57	Dimethyl ellagic acid	$C_{16}H_9O_8^-$	329.03194	31.94	95.14	125.18	31.94–125.18
20	10.85	Trimethyl ellagic acid	$C_{17}H_{11}O_8^-$	343.04668	-	75.52	111.78	75.52–111.78
21	6.87	Ellagic acid hexoside	$C_{20}H_{15}O_{13}^-$	463.05601	9.51	12.21	13.09	9.51–13.09
22	7.55	Methyl ellagic acid hexoside	$C_{21}H_{17}O_{13}^-$	477.07058	38.10	43.04	43.03	38.10–43.04
		∑			33.32	44.81	48.03	33.32–48.03
		Other phenolic acids and their glycosides						
23	3.09	Hydroxybenzoic acid	$C_7H_5O_3^-$	137.02422	66.54	75.62	67.07	66.54–75.62
24	1.88	Dihydroxybenzoic acid isomer I	$C_7H_5O_4^-$	153.01946	0	0	0	0
25	5.12	Dihydroxybenzoic acid isomer II	$C_7H_5O_4^-$	153.01911	26.70	-	56.35	26.70–56.35
26	2.36	Hydroxybenzoic acid hexoside	$C_{13}H_{15}O_9^-$	315.07520	79.52	59.13	32.25	32.25–79.52
27	2.96	Vanillic acid hexoside	$C_{14}H_{17}O_9^-$	329.08958	25.02	29.84	0	0–29.84
		∑			48.01	48.25	50.19	48.01–50.19
		∑ Total recovery of phenolic acid and derivatives			76.40	56.53	86.30	56.53–86.30
		Flavonoids and derivatives						
		Flavan-3-ols and procyanidins						
28	5.29	Catechin	$C_{15}H_{13}O_6^-$	289.07260	93.57	77.26	50.61	50.61–93.57
29	6.63	Epicatechin	$C_{15}H_{13}O_6^-$	289.07259	67.61	67.86	41.95	41.95–67.86
30	6.54	Methyl epigallocatechin	$C_{16}H_{15}O_7^-$	319.08293	12.38	0	-	0–12.38
31	7.68	Epicatechin-gallate	$C_{22}H_{17}O_{10}^-$	441.08941	80.00	0	-	0–80.00
32	4.18	Catechin hexoside	$C_{21}H_{23}O_{11}^-$	451.12584	68.83	93.38	69.09	69.09–93.38
33	5.73	Epicatechin-hexoside	$C_{21}H_{25}O_{11}^+$	453.14384	56.80	75.10	-	56.80–75.10
34	4.51	B-type procyanidin dimer isomer I	$C_{30}H_{25}O_{12}^-$	577.13795	83.56	21.80	39.07	21.80–83.56
35	6.33	B-type procyanidin dimer isomer II	$C_{30}H_{25}O_{12}^-$	577.13723	73.12	91.33	63.74	63.74–91.33
36	6.63	Chalcan flavan-3-ols dimer iso. II	$C_{30}H_{27}O_{12}^-$	579.15511	76.98	57.41	-	57.41–76.98
37	5.29	Chalcan flavan-3-ol dimer isomer I	$C_{30}H_{27}O_{12}^-$	579.15287	94.87	68.67	33.12	33.12–94.87
38	6.19	Methyl B-type prodelphinidin	$C_{31}H_{27}O_{13}^-$	607.14904	0	0	-	0
39	6.02	Procyanidin trimer B-type isomer I	$C_{45}H_{37}O_{18}^-$	865.19890	74.33	87.76	75.93	74.33–87.76
40	6.93	Procyanidin trimer B-type isomer II	$C_{45}H_{37}O_{18}^-$	865.19733	31.38	0	-	0–31.38
		∑			85.00	65.65	49.75	49.57–85.00
		Other detected flavonoids						
41	10.16	Kaempferol	$C_{15}H_9O_6^-$	285.04097	0	54.56	52.58	0–54.56
42	9.91	Naringenin	$C_{15}H_{11}O_5^-$	271.06201	102.19	103.78	116.53	102.19–116.53
43	8.49	Phloridzin	$C_{21}H_{23}O_{10}^-$	435.12768	128.75	122.32	98.08	98.08–128.75
		∑			103.34	109.27	98.78	98.78–109.27
		∑ Total recovery of flavonoids and derivatives			85.14	66.16	53.07	53.07–85.14
		Paeonia root terpenoids						
44	9.97	Nor-paeonilactone	$C_9H_{15}O_2^+$	155.10880	-	37.72	-	37.72
45	6.40	Paeoveitol D	$C_{10}H_{11}O_3^+$	179.07217	63.25	0	-	0–63.25
46	6.93	Paeonisothujone	$C_{10}H_{15}O_3^+$	183.10219	4.85	0	-	0–4.85
47	6.60	Paeonilactone B	$C_{10}H_{13}O_4^+$	197.08347	27.44	46.58	25.02	25.02–46.58
48	3.50	Paeonilactone A	$C_{10}H_{15}O_4^+$	199.09852	-	56.27	-	56.27
49	2.62	9-Hydroxypaeonilactone A	$C_{10}H_{15}O_5^+$	215.09411	0	26.31	-	0–26.31
50	10.31	Paeoniflorigenone	$C_{17}H_{19}O_6^+$	319.12118	56.97	170.17	73.95	56.97–170.17

Table 9. *Cont.*

No	RT	Compound Name	Formula	*m/z* Exact Mass	Recovery after In Vitro GID (%)			Recovery Range (%)
					DPT	DPP	DPO	
51	5.82	Oxypaeoniflorin	$C_{23}H_{27}O_{12}^-$	495.15174	89.52	86.15	92.85	86.15–92.85
52	8.90	Mudanpioside D	$C_{24}H_{29}O_{12}^-$	509.17478	-	94.92	-	94.92
53	7.07	Paeoniflorin + HCOOH	$C_{24}H_{29}O_{13}^-$	525.16398	66.69	93.73	65.16	65.16–93.73
54	7.75	Albiflorin + HCOOH	$C_{24}H_{29}O_{13}^-$	525.16361	119.68	103.46	111.85	103.46–119.68
55	2.59	Galloyl desbenzoyl paeoniflorin	$C_{23}H_{27}O_{14}^-$	527.14182	47.83	30.60	-	30.60–47.83
56	10.17	Benzoyl paeoniflorin	$C_{30}H_{33}O_{12}^+$	585.20263	-	-	53.04	53.04
57	9.91	Mudanpioside J	$C_{31}H_{33}O_{14}^-$	629.19505	107.32	91.87	93.54	91.87–107.32
58	7.87	Galloyl-paeoniflorin	$C_{30}H_{31}O_{15}^-$	631.16919	95.80	50.35	77.00	50.35–95.80
		$\sum$ Total recovery of terpenoids			80.09	90.25	63.56	63.56–90.25
		$\sum\sum$ Total recovery of detected bioactive compounds			81.91	72.47	71.75	71.75–81.91

GID: digestion in the gastrointestinal tract; DPT: digested of *Paeonia tenuifola* tea; DPP: digested of *Paeonia peregrina* tea; DPO: digested of *Paeonia officinallis* tea. ** Compound identified also in digested sample. The recovery of total and individual compounds was calculated as the ratio of areas before and after *in vitro* GID. "-" not an identified compound.

3. Materials and Methods

3.1. Origin of Plant Material

The fresh roots of PT, PP, and PO were collected from eleven localities in Serbia. PT were collected from Gulenovci, Deliblato sands, and Bogovo gumno, PP from Pirot, Južni Kučaj, Golina, Bogovo gumno, Krivi vir, and Pančevo while PO were from Rujevica and Božurna. The roots were collected at the end of the vegetation, in September 2022. As all peonies in the Republic of Serbia are protected by law, their collection was conducted with appropriate permission (353–01-162/2022–04, issued on 24 February, Ministry of Environmental Protection of the Republic of Serbia). The voucher specimens of these medicinal plant species were deposited in the herbarium BUNS of the Department of Biology and Ecology at the University of Novi Sad, Faculty of Sciences (Novi Sad, Serbia), where the identification confirmation was performed. Prior to extraction, the collected roots were left to dry in a shaded room for 30 days at 20 °C. Dried roots were ground in the mill (M-20, IKA Universal mill, IKA®, GmbH&Co., Königswinter, Germany) and separated by a sieve to obtain fine particles with a size of 0.75 mm. The powdered roots were stored in a refrigerator (4 °C).

3.2. Chemicals and Reagents

Ethyl alcohol (Zorka Pharma, Šabac, Serbia, 96%, v/v) and distilled water, as a mixture, were used as extraction agents. Methyl alcohol (HPLC grade), Folin-Ciocalteu reagent, gallic acid, catechin hydrate, aluminum chloride, hydrochloric acid, sodium nitrate, sodium chloride, sodium hydroxide, sodium hydrogen carbonate, 6-hydroxy-2,5,7,8-tetramethylchroman-2-carboxylic acid (Trolox), potassium persulfate, salivary α-amylase solution, pancreatin from porcine pancreas, bile acid mixture from bovine and ovine mucin, mucin, and pepsin from porcine stomach were purchased from Sigma-Aldrich, Darmstadt, Germany. L-3,4-dihydroxyphenylalanine, 5,5′-Dithiobis(2-nitrobenzoic acid), acetylcholinesterase from *Electrophorus electricus* (electric eel) Type-VI-S (EC 3.1.1.7), butyrylcholinesterase from equine serum (EC 3.1.1.8), acetylthiocholine iodide, butyrylthiocholine chloride, kojic acid, alpha-amylase *ex-porcine* pancreas (EC 3.2.1.1), acarbose, *p*-iodonitrotetrazoliumviolet (>95%), α-glucosidase solution from *Saccharomyces cerevisiae* (EC 3.2.1.20), Lugol reagents (diluted iodine-potassium iodide solution), ABTS, DPPH, tryptic soy broth (TSB), and formic acid were obtained by Sigma Aldrich, St. Louis, MO, USA. Gentamicin (solution for injection, 40 mg/mL) was bought from Panfarma (Belgrade, Serbia).

3.3. Extraction

3.3.1. MAE

MAE was performed using a method previously reported by Batinić et al. [17]. MAE was carried out at 100 °C using a microwave reactor (Milestone ETHOS X, 2.45 GHz, Milestone, Italy) equipped with a digital infrared temperature sensor that monitors the process temperature and two magnetrons with a maximum operative power of 1.8 kW. All experiments were conducted in three cycles, in the SR-15 rotor with a power of 0.7 kW, in a closed poly(tetrafluoroethylene) Teflon vessel (0.1 L), using a magnetic stirring bar (12 × 30 mm) for uniform mixing (the mixing speed was software-controlled; magnetic stirring of solution up to a speed of 3400 rpm). Ethyl alcohol with 50% water, an extraction time of 2 min, and a solid-to-solvent ratio of 1:10 were employed in the MAE. Following the extraction process, permeate was separated from retentate using a laboratory glass funnel and cellulose-acetate filter (25 mm, 0.45 μm). The solvent was removed using vacuum evaporation (Rotavapor Heidolph 4001-efficient, Heidolph Instruments, Schwabach, Germany) at a temperature of 45 °C and a pressure of 0.180 ± 0.05 bar. The extracts were stored in the refrigerator at 4 °C before analysis.

3.3.2. UAE

UAE was performed in the ultrasound bath (Digital ultrasonic cleaner bath, DU-32, 40 kHz, 100 W, Argo LAB, Carpi—MO, Italy) with a maximal useful volume of 3.2 L. The method was previously described by Batinić et al. [17]. The roots were placed in a 0.1 L flask, and an extraction agent, ethyl alcohol (50%, *v*/*v*), was added (the solid-to-solvent ratio was 1:10). The Erlenmeyer flask with a sample was immersed in the ultrasonic bath and sonicated for 30 min at 30 °C. After sonication, the extracts were filtered through the cellulose-acetate filter (25 mm, 0.45 μm), while the solvent was removed using a rotary vapor evaporator at 45 °C at 0.180 ± 0.05 bar. The extracts were stored at 4 °C prior to analysis.

3.3.3. M Method

The M method in an Erlenmeyer flask (0.1 L) was performed on a tube roller mixer (Stuart, SRT-6, Germany) with agitation fixed at 200 rpm, at 30 °C [17]. The volume of extraction agent (ethyl alcohol, 50%, *v*/*v*) was 0.01 L, the solid-to-solvent ratio was 1:10, and the extraction time was 30 min. Dry extracts were obtained using vacuum evaporation, as described in the previous section. The extracts were stored at 4 °C until further measurements.

3.3.4. Preparation of Hot Water Extracts (Teas)

PT (Gulenovci), PP (Pirot), and PO (Rujevica) were selected for the study of *in vitro* simulated GID as they proved to be most effective against tested pathogens, and they also have significant enzyme-inhibitory potential. Also, as previous tests show, they possess a prominent potential to neutralize ABTS and DPPH radicals. Finely ground root samples (4 g) were mixed with 40 mL of boiling water and gently stirred on a mechanical shaker for 30 min. The hot water extracts were prepared according to the standard procedure for the preparation of teas from the roots of *Althaea officinalis* [92]. The samples were then centrifuged at 4000 rpm for 5 min, and liquid fractions (teas) were freeze-dried and used for *in vitro* gastrointestinal digestion.

3.4. Chemical and Structural Analysis

3.4.1. UHPLC-LTQ-OrbiTrap MS Analysis

Selected *Paeonia* extracts obtained using the UAE method are included in the UHPLC-LTQ-OrbiTrap MS analysis with the aim of identifying and quantifying their individual compounds. The experiments were performed using a liquid chromatography system (Thermo Fisher Scientific, Karlsruhe, Germany), which consisted of an Accela autosampler and quaternary Accela 600 pump connected to the orbitrap hybrid mass spectrometer (LTQ

OrbiTrap XL, Thermo Fisher Scientific, Karlsruhe, Germany) with heated electrospray ionization, operating in positive and negative ionization modes. Separations were conducted on a Syncronis™ C18 reversed-phase column (50 × 2.1 mm, 1.7 μm) from Thermo Fisher Scientific (Karlsruhe, Germany). The molecular editor software ChemDraw (ChemDraw 12.0, Waltham, MA, USA) was used for drawing the structure of organic molecules and for calculating the molecular masses of the active compounds of interest. The software Xcalibur (Xcalibur 2.1, Thermo Fisher Scientific, Waltham, MA, USA) was used for instrument control, data acquisition, and data analysis. Deprotonated molecule mass $[M-H]^-$ and MS^2, MS^3, and MS^4 fragmentation patterns were used for the identification of active compounds in the extract with the assistance of the available spectroscopic, accurate mass, and MS fragmentation data from the literature [15,16,19,20,93].

3.4.2. FTIR Analysis

FTIR spectroscopy is an effective and non-destructive method of instrumental analysis for the differentiation and characterization of organic or inorganic materials, natural products, drugs, etc. by observing the individual bands or functional groups to precisely identify the molecular conformations, bonding types, and physical or chemical interactions that compose the sample. FTIR spectral analysis was recorded using an ATR-IR spectrometer (Nicolet™ iS™, Thermo Fisher Scientific, Waltham, MA, USA) in the wavenumber range between 500 and 4000 cm^{-1}, with 64 accumulations, and a resolution of 4 cm^{-1}, at 25 ± 5 °C. The method was previously described by Batinić et al. [17]. The FTIR analysis was performed by fixing 20 mg of dry root extract (prepared by vacuum evaporation as previously described) to a brazed diamond crystal plate for smart orbit (Thermo Fischer Scientific, Waltham, MA, USA). FTIR spectra were recorded in ATR mode and corrected by the OMNIC spectroscopy software (OMNIC™ Series software 9.8.635, Thermo Fisher Scientific, Waltham, MA, USA). A graphic view of spectra and deconvolution were conducted in the OriginPro 9.0 software (OriginLab Co., Northampton, MA, USA).

3.4.3. Determination of TPC

The TPC in the dry root extracts of PT, PP, and PO was determined by a modified Folin-Ciocalteu method [16,94]. The extract (0.02 mL, 1 mg/mL) was mixed with 0.1 mL of Folin-Ciocalteu phenol reagent (previously diluted 2-fold with distilled water), after which 0.3 mL of sodium carbonate solution (20%, *w/v*) was added, and the mixture was made up to 2 mL with distilled water. After 120 min of incubation at 25 ± 5 °C, the absorbance (λ_{max} = 765 nm) was read against a blank using a UV/Visible scanning spectrophotometer (UV/Vis 1800, Shimadzu, Tokyo, Japan). The analytical standard of gallic acid (GA) was used for the construction of the calibration curve (0.1–1.6 mg/mL), while the amount of polyphenols was expressed as milligrams of GA equivalents per gram of dry extract (mg GAE/g).

3.4.4. Determination of TFC

The TFC in the dry root extracts of PT, PP, and PO was estimated colorimetrically using the aluminum chloride colorimetric assay based on the experimental procedure given by Shraim et al. [95]. In brief, an aliquot of 0.25 mL of extract (1 mg/mL) was mixed with 0.075 mL of sodium nitrite solution (5%, *w/v*) and 1.25 mL of distilled water. After 5 min, 0.15 mL of aluminum chloride solution (10%, *w/v*) was added to the mixture, and 1 min later, 0.5 mL of sodium hydroxide solution (1 mol/L) was also added to complete the reaction. The final volume was made up of 3 mL of distilled water. Then, the mixture was gently mixed (Vortex 3, IKA®, Königswinter, Germany) and the tube containing the mixture was kept in the dark for 30 min prior to UV/Vis analysis. The analytical standard of catechin (CA) was used for the construction of the calibration curve (0.037–0.3 mg/mL). The absorbance (λ_{max} = 510 nm) was measured against a blank using a UV/visible scanning spectrophotometer, while TFC was expressed as CA equivalents per gram of dry extract (mg CAE/g).

3.5. Determination of Free Radical Scavenging Activity

ABTS and DPPH Assays

The free radical scavenging activity of the liquid root extracts (obtained at different extraction methods) was determined using two assays—ABTS and DPPH tests. The basis of the ABTS assay is the interaction between polyphenol antioxidants and the pregenerated $ABTS^{\bullet+}$ radical cation. $ABTS^{\bullet+}$ can be easily quantitatively detected due to the bleaching of absorption spectrum characteristic maxima at 734–757 nm, depending on the solvatochromic effects of the solvent used for extraction. Usually, $ABTS^{\bullet+}$ is pregenerated a day before by mixing $ABTS^{\bullet+}$ solution (4×10^{-3} g/mL) with 0.088 mL of potassium persulfate (2.45×10^{-3} mol/L) and standing overnight (12–16 h) at 0–4 °C to complete the reaction of radical activation (the end of the reaction can be easily observed by a color change from deep to bluish-green). Following activation, the ABTS stock solution was diluted with ethyl alcohol (50%, v/v) to reach an absorbance of 0.700 ± 0.020 at 753 nm. Then, 2.8 mL of ABTS stock solution was mixed with 0.2 mL of extract, while the blank was prepared by mixing the same amount of ABTS stock solution with 0.2 mL of extraction agent (ethyl alcohol, 50% v/v). After 30 min of incubation in the dark at 20 ± 5 °C, the antioxidant activity of the extracts was determined by measuring the absorbance compared to the blank. The radical scavenging activity (RSA_{ABTS}) was calculated according to the following equation:

$$RSA_{ABTS}\ (\%) = \frac{A_0 - Ax}{A_0} \times 100 \tag{1}$$

where A_0 represents the absorbance of $ABTS^{\bullet+}$ solution, while A_x is the absorbance of $ABTS^{\bullet+}$ solution and the extract. Trolox was used as a standard for the calibration curve (0.030–1.0 mg/mL). The RSA_{ABTS} was expressed as µg Trolox equivalents (TE) per mL of extract (µg TE/mL).

The principle of the DPPH assay is based on the reduction of $DPPH^{\bullet}$, which has an absorption maximum at 517 nm. The $DPPH^{\bullet}$ stock solution was prepared by dissolving 0.252 mg of DPPH in 9 mL of ethyl alcohol (96%, v/v). For the photometric assay, 2.8 mL of $DPPH^{\bullet}$ stock solution and 0.2 mL of extract were mixed. The blank was prepared by mixing 2.8 mL of $DPPH^{\bullet}$ stock solution with 0.2 mL of ethyl alcohol (50% v/v). The absorbance reading was taken after 30 min of incubation in a dark place (20 ± 5 °C) against a blank at 517 nm. The radical scavenging activity (RSA_{DPPH}) was calculated according to the following equation:

$$RSA_{DPPH}\ (\%) = \frac{A_0 - Ax}{A_0} \times 100 \tag{2}$$

where A_0 represents the absorbance of $DPPH^{\bullet}$ solution and extraction solvent, while A_x is the absorbance of $DPPH^{\bullet}$ solution and the extract. The results were expressed as the concentration of extract required to neutralize 50% of $DPPH^{\bullet}$ (IC_{50}, mg/mL).

3.6. Determination of Enzyme Inhibitory Activities

3.6.1. AChE and BuChE Enzymatic Assays

According to Grochowski et al. [96], the reaction mixture composed of 0.05 mL of root extract (1 mg/mL), 0.125 mL of 5,5′-dithiobis(2-nitrobenzoic acid) (3×10^{-3} mol/L), and 0.025 mL of AChE (0.265 U/mL), or BuChE (0.026 U/mL) Tris-hydrochloride buffer solution (pH 8.0) was added to the substrates (ACh, 0.015 mol/L or butyrylthiocholine, 1.5×10^{-3} mol/L). Moreover, a blank (prepared in the same manner but without the root extract) was prepared, and all absorbances were read at 405 nm after 15 min. The standard inhibitor for cholinesterases was galantamine, and milligrams of galantamine equivalents per gram of extract (mg GALAE/g) was the measurement unit.

3.6.2. HPA Enzymatic Assay

According to Sut et al. [19], after 10 min of incubation at 37 °C, the reaction mixture comprising the root extract (0.05 mL, 1 mg/mL) and HPA solution *ex-porcine* pancreas

(0.05 mL, 10 U/mL) in phosphate buffer (pH 6.9, with 6×10^{-3} mol/L of sodium chloride) was added to a starch solution (0.05 mL, 0.05% w/v). A blank was made by adding the test solution to all reagents without root extract. The reaction was ended with the addition of 0.025 mL of hydrochloric acid (1 mol/L) and 0.1 mL of iodine-potassium iodide (Lugol's reagent). After 10 min of incubation at 37 °C, all of the absorbances were recorded at 630 nm. The results were expressed as millimoles of acarbose equivalents per gram of extract (ACAE/g).

3.6.3. HIG Enzymatic Assay

The HIG enzymatic assay was performed following the experimental procedure given by Grochowski et al. [96]. In brief, 0.05 mL of the root extract (1 mg/mL) was mixed with 0.05 mL of glutathione (0.5 mg/mL), 0.05 mL of HIG (0.2 U/mL) in phosphate buffer (pH 6.8, 1 mol/L), and 0.05 mL of 4-N-trophenyl-α-D-glucopyranoside (0.1 mol/L). The reaction was stopped with the addition of 0.05 mL of sodium carbonate (0.2 mol/L). Moreover, the blank was prepared in the same manner but without root extract. The absorbances were recorded at 400 nm (with a 96-well microplate reader, Agilent Technologies Epoch, Winooski, VT, USA) after 15 min of incubation at 37 °C. Millimoles of acarbose equivalents per gram of extract (mmol ACAE/g) were the measurement unit.

3.6.4. Tyrosinase Enzymatic Assay

The tyrosinase enzymatic assay was carried out following the instructions provided by Grochowski et al. [96]. Specifically, 0.025 mL of extract solution of root extract (1 mg/mL) was mixed with 0.04 mL of tyrosinase (200 U/mL) and 0.1 mL of phosphate buffer (pH 6.8, 0.04 mol/L) in a 96-well microplate and incubated for 15 min at 25 °C. Then, the reaction was initiated using L-3,4-dixydroxyphenylalanine (0.04 mL, 0.01 mol/L), and after 10 min of incubation at 25 °C, the absorbance was read at 492 nm. A control was prepared in the same manner, but without tyrosinase. The tyrosinase enzymatic assay was determined by subtracting the absorbance of the control from that of the test solution, and the results were expressed as milligrams of kojic acid equivalents per gram of extract (mg KAE/g).

3.7. *Molecular Docking*

The initial structures of macromolecular targets in complexes with corresponding inhibitors were downloaded from the Protein Databank (PDB). Specifically, the following PDB structures were utilized: 4 TPK for AChE [97], BuChE [98], 4EY5 for 1OSE for HPA [99], 5NN8 for HIG [100], and 3NQ1 for tyrosinase [101]. The ionization states of the enzymes were adjusted to pH 7.40 using PROPKA [102]. Prior to simulations, we removed all water molecules and co-crystallized small molecules, creating space for the binding of the studied compounds. Vega ZZ 3.2.3. was used as the GUI [103]. The 2D structures of all compounds identified in the root extracts of three *Paeonia* species were either downloaded from PubChem or sketched in ChemDraw. Initial conformations of these compounds were generated using the MMFF94s force field in LigandScout 4.4 [104]. Subsequently, the final structures were optimized using the semiempirical PM7 method [105] implemented in MOPAC2016 [106], incorporating the COSMO solvation model of water and applying the PRECISE option to increase the accuracy. The final structures of all ligands were stored in the .sdf database. To identify the active site of each protein for molecular docking, we selected all residues within 10 Å from the co-crystallized inhibitor. AutoDock Vina 1.1 was chosen for the molecular docking process [107]. The virtual screening module within Vega ZZ 3.2.3 was used to study the binding affinities of the natural product database against each of the five enzymes. The exhaustiveness was set to 25, and 5 binding modes were saved for each ligand.

3.8. Determination of Antibacterial Activity

3.8.1. Selection of Microorganisms and Culture Conditions

Antibacterial activity was tested against six bacterial strains from the National Collection of Type Cultures (NCTC) and the American Type Culture Collection (ATCC). For the bioassays, three Gram-positive bacteria species, namely, *L. monocytogenes* NCTC 7973, *S. aureus* ATCC 11632, and *B. cereus* human isolate, and three Gram-negative bacteria species, namely, *S.* Typhimurium ATCC 13311, *P. aeruginosa* ATCC 27853, and *E. coli* ATCC 25922, were used. All tested bacteria were from the Laboratory of Mycology, Department of Plant Physiology, University of Belgrade, Institute for Biological Research "Siniša Stanković", Belgrade, Serbia. Bacteria were maintained on Mueller–Hinton agar and stored at 4 °C.

3.8.2. Broth Microdilution Method

In order to investigate the antibacterial activity of the root extracts, the modified broth microdilution method was used [15,16]. Bacterial species were cultured for 24 h at 37 °C in a Tryptic soy broth (TSB) medium. The fresh bacterial suspension was adjusted with sterile saline to a concentration of 1.0×10^8 per well. All root extracts were dissolved in ethyl alcohol (30%, *v*/*v*) to prepare a root extract (CFU) colony-forming unit stock solution with a concentration of 10 mg/mL. Minimal inhibitory concentration (MIC) and minimal bactericidal concentration (MBC) determinations were conducted by a serial dilution method using 96-well microtiter polystyrene plates. The MIC and MBC were conducted by serial subcultivation of 0.16 mL of extract into microtiter plates containing 0.04 mL of broth per well, followed by the addition of 0.01 mL of bacterial suspension and further incubation for 24 h at 37 °C; the MIC/MBC values were obtained following the addition of 0.02 mL of *p*-iodonitrotetrazolium violet (0.2 mg/mL) and incubation at 37 °C for 30 min. The lowest concentrations without visible growth were taken as MIC values, while the MBC indicates the lowest concentrations of root extracts at which the original inoculum was killed by 99.5%. A positive control, the antibiotic Gentamicin®, was used in the experiment.

3.9. Simulated In Vitro GID and Bioaccessibility

Prepared teas of selected *Peaonie* root samples (PO, PP, and PT) were subjected to a static *in vitro* GID with the aim of determining the recovery of specific bioactive compounds. The lyophilized powders from each infusion were completely dissolved in 5 mL of milli-Q water (dissolved teas) and further used for control and *in vitro* GID. *In vitro* GID was performed following the protocol previously reported by Aura and Härkönen [108]. In brief, dissolved tea (5 mL) was first subjected to the oral digestion phase by mixing it with 15 mL of milli-Q water, 10 mL of 0.85% NaCl, and salivary amylase solution (50 U), with the pH adjusted to 6.9. At this phase, the mixture was shaken on an orbital shaker (120 rpm) and incubated at 37 °C for 5 min. Then, the entire amount of the oral bolus was mixed with 4.5 mL of 150 mM HCl and 1 mL of pepsin (2 mg/mL). In the gastric phase, the pH of all mixtures was adjusted to 2.5, with continuous mixing at 37 °C for 2 h. After this time, the gastric chyme of all samples was mixed with 4 mL of bile acids (deoxycholic and cholic acid), 4 mL of pancreatin solution (18.75 mg/mL), and 1 mL of mucins, and the pH was immediately adjusted to 7.0 in all samples. In the intestinal phase, the mixtures were incubated at 37 °C for 3 h. At the end of digestion, milli-Q water was added to all mixtures to achieve a final volume of 45 mL. Thereafter, the digested mixtures were centrifuged (4000 rpm, 10 min), while the supernatants obtained were filtered through 0.45 μm filters (digeste) (samples were labeled as DPT, DPP, and DPO). Dissolved lyophilized tea (5 mL) mixed with milli-Q water to a final volume of 45 mL was used as a control for digestion (labeled as PTc, PPc, and POc). The control samples and digested samples were passed through SPE cartridges and 0.22 μm filters, to prepare for UHPLC Q-ToF MS analysis. The SPE cartridge was conditioned by washing with 5 mL of acidified methyl alcohol and milli-Q water, while the absorbed bioactive compounds were eluted with 1.5 mL of acidified methyl alcohol (0.1% methyl alcohol).

UHPLC Q-ToF MS Analysis Digested Samples

Separation and identification of bioactive compounds were performed on an Agilent 1290 Infinity ultra-high-performance liquid chromatography (UHPLC) system coupled to a quadrupole time-of-flight mass spectrometer (6530C Q-ToF-MS) (Agilent Technologies, Inc., Stevens Creek Blvd, Santa Clara, CA, USA), as previously described in detail by Kostić et al. [109]. Spectra were recorded in the m/z range from 100 to 1700 in both operating ionization modes (ESI+/ESI−), using auto-MS/MS acquisition. Agilent MassHunter software (version B.10.00)was used for instrument control and data analysis. Bioactive compounds were identified based on their exact m/z mass, MS fragmentation (Table S2), and date from the literature [2,22,24,29,45].

The bioaccessibility of the individual and total identified bioactive compounds (BCs) was presented as the percentage recovery (%) and calculated according to the following Equation (3):

$$Recovery\ (\%) = \frac{\sum BCd}{\sum BCc} \times 100 \quad (3)$$

where *BCd* is the area of each identified compound and sum of identified compounds in the digested tea samples, and *BCc* is the area of each identified compound and sum of identified compounds in the control teas.

The relative content (%) of bioactive compounds in each sample (before and after *in vitro* GID) was calculated as the ratio of the areas of individual and total BCs identified (the percentage of total area is defined as 100% for each sample—Equation (4)).

$$Relative\ content\ (\%) = \frac{\sum Area\ of\ individual\ BC}{\sum Total\ area\ of\ all\ identified\ BCs} \times 100 \quad (4)$$

3.10. Statistical Analysis

With the aim of investigating the statistical significance of the factors' influence (locality and extraction method) and the interaction between factors, as well as the combination of the factors for obtaining the highest TPC in all employed *Paeonia* species, the statistical analysis was performed employing one-way analysis of variance (ANOVA), Duncan's post hoc test, and experimental design (software STATISTIC 7.0.). The results are presented as mean value ± standard deviation (except in the case of antibacterial analysis), and the differences were considered statistically significant at $p < 0.05$, $n = 3$ (one-way ANOVA and Duncan's post hoc test). The antibacterial analysis was also performed in triplicate, but the highest value obtained was taken as MIC and MBC ("stricter criteria" rule was applied, which is common in antimicrobial assays).

4. Conclusions

This study offered insight into the chemical profile and *in vitro* biological activities of water–ethanolic extracts of the roots of PT, PP, and PO wild plants growing at different localities in Serbia. The results of chemical characterization show that *Paeonia* terpenes are the most dominant class of molecules presented in root extracts; hot water extracts are the source of different classes of bioactives, such as gallic and ellagic acid derivatives, flavonoids, procyanidins, and *Paeonia* root terpenoids. Among the tested root extracts, the highest TPC was observed in the PP extract obtained by MAE (Pirot) and in the PO extract obtained by method M (Rujevica). Antioxidant activity varied depending on the species and origin of the tested peony roots, as well as the extraction method implemented. According to that, the results showed that the highest ABTS scavenging potential was obtained in the PT extracts from Pančevo (MAE). The antioxidant activity of the extracts measured by the DPPH method also varied, depending on both the locality and extraction method. The extracts show various enzyme-inhibitory potentials on both AChE/BuChE, HPA, HIG, and tyrosinase, being the most effective in the inhibition of the AChE/BuChE enzymes. On the other hand, all root extracts show very similar and moderate antibacterial activity against two Gram-positive (*B. cereus* and *L. monocytogenes*) and one Gram-negative

(*P. aeruginosa*) bacteria strains; the most effective samples were macerates of PP (Južni Kučaj) and PO (Rujevica). The molecular docking analysis on five enzymes provided a detailed overview of the protein–ligand interactions contributing to the observed activities of the compounds from *Peaonia* root extracts. In addition, the GID results showed the dominant presence of methyl gallate and digallate in digests, probably originating from tannin derivatives, which may have potentially strong activity, making the hot water extracts (teas) eligible for use as food supplements.

In summary, the PT, PP, and PO extracts, as well as hot water extracts (teas), proved to be great sources of bioactives due to their unique chemical composition and demonstrated biological potential, which makes them promising constituents to include in many novel products of the pharmaceutical, cosmetic, and food industries. In most cases, PT from Gulenovci, PP from Pirot, and PO from Rujevica have strong activity in the assays used. The results of antioxidant, enzyme-inhibitory, and antibacterial activities, as well as the content of the extracted polyphenols, varied depending on the extraction method used, and they showed that the use of MAE is the most beneficial for the extraction of bioactive molecules from PP root extracts. In the analyzed extracts of the roots of the other two *Paoenia* species, UAE and method M alternated, without favoring either one. The mentioned plant resources could be highly recommended for further cultivation, which will enable the continuous supply of industries with herbal raw materials (the roots) of standardized quality.

Supplementary Materials: The following supporting information can be downloaded at: https://www.mdpi.com/article/10.3390/ph17040518/s1, Figure S1 (Supp. 1): Preliminary screening of factor level's impact (locality and extraction procedure) on the total polyphenolic concentration (TPC) of *Paeonia tenuifolia* L; Figure S2 (Supp. 2): ATR-FTIR spectra of the root extracts of *Paeonia tenuifolia* L. (PT), *Paeonia peregrina* Mill. (PP), and *Paeonia officinalis* L. (PO); UAE—ultrasound-assisted extraction; Figure S3 (Supp. 2): ATR-FTIR spectra of the root extracts of *Paeonia tenuifolia* L. (PT), *Paeonia peregrina* Mill. (PP), and *Paeonia officinalis* L. (PO); M—maceration; Table S1 (Supp. 3): Full factorial design for screening of factors' influence on total polyphenolic concentration (TPC) of root extracts of *Paeonia tenuifolia* L., *Paeonia peregrina* Mill., and *Paeonia officinalis* L., with the measured and predicted values; Table S2 (Supp. 3): Characterisation of detected bioactive compounds in selected peony root teas before and after *in vitro* GID, using UHPLC-QToF-MS. Target compounds, expected retention time (RT), base peak, molecular formula, calculated mass, exact mass and MS^2 fragments are presented.

Author Contributions: Conceptualization: P.B.; methodology: P.B., A.J., D.S., G.Z., I.C., U.G., N.Č., M.B.P., D.D.M., T.C. and A.M.; software: P.B., A.J., G.Z., I.C., U.G., N.Č. and D.D.M.; validation: A.J., D.S., G.Z., I.C., U.G., N.Č., M.B.P., B.B. and T.M.; formal analysis: A.J., D.S., I.C., U.G., B.B. and T.M.; investigation: P.B., A.J., D.S., G.Z., I.C., U.G., N.Č., M.B.P., D.D.M. and T.C.; resources: D.S., G.Z., I.C., U.G., M.B.P., D.D.M., T.C., B.B. and T.M.; data curation: P.B., A.J., G.Z. and I.C.; writing-original draft preparation: P.B., A.J., I.C., U.G., N.Č., M.B.P., D.D.M. and T.M.; writing-review and editing: A.J., D.S., G.Z., I.C., U.G., N.Č., M.B.P., D.D.M., T.C., B.B. and T.M.; visualization: T.M., supervision: A.J., D.S., G.Z., A.M., B.B. and T.M.; project administration: T.M.; funding acquisition: B.B. and T.M. All authors have read and agreed to the published version of the manuscript.

Funding: This research was funded by the Ministry of Science, Technological Development, and Innovation of the Republic of Serbia (#Grant Nos: 451-03-1202/2021-09/3, 451-03-66/2024-03/200003, 451-03-47/2024-01/200007, 451-03-47/2024-01/200019, 451-03-47/2024-01/200168, and 451-03-65/2024-03/200116) and the Science Fund of the Republic of Serbia (#Grant No. 7744714 and #Grant No. 7751519, MultiPromis).

Institutional Review Board Statement: Not applicable.

Informed Consent Statement: Not applicable.

Data Availability Statement: Data are contained within the article and Supplementary Materials.

Acknowledgments: The authors would like to express their gratitude to Milica Rat, curator of Herbarium BUNS, University of Novi Sad, Faculty of Science, Novi Sad, Serbia, who identified the plant material, as well as to Željana Prijić and Stefan Gordanić, researchers from the Institute for Medicinal Plant Research "Dr Josif Pančić", Belgrade, Serbia, Department for Agricultural Research and Development, for providing help during sample collection.

Conflicts of Interest: The authors declare no conflicts of interest.

References

1. Li, P.; Shen, J.; Wang, Z.; Liu, S.; Liu, Q.; Li, Y.; He, C.; Xiao, P. Genus *Paeonia*: A Comprehensive Review on Traditional Uses, Phytochemistry, Pharmacological Activities, Clinical Application, and Toxicology. *J. Ethnopharmacol.* **2021**, *269*, 113708. [CrossRef] [PubMed]
2. Yang, Y.; Li, S.; da Silva, J.A.T.; Yu, X.; Wang, L. Characterization of Phytochemicals in the Roots of Wild Herbaceous Peonies from China and Screening for Medicinal Resources. *Phytochemistry* **2020**, *174*, 112331. [CrossRef] [PubMed]
3. Parker, S.; May, B.; Zhang, C.; Zhang, A.L.; Lu, C.; Xue, C.C. A Pharmacological Review of Bioactive Constituents of *Paeonia lactiflora* Pallas and *Paeonia veitchii* Lynch. *Phytother. Res.* **2016**, *30*, 1445–1473. [CrossRef] [PubMed]
4. Oancea, S.; Perju, M.; Olosutean, H. Influence of Enzyme-Aided Extraction and Ultrasonication on the Phenolics Content and Antioxidant Activity of *Paeonia officinalis* L. Petals. *J. Serbian Chem. Soc.* **2020**, *85*, 845–856. [CrossRef]
5. Oancea, S.; Perju, M.; Coman, D.; Olosutean, H. Optimization of Conventional and Ultrasound-Assisted Extraction of *Paeonia officinalis* Anthocyanins, as Natural Alternative for a Green Technology of Cotton Dyeing. *Rom. Biotechnol. Lett.* **2021**, *26*, 2527–2534. [CrossRef]
6. Jovanović, A.; Petrović, P.; Đorđević, V.; Zdunić, G.; Šavikin, K.; Bugarski, B. Polyphenols Extraction from Plant Sources. *Lek. Sirovine* **2017**, *37*, 45–49. [CrossRef]
7. Jovanović, A.A.; Mosurović, M.; Bugarski, B.; Batinić, P.; Čutović, N.; Gordanić, S.; Marković, T. *Melissa officinalis* Extracts Obtained Using Maceration, Ultrasoundand Microwave-Assisted Extractions: Chemical Composition, Antioxidant Capacity, and Physical Characteristics. *Lek. Sirovine* **2022**, 51–59. [CrossRef]
8. Jovanović, A.A.; Đorđević, V.B.; Zdunić, G.M.; Pljevljakušić, D.S.; Šavikin, K.P.; Gođevac, D.M.; Bugarski, B.M. Optimization of the Extraction Process of Polyphenols from *Thymus serpyllum* L. Herb Using Maceration, Heat- and Ultrasound-Assisted Techniques. *Sep. Purif. Technol.* **2017**, *179*, 369–380. [CrossRef]
9. Jovanović, A.A.; Vajić, U.-J.V.; Mijin, D.Z.; Zdunić, G.M.; Šavikin, K.P.; Branković, S.; Kitić, D.; Bugarski, B.M. Polyphenol Extraction in Microwave Reactor Using By-Product of *Thymus serpyllum* L. and Biological Potential of the Extract. *J. Appl. Res. Med. Aromat. Plants* **2022**, *31*, 100417. [CrossRef]
10. Liazid, A.; Palma, M.; Brigui, J.; Barroso, C.G. Investigation on Phenolic Compounds Stability during Microwave-Assisted Extraction. *J. Chromatogr. A* **2007**, *1140*, 29–34. [CrossRef]
11. Ahmad, F.; Tabassum, N.; Rasool, S. Medicinal Uses and Phytoconstituents of *Paeonia officinalis*. *Int. Res. J. Pharm.* **2012**, *3*, 85–87.
12. Ahmad, F.; Tabassum, N. Effect of 70% Ethanolic Extract of Roots of *Paeonia officinalis* Linn. on Hepatotoxicity. *J. Acute Med.* **2013**, *3*, 45–49. [CrossRef]
13. Kostova, I.N.; Simeonov, M.F.; Todorova, D.I. A Monoterpene Glucoside from *Paeonia peregrina* Roots. *Phytochemistry* **1998**, *47*, 1303–1307. [CrossRef]
14. Nikolova, P.; Ivanovska, N. Estimation of Immunological Properties of Flower and Root Extracts from *Paeonia peregrina*. *J. Herbs Spices Med. Plants* **2000**, *6*, 1–9. [CrossRef]
15. Marković, T.; Čutović, N.; Carević, T.; Gašić, U.; Stojković, D.; Xue, J.; Jovanović, A. *Paeonia peregrina* Mill Petals as a New Source of Biologically Active Compounds: Chemical Characterization and Skin Regeneration Effects of the Extracts. *Int. J. Mol. Sci.* **2023**, *24*, 11764. [CrossRef]
16. Čutović, N.; Marković, T.; Kostić, M.; Gašić, U.; Prijić, Ž.; Ren, X.; Lukić, M.; Bugarski, B. Chemical Profile and Skin-Beneficial Activities of the Petal Extracts of *Paeonia tenuifolia* L. from Serbia. *Pharmaceuticals* **2022**, *15*, 1537. [CrossRef] [PubMed]
17. Batinić, P.; Cutovic, N.; Jovanović, A.; Stojković, D.; Zengin, G.; Carević, T.; Prijić, Ž.; Marinković, A.; Marković, T. Antioxidant, Antibacterial and Anti-Enzymatic Activity of the Leaf Extracts of *Paeonia daurica* Andrews Grown in Serbia. *Lek. Sirovine* **2023**, *43*, 1–8. [CrossRef]
18. Robin, T.; Reuveni, S.; Urbakh, M. Single-Molecule Theory of Enzymatic Inhibition. *Nat. Commun.* **2018**, *9*, 779. [CrossRef]
19. Sut, S.; Zengin, G.; Dall'Acqua, S.; Gazdová, M.; Šmejkal, K.; Bulut, G.; Dogan, A.; Haznedaroglu, M.Z.; Aumeeruddy, M.Z.; Maggi, F. *Paeonia arietina* and *Paeonia kesrounansis* Bioactive Constituents: NMR, LC-DAD-MS Fingerprinting and *in vitro* Assays. *J. Pharm. Biomed. Anal.* **2019**, *165*, 1–11. [CrossRef]
20. Pan, Y.; Gao, Z.; Huang, X.-Y.; Chen, J.-J.; Geng, C.-A. Chemical and Biological Comparison of Different Parts of *Paeonia suffruticosa* (Mudan) Based on LCMS-IT-TOF and Multi-Evaluation *in vitro*. *Ind. Crops. Prod.* **2020**, *144*, 112028. [CrossRef]
21. Liu, J.; Sun, H.; Zhang, A.; Yan, G.; Han, Y.; Xue, C.; Zhou, X.; Shi, H.; Wang, X. Serum Pharmacochemistry Combined with Multiple Data Processing Approach to Screen the Bioactive Components and Their Metabolites in Mutan Cortex by Ultra-performance Liquid Chromatography Tandem Mass Spectrometry. *Biomed. Chromatogr.* **2014**, *28*, 500–510. [CrossRef]
22. Li, B.; Ge, J.; Liu, W.; Hu, D.; Li, P. Unveiling Spatial Metabolome of *Paeonia suffruticosa* and *Paeonia lactiflora* Roots Using MALDI MS Imaging. *New Phytol.* **2021**, *231*, 892–902. [CrossRef] [PubMed]
23. Nishizawa, M.; Yamagishi, T.; Nonaka, G.; Nishioka, I.; Nagasawa, T.; Oura, H. Tannins and Related Compounds. XII. Isolation and Characterization of Galloylglucoses from *Paeoniae* Radix and Their Effect on Urea-Nitrogen Concentration in Rat Serum. *Chem. Pharm. Bull.* **1983**, *31*, 2593–2600. [CrossRef]
24. Yan, Z.; Xie, L.; Li, M.; Yuan, M.; Tian, Y.; Sun, D.; Zhang, Y.; Niu, L. Phytochemical Components and Bioactivities of Novel Medicinal Food–Peony Roots. *Food Res. Int.* **2021**, *140*, 109902. [CrossRef] [PubMed]

25. Nie, R.; Zhang, Y.; Jin, Q.; Zhang, S.; Wu, G.; Chen, L.; Zhang, H.; Wang, X. Identification and Characterisation of Bioactive Compounds from the Seed Kernels and Hulls of *Paeonia lactiflora* Pall by UPLC-QTOF-MS. *Food Res. Int.* **2021**, *139*, 109916. [CrossRef] [PubMed]
26. Fan, F.-Y.; Huang, C.-S.; Tong, Y.-L.; Guo, H.-W.; Zhou, S.-J.; Ye, J.-H.; Gong, S.-Y. Widely Targeted Metabolomics Analysis of White Peony Teas with Different Storage Time and Association with Sensory Attributes. *Food Chem.* **2021**, *362*, 130257. [CrossRef] [PubMed]
27. Xu, Y.; Liang, P.-L.; Chen, X.-L.; Gong, M.-J.; Zhang, L.; Qiu, X.-H.; Zhang, J.; Huang, Z.-H.; Xu, W. The Impact of Citrus-Tea Cofermentation Process on Chemical Composition and Contents of Pu-Erh Tea: An Integrated Metabolomics Study. *Front Nutr.* **2021**, *8*, 737539. [CrossRef]
28. Osuntokun, O.T.; Idowu, T.O.; Gamberini, M.C. Bio-Guided Isolation, Purification and Chemical Characterization of Epigallocatechin; Epicatechin, Stigmasterol, Phytosterol from of Ethyl Acetate Stem Bark Fraction of *Spondias mombin* (Linn.). *Biochem. Pharmacol.* **2018**, *7*, 1–9. [CrossRef]
29. Li, P.; Zhang, Z.-M.; Li, T.; Zhang, Y.-B.; Sze, S.C.W.; Wang, G.-C.; Li, Y.-L.; Ye, W.-C. Monoterpene Derivatives from the Roots of *Paeonia lactiflora* and Their Anti-Proliferative Activity. *Fitoterapia* **2014**, *98*, 124–129. [CrossRef]
30. Yoshikawa, M.; Harada, E.; Minematsu, T.; Muraoka, O.; Yamahara, J.; Murakami, N.; Kitagawa, I. Absolute Stereostructures of Paeonisothujone, a Novel Skeletal Monoterpene Ketone, and Deoxypaeonisuffrone, and Isopaeonisuffral, Two New Monoterpenes, from Moutan Cortex. *Chem. Pharm. Bull.* **1994**, *42*, 736–738. [CrossRef]
31. Shimizu, M.; Hayashi, T.; Morita, N.; Kimura, I.; Kimura, M.; Kiuchi, F.; Noguchi, H.; Iitaka, Y.; Sankawa, U. Paeoniflorigenone, a New Monoterpene from *Paeony* Roots. *Tetrahedron Lett.* **1981**, *22*, 3069–3070. [CrossRef]
32. Chen, P.-C.; Dlamini, B.S.; Chen, C.-R.; Shih, W.-L.; Lee, C.-H.; Chang, C.-I. Inhibitory Potential of Chemical Constituents from *Paeonia suffruticosa* Against α-glucosidase and α-amylase. *Pharm. Chem. J.* **2022**, *56*, 821–826. [CrossRef]
33. Xie, A.; Lv, M.; Zhang, D.; Shi, Y.; Yang, L.; Yang, X.; Du, J.; Sun, L.; Sun, X. Effects of Slight Shading in Summer on the Leaf Senescence and Endogenous Hormone and Polyamine Contents in Herbaceous Peony. *Sci. Rep.* **2023**, *13*, 18714. [CrossRef] [PubMed]
34. Seneme, E.F.; Dos Santos, D.C.; Silva, E.M.R.; Franco, Y.E.M.; Longato, G.B. Pharmacological and Therapeutic Potential of Myristicin: A Literature Review. *Molecules* **2021**, *26*, 5914. [CrossRef]
35. Yayli, N.; Yaşar, A.; Yayli, N.; Albay, M.; Coşkunçelebi, K. Essential Oil Analysis and Antimicrobial Activity of *Paeonia mascula* from Turkey. *Nat. Prod. Commun.* **2008**, *3*, 1934578X0800300624. [CrossRef]
36. Jiang, H.; Zhou, R.; An, L.; Guo, J.; Hou, X.; Tang, J.; Wang, F.; Du, Q. Exploring the Role and Mechanism of Astragalus Membranaceus and Radix *Paeoniae* Rubra in Idiopathic Pulmonary Fibrosis through Network Pharmacology and Experimental Validation. *Sci. Rep.* **2023**, *13*, 10110. [CrossRef]
37. Sun, L.; Kong, C.; Zhao, H.; Wu, D.; Xu, F. Two New Disaccharide Glycosides from the Root Cortex of *Paeonia ostii*. *Rec. Nat. Prod.* **2022**, *35*, 2564–2568. [CrossRef] [PubMed]
38. Zhang, T.; Si, F.; Zhang, Y.; Gai, S. Effect of Exogenous Gibberellin on DNA Methylation Level and Expression of Related Enzyme Genes in Tree Peony Floral Buds. *Sci. Agric. Sin.* **2018**, *51*, 3561–3569.
39. Yuxi, Z.; Yanchao, Y.; Zejun, L.; Tao, Z.; Feng, L.; Chunying, L.; Shupeng, G. GA 3 Is Superior to GA 4 in Promoting Bud Endodormancy Release in Tree Peony (*Paeonia suffruticosa*) and Their Potential Working Mechanism. *BMC Plant. Biol.* **2021**, *21*, 323. [CrossRef]
40. Bai, Z.-Z.; Ni, J.; Tang, J.-M.; Sun, D.-Y.; Yan, Z.-G.; Zhang, J.; Niu, L.-X.; Zhang, Y.-L. Bioactive Components, Antioxidant and Antimicrobial Activities of *Paeonia rockii* Fruit during Development. *Food Chem.* **2021**, *343*, 128444. [CrossRef]
41. Zhang, Q.; Lei, H.-M.; Wang, P.-L.; Ma, Z.-Q.; Zhang, Y.; Wu, J.-J.; Nie, J.; Chen, S.-J.; Han, W.-J.; Wang, Q. Bioactive Components from *Qingwen baidu* Decoction against LPS-Induced Acute Lung Injury in Rats. *Molecules* **2017**, *22*, 692. [CrossRef] [PubMed]
42. Yan, Z.; Xie, L.; Tian, Y.; Li, M.; Ni, J.; Zhang, Y.; Niu, L. Insights into the Phytochemical Composition and Bioactivities of Seeds from Wild Peony Species. *Plants* **2020**, *9*, 729. [CrossRef] [PubMed]
43. Tanaka, T.; Kataoka, M.; Tsuboi, N.; Kouno, I. New Monoterpene Glycoside Esters and Phenolic Constituents of *Paeoniae* Radix, and Increase of Water Solubility of Proanthocyanidins in the Presence of Paeoniflorin. *Chem. Pharm. Bull.* **2000**, *48*, 201–207. [CrossRef]
44. Shi, Y.-H.; Zhu, S.; Ge, Y.-W.; Toume, K.; Wang, Z.; Batkhuu, J.; Komatsu, K. Characterization and Quantification of Monoterpenoids in Different Types of Peony Root and the Related *Paeonia* Species by Liquid Chromatography Coupled with Ion Trap and Time-of-Flight Mass Spectrometry. *J. Pharm. Biomed. Anal.* **2016**, *129*, 581–592. [CrossRef]
45. Li, H.; Shi, Y.; Pang, Q.; Mei, Y.; Su, Z.; Yao, X.-S.; Yu, Y. Monoterpene Glycosides with Anti-Inflammatory Activity from *Paeoniae* Radix. *Fitoterapia* **2019**, *138*, 104290. [CrossRef] [PubMed]
46. Liang, W.-J.; Ma, Y.-B.; Geng, C.-A.; Huang, X.-Y.; Xu, H.-B.; Zhang, X.-M.; Chen, J.-J. Paeoveitols A–E from *Paeonia veitchii*. *Fitoterapia* **2015**, *106*, 36–40. [CrossRef]
47. Bai, Z.-Z.; Tang, J.-M.; Ni, J.; Zheng, T.-T.; Zhou, Y.; Sun, D.-Y.; Li, G.-N.; Liu, P.; Niu, L.-X.; Zhang, Y.-L. Comprehensive Metabolite Profile of Multi-Bioactive Extract from Tree Peony (*Paeonia ostii* and *Paeonia rockii*) Fruits Based on MS/MS Molecular Networking. *Food Res. Int.* **2021**, *148*, 110609. [CrossRef]

48. Klaus, A.; Kozarski, M.; Vunduk, J.; Todorovic, N.; Jakovljevic, D.; Zizak, Z.; Pavlovic, V.; Levic, S.; Niksic, M.; Van Griensven, L.J.L.D. Biological Potential of Extracts of the Wild Edible Basidiomycete Mushroom Grifola Frondosa. *Food Res. Int.* **2015**, *67*, 272–283. [CrossRef]
49. Mathlouthi, M.; Koenig, J.L. Vibrational Spectra of Carbohydrates. *Adv. Carbohydr. Chem. Biochem.* **1987**, *44*, 7–89.
50. Jovanović, A.; Đorđević, V.; Zdunić, G.; Šavikin, K.; Pljevljakusić, D.; Bugarski, B. Ultrasound-Assisted Extraction of Polyphenols from *Thymus serpyllum* and Its Antioxidant Activity. *Hem. Ind.* **2016**, *70*, 391–398. [CrossRef]
51. Jovanović, A.A.; Petrović, P.M.; Zdunić, G.M.; Šavikin, K.P.; Kitić, D.; Đorđević, V.B.; Bugarski, B.M.; Branković, S. Influence of Lyophilized Thymus Serpyllum L. Extracts on the Gastrointestinal System: Spasmolytic, Antimicrobial and Antioxidant Properties. *S. Afr. J. Bot.* **2021**, *142*, 274–283. [CrossRef]
52. Čutović, A.; Marković, T.; Žugić, A.; Batinić, P.; Bugarski;, B.; Jovanović, A. Antioxidant Activity of *Paeonia tenuifolia* L. Petal Extract-Loaded Liposomes. *Lekovite sirovine* **2023**, *43*, e167. [CrossRef]
53. Hidalgo, M.; Sánchez-Moreno, C.; de Pascual-Teresa, S. Flavonoid–Flavonoid Interaction and Its Effect on Their Antioxidant Activity. *Food Chem.* **2010**, *121*, 691–696. [CrossRef]
54. Wang, L.; Weller, C.L. Recent Advances in Extraction of Nutraceuticals from Plants. *Trends Food Sci. Technol.* **2006**, *17*, 300–312. [CrossRef]
55. Hirano, R.; Sasamoto, W.; Matsumoto, A.; Itakura, H.; Igarashi, O.; Kondo, K. Antioxidant Ability of Various Flavonoids against DPPH Radicals and LDL Oxidation. *J. Nutr. Sci. Vitaminol.* **2001**, *47*, 357–362. [CrossRef] [PubMed]
56. Ji, H.-F.; Zhang, H.-Y. Theoretical Evaluation of Flavonoids as Multipotent Agents to Combat Alzheimer's Disease. *J. Mol. Struct. THEOCHEM* **2006**, *767*, 3–9. [CrossRef]
57. Karim, N.; Khan, H.; Khan, I.; Guo, O.; Sobarzo-Sánchez, E.; Rastrelli, L.; Kamal, M.A. An Increasing Role of Polyphenols as Novel Therapeutics for Alzheimer's: A Review. *Med. Chem.* **2020**, *16*, 1007–1021. [CrossRef]
58. Navarrete-Yañez, V.; Garate-Carrillo, A.; Rodriguez, A.; Mendoza-Lorenzo, P.; Ceballos, G.; Calzada-Mendoza, C.; Hogan, M.C.; Villarreal, F.; Ramirez-Sanchez, I. Effects of (−)-Epicatechin on Neuroinflammation and Hyperphosphorylation of Tau in the Hippocampus of Aged Mice. *Food Funct.* **2020**, *11*, 10351–10361. [CrossRef] [PubMed]
59. Ramkumar, K.M.; Thayumanavan, B.; Palvannan, T.; Rajaguru, P. Inhibitory Effect of Gymnema Montanum Leaves on α-glucosidase Activity and α-amylase Activity and Their Relationship with Polyphenolic Content. *Med. Chem. Res.* **2010**, *19*, 948–961. [CrossRef]
60. Xiao, J. Natural Polyphenols and Diabetes: Understanding Their Mechanism of Action. *Curr. Med. Chem.* **2015**, *22*, 2–3. [CrossRef]
61. Abdel-Moneim, A.; Abd El-Twab, S.M.; Yousef, A.I.; Ashour, M.B.; Reheim, E.S.A.; Hamed, M.A.A. New Insights into the *in vitro*, *in situ* and *in vivo* Antihyperglycemic Mechanisms of Gallic Acid and p-coumaric Acid. *Arch. Physiol. Biochem.* **2022**, *128*, 1188–1194. [CrossRef]
62. Sourris, K.C.; Watson, A.; Jandeleit-Dahm, K. Inhibitors of Advanced Glycation End Product (AGE) Formation and Accumulation. In *Reactive Oxygen Species: Network Pharmacology and Therapeutic Applications*; Springer: Cham, Switzerland, 2021; pp. 395–423. [CrossRef]
63. Zengin, G.; Bulut, G.; Mollica, A.; Haznedaroglu, M.Z.; Dogan, A.; Aktumsek, A. Bioactivities of *Achillea phrygia* and *Bupleurum croceum* Based on the Composition of Phenolic Compounds: *In vitro* and *in silico* Approaches. *Food Chem. Toxicol.* **2017**, *107*, 597–608. [CrossRef]
64. Zolghadri, S.; Bahrami, A.; Hassan Khan, M.T.; Munoz-Munoz, J.; Garcia-Molina, F.; Garcia-Canovas, F.; Saboury, A.A. A Comprehensive Review on Tyrosinase Inhibitors. *J. Enzyme Inhib. Med. Chem.* **2019**, *34*, 279–309. [CrossRef]
65. Dogra, S.; Sarangal, R. Pigmentary Disorders: An Insight. *Pigment Int.* **2014**, *1*, 5–7. [CrossRef]
66. Talebi, M.; Majidi, K.; Bassam, K.; Abdi, M.; Daneshvar, M.; Moayedi, S.S.; Pourhesabi, S.; Attarroshan, M.; Boumi, S.; Kabiri, M. Synthesis, Biological Evaluation, and Molecular Docking Analysis of Novel 1, 3, 4-Thiadiazole-Based Kojic Acid Derivatives as Tyrosinase Inhibitors. *J. Mol. Struct.* **2022**, *1268*, 133707. [CrossRef]
67. Chaita, E.; Lambrinidis, G.; Cheimonidi, C.; Agalou, A.; Beis, D.; Trougakos, I.; Mikros, E.; Skaltsounis, A.-L.; Aligiannis, N. Anti-Melanogenic Properties of Greek Plants. A Novel Depigmenting Agent from Morus Alba Wood. *Molecules* **2017**, *22*, 514. [CrossRef] [PubMed]
68. Kaper, J.B.; O'Brien, A.D. Overview and Historical Perspectives. *Microbiol. Spectr.* **2014**, *2*. [CrossRef]
69. Mühldorfer, I.; Ziebuhr, W.; Hacker, J. Escherichia coli in Urinary Tract Infections. In *Molecular Medical Microbiology*; Elsevier: Amsterdam, The Netherlands, 2002; pp. 1515–1540.
70. Cowan, M.M. Plant Products as Antimicrobial Agents. *Clin. Microbiol. Rev.* **1999**, *12*, 564–582. [CrossRef] [PubMed]
71. Rios, J.-L.; Recio, M.C. Medicinal Plants and Antimicrobial Activity. *J. Ethnopharmacol.* **2005**, *100*, 80–84. [CrossRef]
72. Ngan, L.T.M.; Moon, J.-K.; Kim, J.-H.; Shibamoto, T.; Ahn, Y.-J. Growth-Inhibiting Effects of *Paeonia lactiflora* Root Steam Distillate Constituents and Structurally Related Compounds on Human Intestinal Bacteria. *World J. Microbiol. Biotechnol.* **2012**, *28*, 1575–1583. [CrossRef]
73. Davidson, P.M.; Taylor, T.M.; Schmidt, S.E. Chemical Preservatives and Naturally Antimicrobial Compounds. In *Food Microbiology: Fundamentals and Frontiers*; ASM Press: Washington, DC, USA, 2012.
74. Stojković, D.; Soković, M.; Glamočlija, J.; Džamić, A.; Ćirić, A.; Ristić, M.; Grubišić, D. Chemical Composition and Antimicrobial Activity of *Vitex agnus-castus* L. Fruits and Leaves Essential Oils. *Food Chem.* **2011**, *128*, 1017–1022. [CrossRef]

75. Yi, S.; Zhu, J.; Fu, L.; Li, J. Tea Polyphenols Inhibit *Pseudomonas aeruginosa* through Damage to the Cell Membrane. *Int. J. Food Microbiol.* **2010**, *144*, 111–117. [CrossRef]
76. Bouarab-Chibane, L.; Forquet, V.; Lantéri, P.; Clément, Y.; Léonard-Akkari, L.; Oulahal, N.; Degraeve, P.; Bordes, C. Antibacterial Properties of Polyphenols: Characterization and QSAR (Quantitative Structure–Activity Relationship) Models. *Front. Microbiol.* **2019**, *10*, 829. [CrossRef] [PubMed]
77. Widyaningrum, I.; Wibisono, N.; Kusumawati, A.H. Effect of Extraction Method on Antimicrobial Activity against *Staphylococcus aureus* of Tapak Liman (*Elephantopus scaber* L.) Leaves. *Int. J. Med. Health Sci.* **2020**, *3*, 105–110.
78. Aligiannis, N.; Kalpoutzakis, E.; Mitaku, S.; Chinou, I.B. Composition and Antimicrobial Activity of the Essential Oils of Two Origanum Species. *J. Agric. Food Chem.* **2001**, *49*, 4168–4170. [CrossRef]
79. Qin, W.; Ketnawa, S.; Ogawa, Y. Effect of Digestive Enzymes and pH on Variation of Bioavailability of Green Tea during Simulated *in vitro* Gastrointestinal Digestion. *Food Sci. Hum. Wellness* **2022**, *11*, 669–675. [CrossRef]
80. Koláčková, T.; Sumczynski, D.; Minařík, A.; Yalçin, E.; Orsavová, J. The Effect of *in vitro* Digestion on Matcha Tea (*Camellia sinensis*) Active Components and Antioxidant Activity. *Antioxidants* **2022**, *11*, 889. [CrossRef]
81. Chen, G.-L.; Chen, S.-G.; Xie, Y.-Q.; Chen, F.; Zhao, Y.-Y.; Luo, C.-X.; Gao, Y.-Q. Total Phenolic, Flavonoid and Antioxidant Activity of 23 Edible Flowers Subjected to *in vitro* Digestion. *J. Funct. Foods* **2015**, *17*, 243–259. [CrossRef]
82. Huang, W.; Mao, S.; Zhang, L.; Lu, B.; Zheng, L.; Zhou, F.; Zhao, Y.; Li, M. Phenolic Compounds, Antioxidant Potential and Antiproliferative Potential of 10 Common Edible Flowers from China Assessed Using a Simulated *in vitro* Digestion–Dialysis Process Combined with Cellular Assays. *J. Sci. Food Agric.* **2017**, *97*, 4760–4769. [CrossRef] [PubMed]
83. Kelebek, H.; Sasmaz, H.K.; Aksay, O.; Selli, S.; Kahraman, O.; Fields, C. Exploring the Impact of Infusion Parameters and *in vitro* Digestion on the Phenolic Profile and Antioxidant Capacity of Guayusa (*Ilex guayusa* Loes.) Tea Using Liquid Chromatography, Diode Array Detection, and Electrospray Ionization Tandem Mass Spectrometry. *Foods* **2024**, *13*, 694. [CrossRef] [PubMed]
84. Ćirkovic Veličković, T.D.; Stanić-Vučinić, D.J. The Role of Dietary Phenolic Compounds in Protein Digestion and Processing Technologies to Improve Their Antinutritive Properties. *Compr. Rev. Food Sci. Food Saf.* **2018**, *17*, 82–103. [CrossRef] [PubMed]
85. Jakobek, L. Interactions of Polyphenols with Carbohydrates, Lipids and Proteins. *Food Chem.* **2015**, *175*, 556–567. [CrossRef] [PubMed]
86. Pešić, M.B.; Milinčić, D.D.; Kostić, A.Ž.; Stanisavljević, N.S.; Vukotić, G.N.; Kojić, M.O.; Gašić, U.M.; Barać, M.B.; Stanojević, S.P.; Popović, D.A. *In vitro* Digestion of Meat-and Cereal-Based Food Matrix Enriched with Grape Extracts: How Are Polyphenol Composition, Bioaccessibility and Antioxidant Activity Affected? *Food Chem.* **2019**, *284*, 28–44. [CrossRef] [PubMed]
87. Liang, H.; Huang, Q.; Zou, L.; Wei, P.; Lu, J.; Zhang, Y. Methyl Gallate: Review of Pharmacological Activity. *Pharmacol. Res.* **2023**, *194*, 106849. [CrossRef] [PubMed]
88. Milinčić, D.D.; Stanisavljević, N.S.; Kostić, A.Ž.; Gašić, U.M.; Stanojević, S.P.; Tešić, Ž.L.; Pešić, M.B. Bioaccessibility of Phenolic Compounds and Antioxidant Properties of Goat-Milk Powder Fortified with Grape-Pomace-Seed Extract after *in vitro* Gastrointestinal Digestion. *Antioxidants* **2022**, *11*, 2164. [CrossRef] [PubMed]
89. Oh, J.-H.; Lee, C.-Y.; Lee, Y.-E.; Yoo, S.-H.; Chung, J.-O.; Rha, C.-S.; Park, M.-Y.; Hong, Y.-D.; Shim, S.-M. Profiling of *in vitro* Bioaccessibility and Intestinal Uptake of Flavonoids after Consumption of Commonly Available Green Tea Types. *Molecules* **2021**, *26*, 1518. [CrossRef] [PubMed]
90. Yu, J.-B.; Wang, Y. Gut Microbiota-Based Pharmacokinetics and the Antidepressant Mechanism of Paeoniflorin. *Front. Pharmacol.* **2019**, *10*, 442126. [CrossRef] [PubMed]
91. Liu, Z.Q.; Jiang, Z.H.; Liu, L.; Hu, M. Mechanisms Responsible for Poor Oral Bioavailability of Paeoniflorin: Role of Intestinal Disposition and Interactions with Sinomenine. *Pharm. Res.* **2006**, *23*, 2768–2780. [CrossRef]
92. Institute for Medicinal Plant Research Dr. Josif Pančić Čaj Od Korena Belog Sleza (Tea of Root of *Althaea officinalis*). Available online: https://www.mocbilja.rs/proizvod/caj-od-korena-belog-sleza/ (accessed on 1 April 2024).
93. Wang, X.; Xiong, H.; Wang, S.; Zhang, Y.; Song, Z.; Zhang, X. Physicochemical Analysis, Sensorial Evaluation, Astringent Component Identification and Aroma-Active Compounds of Herbaceous Peony (*Paeonia lactiflora* Pall.) Black Tea. *Ind. Crops Prod.* **2023**, *193*, 116159. [CrossRef]
94. Classics Lowry, O.; Rosebrough, N.; Farr, A.; Randall, R. Protein Measurement with the Folin Phenol Reagent. *J. Biol. Chem.* **1951**, *193*, 265–275. [CrossRef]
95. Shraim, A.M.; Ahmed, T.A.; Rahman, M.M.; Hijji, Y.M. Determination of Total Flavonoid Content by Aluminum Chloride Assay: A Critical Evaluation. *Lwt* **2021**, *150*, 111932. [CrossRef]
96. Grochowski, D.M.; Uysal, S.; Aktumsek, A.; Granica, S.; Zengin, G.; Ceylan, R.; Locatelli, M.; Tomczyk, M. *In vitro* Enzyme Inhibitory Properties, Antioxidant Activities, and Phytochemical Profile of *Potentilla thuringiaca*. *Phytochem. Lett.* **2017**, *20*, 365–372. [CrossRef]
97. Cheung, J.; Rudolph, M.J.; Burshteyn, F.; Cassidy, M.S.; Gary, E.N.; Love, J.; Franklin, M.C.; Height, J.J. Structures of Human Acetylcholinesterase in Complex with Pharmacologically Important Ligands. *J. Med. Chem.* **2012**, *55*, 10282–10286. [CrossRef] [PubMed]
98. Brus, B.; Kosak, U.; Turk, S.; Pislar, A.; Coquelle, N.; Kos, J.; Stojan, J.; Colletier, J.-P.; Gobec, S. Discovery, Biological Evaluation, and Crystal Structure of a Novel Nanomolar Selective Butyrylcholinesterase Inhibitor. *J. Med. Chem.* **2014**, *57*, 8167–8179. [CrossRef] [PubMed]

99. Gilles, C.; Astier, J.; Marchis-Mouren, G.; Cambillau, C.; Payan, F. Crystal Structure of Pig Pancreatic α-amylase Isoenzyme II, in Complex with the Carbohydrate Inhibitor Acarbose. *Eur. J. Biochem.* **1996**, *238*, 561–569. [CrossRef]
100. Roig-Zamboni, V.; Cobucci-Ponzano, B.; Iacono, R.; Ferrara, M.C.; Germany, S.; Bourne, Y.; Parenti, G.; Moracci, M.; Sulzenbacher, G. Structure of Human Lysosomal Acid α-glucosidase–a Guide for the Treatment of Pompe Disease. *Nat. Commun.* **2017**, *8*, 1111. [CrossRef] [PubMed]
101. Sendovski, M.; Kanteev, M.; Ben-Yosef, V.S.; Adir, N.; Fishman, A. First Structures of an Active Bacterial Tyrosinase Reveal Copper Plasticity. *J. Mol. Biol.* **2011**, *405*, 227–237. [CrossRef]
102. Olsson, M.H.M.; Søndergaard, C.R.; Rostkowski, M.; Jensen, J.H. PROPKA3: Consistent Treatment of Internal and Surface Residues in Empirical pKa Predictions. *J. Chem. Theory Comput.* **2011**, *7*, 525–537. [CrossRef]
103. Pedretti, A.; Mazzolari, A.; Gervasoni, S.; Fumagalli, L.; Vistoli, G. The VEGA Suite of Programs: An Versatile Platform for Cheminformatics and Drug Design Projects. *Bioinformatics* **2021**, *37*, 1174–1175. [CrossRef]
104. Halgren, T.A. MMFF VI. MMFF94s Option for Energy Minimization Studies. *J. Comput. Chem.* **1999**, *20*, 720–729. [CrossRef]
105. Stewart, J.J.P. Optimization of Parameters for Semiempirical Methods VI: More Modifications to the NDDO Approximations and Re-Optimization of Parameters. *J. Mol. Model.* **2013**, *19*, 1–32. [CrossRef] [PubMed]
106. Stewart, J.J.P. MOPAC: A Semiempirical Molecular Orbital Program. *J. Comput. Aided Mol. Des.* **1990**, *4*, 1–103. [CrossRef] [PubMed]
107. Trott, O.; Olson, A.J. AutoDock Vina: Improving the Speed and Accuracy of Docking with a New Scoring Function, Efficient Optimization, and Multithreading. *J. Comput. Chem.* **2010**, *31*, 455–461. [CrossRef] [PubMed]
108. Aura, A.-M.; Härkönen, H.; Fabritius, M.; Poutanen, K. Development of An *in vitro* Enzymic Digestion Method for Removal of Starch and Protein and Assessment of Its Performance Using Rye And Wheat Breads. *J. Cereal Sci.* **1999**, *29*, 139–152. [CrossRef]
109. Kostić, A.Ž.; Milinčić, D.D.; Špirović Trifunović, B.; Nedić, N.; Gašić, U.M.; Tešić, Ž.L.; Stanojević, S.P.; Pešić, M.B. Monofloral Corn Poppy Bee-Collected Pollen—A Detailed Insight into Its Phytochemical Composition and Antioxidant Properties. *Antioxidants* **2023**, *12*, 1424. [CrossRef]

pharmaceuticals

Article

Identification of Metabolites from *Catharanthus roseus* Leaves and Stem Extract, and In Vitro and In Silico Antibacterial Activity against Food Pathogens

Qazi Mohammad Sajid Jamal [1,*] and Varish Ahmad [2]

1 Department of Health Informatics, College of Applied Medical Sciences, Qassim University, Buraydah 51452, Saudi Arabia
2 Health Information Technology Department, The Applied College, King Abdulaziz University, Jeddah 21589, Saudi Arabia; vaahmad@kau.edu.sa
* Correspondence: m.quazi@qu.edu.sa

Abstract: The plant produced powerful secondary metabolites and showed strong antibacterial activities against food-spoiling bacterial pathogens. The present study aimed to evaluate antibacterial activities and to identify metabolites from the leaves and stems of *Catharanthus roseus* using NMR spectroscopy. The major metabolites likely to be observed in aqueous extraction were 2,3-butanediol, quinic acids, vindoline, chlorogenic acids, vindolinine, secologanin, and quercetin in the leaf and stem of the *Catharanthus roseus*. The aqueous extracts from the leaves and stems of this plant have been observed to be most effective against food spoilage bacterial strains, followed by methanol and hexane. However, leaf extract was observed to be most significant in terms of the content and potency of metabolites. The minimum inhibitory concentration (20 µg/mL) and bactericidal concentrations (35 g/mL) of leaf extract were observed to be significant as compared to the ampicillin. Molecular docking showed that chlorogenic acid and vindolinine strongly interacted with the bacterial penicillin-binding protein. The docking energies of chlorogenic acid and vindolinine also indicated that these could be used as food preservatives. Therefore, the observed metabolite could be utilized as a potent antibacterial compound for food preservation or to treat their illness, and further research is needed to perform.

Keywords: *Catharanthus roseus*; NMR; indole alkaloids; secondary metabolites; antibacterial; food preservation

1. Introduction

A foodborne infection's symptoms can range from completely asymptomatic to fatal. In the US, foodborne diseases cause 48 million episodes of sickness, 128,000 admitted to hospitals, and 3000 fatalities annually [1]. Proper handling and usage of preservatives have reduced microbial growth and economic loss of food. Infections caused by drug-resistant microorganisms, such as those in water and food, also pose a significant risk to public health [2]. Biosensors have been used to detect, identify, and manage microbial contamination in agricultural and food products for disease prevention and outbreak analysis [3,4]. Metal nanoparticles have the potential to kill numerous drug-resistant bacteria, including those in the Gram-positive and Gram-negative groups [3,4]. Although inorganic nanoparticles have several biocidal capabilities, the method by which they exert their powerful antibacterial efficacy is not as well understood. However, it was thought that releasing ions into solution produces reactive oxygen species that harm bacteria. As other studies show, nanoparticles are so small that they can pass through bacterial cell walls and target their organelles. The inorganic analogs of organic antibiotics are more effective against drug-resistant bacteria because they use many mechanisms of action [5,6].

Inorganic metal oxide nanoparticles, such as the nano-complex of metal oxide, are well admired for their bacteriostatic and bactericidal effects [7].

Similarly, various plants have been described as having significant antimicrobial potential against various pathogens [8]. Recognition and signaling caused by transcription components, alterations in hormone levels, and the creation of secondary metabolites are only a few examples of the many mechanisms involved in stressful reduction reactions. Particularly intriguing are secondary metabolites due to their roles in controlling plant interactions with their environments and subsequent adaptive responses. In a variety of environmental conditions like the lack of moisture and heat, plants increase their production of phenylpropanoid metabolic products like scopolamine, sinapic acid, sinapoyl aldehyde, and flavonoids, all of which support the generation of significant structural substances like lignin while also in reducing oxidative damage and preventing photoinhibition [8,9]. Establishing an equilibrium between the production of the natural therapeutic compounds of attention and the production of the various distress metabolites required by the herb to endure the stress is crucial to the efficacy of the significant molecules [10].

It is widely acknowledged that the *Catharanthus roseus* (L.) *G. Don* (*C. roseus*), or Madagascar periwinkle, is a member of the family *Apocynaceae*, used as a natural remedy in various cultures. For several decades, research and therapy have concentrated on the bioactive compound's potential to be employed as an anticancer as well as an antimicrobial [11]. The plant has also been described for its many pharmacological activities. However, the extraction of bioactive compounds also generates solvent-mediated air, water, and soil pollution. The increase in toxic concentrations in the environment endangers human health, diminishes ecological functioning, and decreases wildlife populations [12]. However, extraction is an important step in the search for phytochemical bioactive molecules and translating their potential into significant therapeutic molecules.

There was also a discussion of more current developments in the application of cell, tissue, or callus cultures to produce desirable phytochemicals from various plants, including *C. roseus* [13,14]. Medications used in chemotherapy are a major part of clinical oncology evaluations. When taken orally, most of these drugs kill tumor cells but have the potential to harm healthy cells as well. These negative effects restrict the use of chemotherapy medications despite their high effectiveness in killing cancer cells.

Therefore, searching for complementary or alternative drugs that would be selectively effective with no adverse effects on health is an active area of research. A lot of these studies are looking into traditional herbal remedies used by different cultures around the world. Moreover, a report from the WHO [15] stated that nearly 80% of the global population relies on medications derived from plants, either entirely or partially. Antimicrobials, cancer, diabetes, fever, hemostasis, and hypertension are only some of the conditions that have been treated using the plant *C. roseus* during traditional medical practices in a number of different societies [16,17]. However, few reports have addressed the effects of *C. roseus* crude aqueous extract in the field of food preservation. This study is aimed to identify the possible primary and secondary metabolites of leaves and stem of *C. roseus* using NMR spectroscopy. We also analyzed the antibacterial potential of different solvents and explored the possible molecular interaction of most interacting molecules with bacterial targets.

2. Results and Discussion

The collected plant leaves and stems were used to prepare their extractions in water, methanol, and hexane. Each extract was checked for its antibacterial activities; leaves and stem extractions with water were observed to be the most significant fraction for antibacterial activities. Therefore, the aqueous fraction underwent NMR analysis to determine the presence of potential metabolites. The analyzed sample fraction peak and its metabolites are shown in Figure 1.

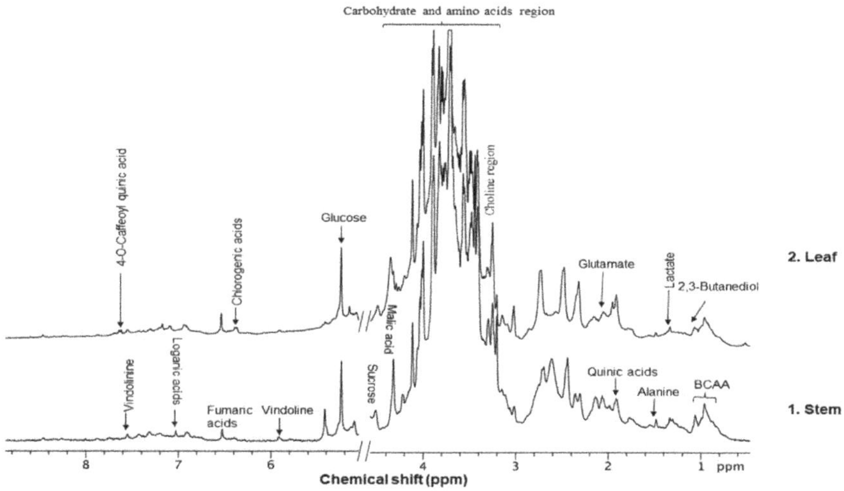

Figure 1. Typical 1 H-NMR spectra of the metabolites of the different sections of *C. roseus*: (1) leaves and (2) stems. Key metabolites: Branch chain amino acids (BCAA), 2,3 butanediol, quinic acids, vindoline, lactate, alanine, pyruvate, glutamate, malic acid, glucose, vindoline, chlorogenic acids, fumaric acid, vindolinine, secologanin, quercetin, respectively.

Metabolite fingerprinting, profiling, and footprinting are the components of methods used for metabolomics studies. Profiling helps to identify and characterize metabolites of a specific metabolic pathway. The main goal of fingerprinting is to compare and distinguish between samples using high-throughput screening and extraction of the metabolite content of different sections of *C. roseus*, like the leaf and stem. Footprinting is the fingerprinting analysis of identified metabolites, which were assigned with the help of NMR one-dimensional spectra of leaf and stem samples. Unlike COSY (homonuclear correlation spectroscopy), which only generates connections between vicinal or geminal protons, TOCSY (Total Correlation Spectroscopy) generates correlations among all protons in a specific spin system. 2D NMR-based methods, mainly TOCSY and COSY, are commonly used for molecule recognition in plant extracts to assign peaks to metabolites accurately. After the identification of the metabolite, a characterization analysis of the NMR spectra assignment of the aliphatic, aromatic, and sugar regions was performed to find discriminating signals in the leaf and stem. They offer an outstanding platform for studying., for example, the anticancer and other medical chemicals, quality control as well as authentication of medicinal plants, their classification at the level of species ecotypes, genotypes, identification of biomarkers for disease diagnosis, and therapeutics. Metabolites including branch chain amino acids (BCAA), 2,3 butanediol, quinic acids, vindoline, lactate, alanine, pyruvate, glutamate, malic acid, glucose, chlorogenic acids, fumaric acid, indoline, secologanin, and quercetin.

2.1. Assessment of the Antimicrobial Impact

The aqueous, methanolic, and hexane extracts were used to analyze the antibacterial effect by agar well diffusion assay against Gram-positive isolates presented as 2, 4, and *S. aureus* and Gram-negative bacteria 1, 3, and *E. coli*. Ampicillin was used as a standard drug. The observed results and the effect of solvent are shown in Figure 2.

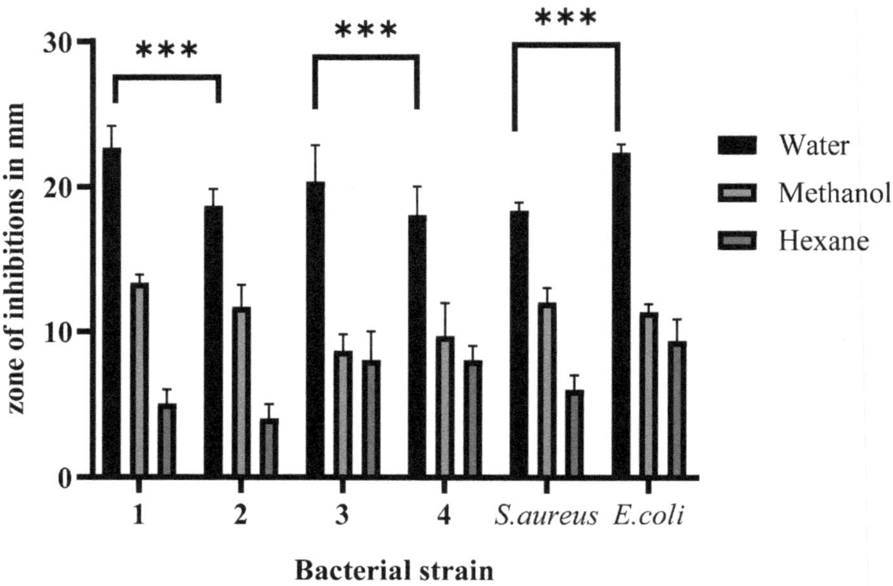

Figure 2. Antibacterial effect of water, methanol, and hexane extracts of *C. roseus* leaves against meat-isolated bacterial pathogens (1, 3 Gram-negative *streptobacilli* and 2, 4 Gram-positive *Streptococcus*). The significant values were expressed as *** p value 0.0001.

The aqueous extracts of leaves have a stronger antimicrobial effect on Gram-negative bacteria than on Gram-positive bacterial isolates, which were subsequently followed by methanol and hexane. Similarly, Gram-negative bacteria are potentially inhibited compared to Gram-positive reference bacteria. Nutrient broth medium was solely utilized as a negative control; Ampicillin was a positive control. *S. aureus* was used as a Gram-positive reference strain, and *E. coli* was used as a Gram-negative reference bacterium strain (Figure 2).

Gram-positive and Gram-negative bacteria isolated from spoiled chicken meat were subjected to the antibacterial effect test. The aqueous extract of leaves has shown stronger inhibition against Gram-negative (22 mm zone of inhibition) bacterial isolates than Gram-positive bacteria. The growth of the standard test indicator *E. coli* has been observed to be inhibited more strongly than that of *S. aureus* (18 mm zone of inhibition). The minimum inhibitory concentrations were 12.5 and 20 g/mL, respectively. The minimum bactericidal concentrations for Gram-negative and Gram-positive bacteria isolates were 20 and 35 g/mL, respectively. The antibacterial effects of stem extract were also analyzed, and hexane and methanol (13 mm zone of inhibition), and hexane (8 mm zone of inhibition) were found to be less significant in comparison to the leaf aqueous extract; the antibacterial effect and significance of extracting solvent are shown in Figures 2 and 3. Significant results were also obtained regarding the stem extract's inhibitory impact and strength against Gram-negative bacteria, but it was less than that of the leaves of the plant.

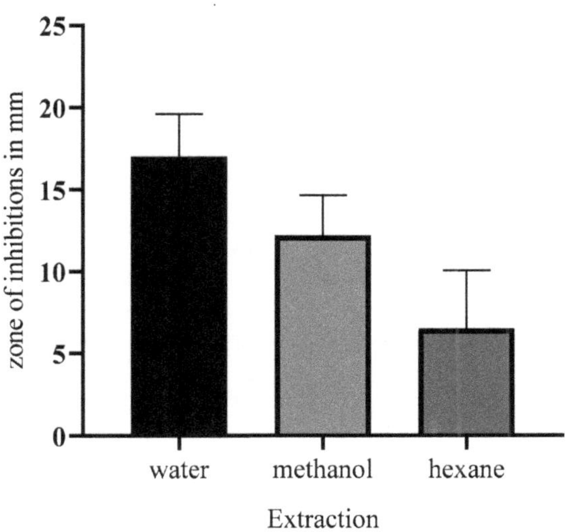

Figure 3. Solvent effect on extraction of metabolites and antimicrobial activity of leaf extract of *C. roseus*. The hexane extract was likely observed to have the least growth inhibitory effect on the bacterium in a medium with methanol, while the optimum extraction had a strong growth inhibitory effect on the bacterium.

2.2. Virtual Screening and Docking Results

The interactions with bacterial receptors were screened via docking studies. The docking scores suggested that the 2exb-Chlorogenic Acid complex showed the best binding energy, i.e., −7.7 kcal/mol, which was supported by six hydrogen bonds (Table 1), which was more than the used control drug (complex: 2exb-Flomoxef) binding energy −7.1 kcal/mol. The interactions through which Chlorogenic Acid could mediate its antibacterial effect are represented in Figure 4A,B (Table 1). Many phenolic molecules have been described as having potential antibacterial and pharmacological activities. Chlorogenic acid (CA), as analyzed in this study by NMR, is a phenolic compound that could be responsible for antibacterial and antibiofilm activities. The high antibacterial efficacy and antibiofilm assays against *S. maltophilia* in both in vitro and in vivo were also examined (MIC > 32 g mL^1), including the TMP/SMX-resistant strain. Chlorogenic acid and plant products containing chlorogenic acid have demonstrated potent antifungal, antibacterial, and antiviral properties. It has been documented that some bacterial pathogens inhibit both Gram-positive (*Streptococcus pneumoniae, Streptococcus mutans, Staphylococcus aureus, Bacillus subtilis,* and others) and Gram-negative (*Shigella dysenteriae, Salmonella typhimurium,* and *E. coli*) [18].

The antibacterial effect of chlorogenic acid has been described against *A. Acidoterrestris* [19] and *Yersinia enterocolitica*. Drugs that target penicillin-binding proteins may inhibit the spread of disease-causing bacteria. Chlorogenic acid destroys bacterial cells, as reported earlier, lending credence to the findings of this investigation. A second compound, 2exb-quercetin, with a docking energy of −7.5 kcal/mol and the formation of two hydrogen bonds, performed similarly well (Figure 4C,D and Table 1). Quercetin is a common flavonoid with antibacterial properties. Researchers have investigated the bacteriostatic effect of quercetin on *E. coli, Salmonella enterica, P. aeruginosa, S. aureus,* and *S typhimurium*, as well as the antibacterial mechanism of quercetin in *S. aureus* and *E. coli*. Quercetin had a more pronounced effect on Gram-positive bacteria than Gram-negative bacteria as a bacteriostatic. *E. coli* (at 50 MIC) and *S. aureus* (at 10 MIC) suffered membrane and wall damage when exposed to quercetin. The other screened molecule was vindolinine, which was shown to interact more strongly but less than chlorogenic acid. Complex 2exb-indoline has been observed to show very near and less binding energy, i.e., −6.9 kcal/mol, than control drug binding energy, and interaction with the bacterial receptor could be mediated through the involvement of two hydrogen bonds (Figure 4E,F and Table 1). It was observed that amino acid residues mainly SER62, ARG361, SER420, GLN422, SER357, SER306, LEU421, ASP155, GLY358, SER306, ASN308, ARG361, and LEU359 were involved in the formation hydrogen bonds during 2exb interaction with selected compounds (Table 1). Meanwhile, amino acid residues ALA61 were found in hydrophobic interaction in all complexes (Table 1).

Table 1. The data was obtained after performing molecular docking against penicillin-binding protein 4 (dacB) from *Escherichia coli* (PDB:2EXB) and selected compounds using the AutoDock 4.0 tool.

Complex	Binding Energy	No. of Hydrogen Bonds	Residues Forming Hydrogen Bond	Residues Involved in Hydrophobic Interaction
2exb-Flomoxef	−7.1	11	SER62, ARG361, SER420,GLN422, SER357,SER306,LEU421,ASP155	PRO152,SER398,THR418, GLY419,ASN308,ALA61, GLY358,LYS65,LEU359,ASP155,LYS417
2exb-Chlorogenic Acid	−7.7	6	SER420,GLY358,SER357,SER306,	LEU421, SER62,LYS305,GLY419, THR418,LEU359,ALA61
2exb-quercetin	−7.5	3	ASN308,ARG361,LEU359	SER398,LYS417,THR418,SER420,LEU421,SER62, ALA61,GLY358,PHE160,LYS305,SER306
2exb-vindolinine	−6.9	2	ASN308,SER420	LYS65,ALA61,GLY358,LEU359, LEU421,LYS305,SER306, SER62,PHE160

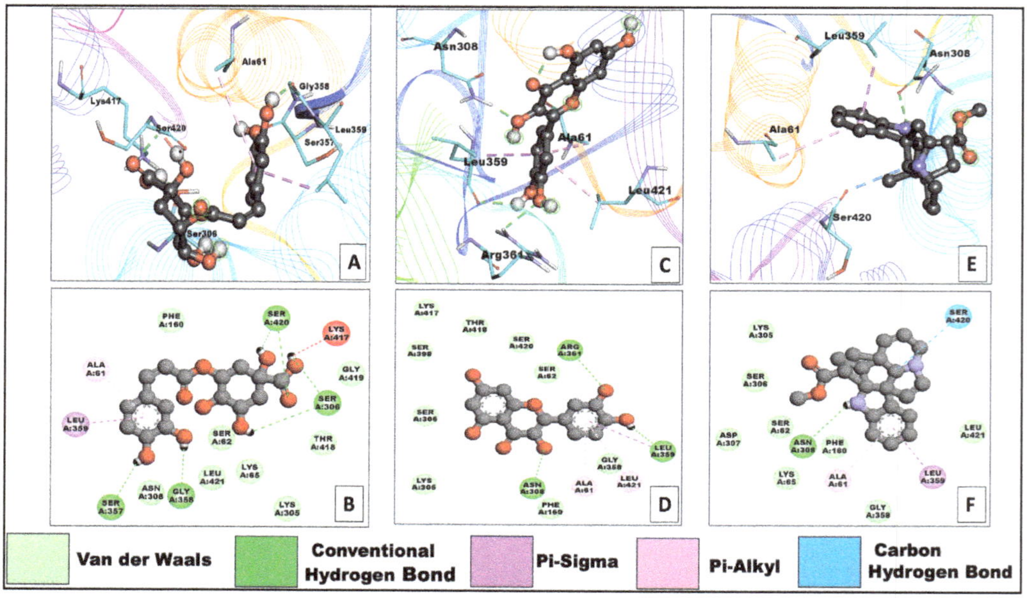

Figure 4. Showing 2D and 3D representations of best-screened compounds and their interaction against penicillin-binding protein 4 (dacB) from *Escherichia coli* (PDB:2EXB). (**A**,**B**) represents 2exb-chlorogenic Acid, (**C**,**D**) represents 2exb-quercetin, and (**E**,**F**) represents 2exb-vindolinine complexes. The receptor molecules (PDB:2EXB) are shown by a rainbow line ribbon pattern, and compounds are in the center, shown by a grey ball and stick shape. In the 3D representation, a cyan stick pattern indicates the most interacting amino acids. In 2D representation, the multicolor spheres show amino acid residues forming different types of interactions.

The binding and interaction patterns of all selected complexes are depicted in the following Figure 4. 3D and 2D graphics have been developed for visual interpretation.

The herbal remedy from *C. roseus* is found in tropical regions. Antibacterial activity in the plant's leaves has been demonstrated against various microorganisms, notably *S. aureus*, *E. coli*, and *C. albicans*. Catharanthine, Vincristine, and vinblastine are only some of the alkaloids found in *C. roseus* leaves, and they're responsible for the plant's antibacterial properties [20]. These alkaloids have been reported to kill bacteria by interfering with their reproduction ability. Moreover, there are phenolic chemicals in *C. roseus*, which have antibacterial effects [21,22].

These chemicals are believed to kill bacteria by causing membrane disruption within their cells. Several bacteria, like *S. aureus*, *E. coli*, and *P. aeruginosa*, were killed by an ethanolic leaf extract. The alcohol-based extract of the leaves was used to treat *S aureus*-induced infection of the skin in rats, as described in vivo research. The medication successfully mitigated the disease's effects [22]. Antibiotic agents, in combination, provided combined benefits for *Candida albicans* who have developed fluconazole resistance. Antimicrobial activities against *E. coli*, *S. aureus*, MRSA strains, and *C. albicans* have also been detected with the ethanol extract of *C. roseus* leaves. Although the precise mechanism(s) by which *C. roseus* inhibited bacterial growth remains unknown, it is likely a combination of several factors. Among these are the alkaloid compounds in *C. roseus*, which can cause the bacterial cell membrane to become permeable and allow vital chemicals to escape. The alkaloids generate free radicals that can cause DNA damage, which stops bacteria from multiplying and interferes with the protein synthesis of bacteria [23]. Studies have shown that the antibacterial effects of *C. roseus* leaves can be attributed to their phenolic and alkaloid content. This plant's ideal dosage and administration method have yet to be determined, and more research is required to establish its efficacy in treating bacterial infections. Being a sensitive analytical technique, NMR is used in the identification of metabolites derived from plants, animals, and microbes.

Fingerprinting circumvents the labeling difficulty caused by the abundance of signals in high-resolution 1H NMR spectra by comparing multiple spectra and, by extension, the specimens that were used when these spectra were produced via the application of multivariate analysis. Metabolites in the living things that were subjected to NMR analysis are the sources of the signals, as seen in the spectra. Finding out whether a collection of samples has similar or dissimilar spectra is more important than determining which metabolites are present. Originally created for use in healthcare applications, this type of pattern detection for analyzing NMR spectra has lately found its way into the examination of plant-based extracts and materials [24].

The phenolic found in plants encompass various categories of chemicals, including simple phenolic, flavonoids, phenolic acids, flavonoids, lignins, and tannins; molecules are characterized by the presence of a minimum one aromatic ring with at least one hydroxyl group attached. The hydroxyl group can either be unbound or involved in another chemical function, such as ether, ester, or glycoside. They are commonly found in plants and are often found in higher concentrations, either as soluble or cell wall-bound chemicals, due to the plant's relation to the atmosphere.

Some primary metabolites like branch chain amino acids (BCAA), lactate, alanine, pyruvate, glutamate, malic acid, glucose, and fumaric acid were likely to be found in *C. roseus* in variable amounts in different parts of the stem and leaf of the plant as we also studied using NMR spectroscopy. Furthermore, some important peaks of secondary metabolites were most likely found in NMR spectra of the leaves aqueous extract of leaves, like 2,3 butanediol, quinic acids, vindoline, chlorogenic acids, vindolinine, secologanin, and quercetin. These metabolites dominated intensity and were detected by NMR in a mixture of plant tissue.

Monoterpenoid Indole Alkaloids, also known as MIAs, are a fascinating class of specialized metabolites that possess a vast array of chemical structures. They are also a source of a number of active biomolecules, including significant pharmacophores like anticancer drugs, camptothecins, and Vinca alkaloids, which are based on this type of structural configuration. The latter substances are found in low concentrations in the leaves of the *C. roseus*. They are the product of a complicated metabolic process, which is the focus of increasing research efforts [25].

The MICAs originate from a one-of-a-kind polyvalent framework that is referred to as strictosamide. This important precursor is the condensed product of an amine derived from tryptophan that has been coupled to a monoterpenoid moiety that has undergone substantial modification. While tryptophan decarboxylase (TDC) facilitates a solitary reaction wherein tryptophan is converted to tryptamine, the organization of the monoterpene secoiridoid moiety needs many reactions to produce secologanin using methyl-erythritol phosphate (MEP) pathway-derived monoterpenoid skeleton [12,26]. Four genes have been identified as being involved in the synthesis of vindoline, a terpenoid indole alkaloid that is an essential component of *C. roseus* leaves. Nevertheless, the information regarding the spatial arrangement of the tabersonine-to-vindoline biosynthetic route still needs to be completed. Previous studies were able to prove the existence of transcripts of the enzyme 16-hydroxytabersonine 16-O-methyltransferase (16OMT), which are specifically localized to the aerial organ epidermis, by using in situ hybridization [27,28]. Acids are a significant group of plant compounds that serve as a crucial layer of defense on leaves to defend against both living and non-living threats. Phenolic chlorogenic acids are prevalent in several plants and exhibit significant antibacterial characteristics. Investigations have shown that chlorogenic acid successfully hinders the growth of many bacteria, including *Shigella dysenteria* and *S. pneumonia* [29], and it was effective against both Gram-negative and Gram-positive bacteria. Furthermore, the coffee bean contains unusually high concentrations of chlorogenic acids, which are extensively dispersed metabolites in plants. The main chemical structure is a conjugate of caffeic acid (3,4-dihydroxy cinnamic acid) and tetrahydroxy-cyclohexane carboxylic acid (quinic acid). Quercetin is the primary phenolic component of this plant and exhibits antimicrobial properties. The antibacterial activity observed in this study could be due to the presence of quercetin, which needs to be explored more in the future [30]. Hydroxylated phenolic molecules with an aromatic ring structure are known as flavonoids. We observed the presence of quercetin, which belongs to this group of chemicals. It is a naturally occurring bioactive chemical with a flavonoid configuration nC6(ring A)-C3(ring C)–C6(ring B). Numerous physiological activities in plants, including pollen proliferation, plant growth, seed germination, photosynthesis, and the formation of antioxidant machinery that confers tolerance against both abiotic and biotic stresses, are all facilitated by quercetin. Consequently, this plant's quercetin has a strong protective effect that has to be investigated further through in vivo research [31,32].

NMR analysis is a useful technique for metabolite analysis despite being somewhat limited by its degree of sensitivity. These analyses can enhance high-throughput system-wide investigations by MS. Utilizing coupled techniques that enable parallel MS and NMR investigations on the same sample is an effective method to expand the portion of the metabolites that can be uncovered through routine study. The latest development in metabolomics has been caused by the need for more in-depth analyses to support the discovery of the metabolic process network and the potential use of metabolomics to reveal gene function. The technique involves utilizing metabolite data to uncover the phenotype of silent mutations by analyzing metabolite signatures by 1H-NMR analysis. Nuclear magnetic resonance spectroscopy (NMR) is commonly used independently to characterize and identify metabolomics samples despite their inherent complementarity. The ability to compare NMR data with references or to use two-dimensional NMR to explain structure is the primary advantage of NMR metabolomic research [33]. This study allows for the investigation of primary metabolites, which include organic acids, sugars, and amino acids, as well as secondary metabolites, which include phenolic compounds, which are frequently abundant in plants. Metabolites such as 2,3 butanediol, quinic acids, vindoline, chlorogenic acids, vindolinine, secologanin, and quercetin in plants extracted from *C. roseus* leaf and stem used as drugs for anticancer other medications used for human health and treatment system. The aerial parts of the plants have shown significant antibacterial activities against bacterial pathogens.

3. Material and Methods

3.1. Plant Material

We collected the cultivated plant material to make 100 g of powder in the months of February and March from the NCR, Ghaziabad, at 28.6692° N and 77.4538° E. At the CSIR-National Botanical Research Institute in Lucknow, India, Dr. K.M. Prabhu Kumar authenticated the cultivated plant (PDSH/LWG/Authentication/Ang./2023-24/47) as *C. roseus* and subsequently deposited it at the same institute under the accession number 119224. The aerial sections of *C. roseus*, such as the leaf and stem, were selected for extraction, in vitro antibacterial activities, and metabolite identification and characterization using NMR spectroscopy. The selected leaves and stems of the plants were collected, kept in the shadows for drying, and powdered. Extraction was carried out at room temperature on a shaker using 10 g/100 mL of water, methanol, and hexane as a solvent in different flasks and used for antimicrobial activities.

3.2. Preparation of Extract

Fresh plant materials were used for metabolite identification. We transferred the fresh and sterilized tubes to the container holding the liquid nitrogen. Frozen tissue was stored for a few hours at −80 °C before drying. However, metabolites may degrade while being stored. The frozen plant parts were ground using a pre-cooled pestle mortar and liquid nitrogen. Transfer the ground leaf and stem into a plastic tube using a spatula. Subsequently, it was mixed and homogenized using the vortex for one minute at 25 °C. Furthermore, 1 to 2 min of room-temperature ultrasonication was performed. After ultracentrifugation, the extract was divided into 2 mL Eppendorf tubes and spun at 4 °C at 10,000 rpm for 10 min. To achieve a clear supernatant, the debris was separated. More time is needed to obtain a clean supernatant with higher-speed centrifugation. More than 1 mL of clear extract was transferred to a 1.5 mL fresh tube. Centrifugation (10,000 rpm, at 4 °C, for 10 min) was again repeated to achieve more clear supernatant and lyophilized. The term "lyophilization" refers to the technique of removing water from frozen products by placing them in a vacuum, resulting in the ice melting and turning into vapor without ever touching a liquid state. Furthermore, 1 to 2 min of room-temperature ultrasonication was also operated.

In preparation for additional NMR analysis, the sample was lyophilized, dried, powdered, and kept at −80 °C. The frozen powder was transferred into Eppendorf tubes. After dissolving the dry powder in 550 µL of D_2O, it was moved to a 5 mm NMR tube. 0.75 mL of potassium dihydrogen phosphate buffer (KH_2 PO_4) in D_2O was added to the tube containing a mixture of the plant sample and 550 µL of D_2O [34,35].

An overview of sample collection, preparation, and crude extraction of leaf and stem from *C. roseus* is given in Figure 5.

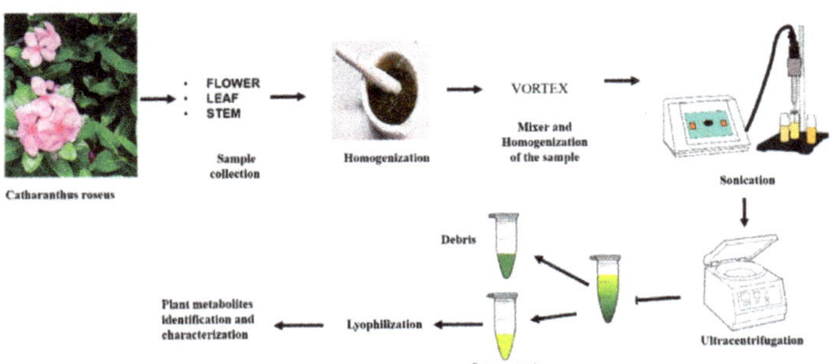

Figure 5. Simple presentation of sample collection, preparation, and metabolite extraction from *Catharanthus roseus* from different parts like flower, leaf, and stem.

3.3. Determination of Antibacterial Activity

To evaluate the antimicrobial significance of the leaves and stem extracts, each extract's antibacterial activity was tested against reference strains and both Gram-positive and Gram-negative meat-derived bacterial isolates. For isolation, the meat sample was suspended in sterile water and kept in open air at room temperature for 2 days for the growth of microbes. The sample was inoculated on a solidified agar medium, grown at 37 °C overnight. From the grown colonies, two Gram-negative and two Gram-positive bacterial isolates were identified by Gram staining and used for a more comprehensive evaluation of the plant extracts' antibacterial properties. The reference bacterial strains were Gram-negative, *E. coli* (ATCC 9637), and Gram-positive, *S. aureus* (ATCC3538). Using agar well diffusion, extracts from the leaves and stems were evaluated for their capacity to regulate the growth of the bacterial indicators [36]. Agar plates were seeded with a bacterial culture that had grown overnight to find the minimal inhibitory concentration and the minimum bactericidal concentration. Antibiotic ampicillin (20 μg) was employed as a benchmark medication to measure the relative antibacterial efficacy of each extract. The statistics were run on GraphPad Prism 9.4.0 (San Diego, CA, USA). The antibacterial activities were analyzed three times. Therefore, the results are the average Standard Deviations for $n = 3$ sample size. A one-way analysis of variance (ANOVA) was used to determine the statistical significance. The p-value was used to evaluate the level of significance. If p is less than 0.05, the result is regarded as significant. The significant values were expressed as *** p value 0.0001.

3.4. Virtual Screening and Docking Studies

The virtual screening was performed with the chemical components of the extracted fraction that showed potent antibacterial activities (water) to find the most interacting molecules with the bacterial drug target (Table 2) directly obtained from the PubChem database [37]. From their SMILS IDs, the 3D structures were generated using the NovoPro online server (https://novoprolabs.com/tools/smiles2pdb) (accessed on 25 December 2023), and 2D structures were generated by Smi2Depict online tool (accessed on 22 February 2024) [38]. Later, the bacterial target crystal structural configuration of penicillin-binding protein 4 (dacB) from *Escherichia coli* (PDB:2EXB) [39] was downloaded from Protein Data Bank (PDB) [40] for molecular docking purposes, and interaction was performed by PyRx tool version 0.8 [41] and AutoDock 4.0 modules as adapted by Jamal et al., 2023 [42,43]. The energy minimization, 3D conformation analysis, and visualization of complexes were performed by Discovery Studio Visualizer 2021 v. 21.1.0.20298 [44] https://discover.3ds.com/discovery-studio-visualizer-download (accessed on 31 December 2023).

Table 2. List of natural compounds selected for virtual screening against penicillin-binding protein 4 (dacB) from *Escherichia coli* (PDB:2EXB).

PubChem IDs	Compound Names	SMILES IDs	2D Structures
CID:262	2,3-Butanediol	CC(C(C)O)O	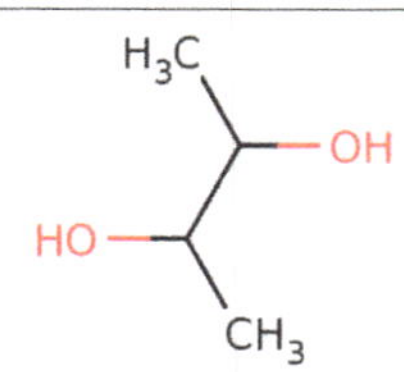
CID:6508	Quinic Acid	C1C(C(C(CC1(C(=O)O)O)O)O)O	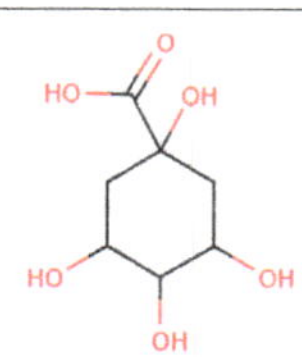

Table 2. *Cont.*

PubChem IDs	Compound Names	SMILES IDs	2D Structures
CID: 260535	Vindoline	CCC12C=CCN3C1C4(CC3)C(C(C2OC(=O)C)(C(=O)OC)O)N(C5=C4C=CC(=C5)OC)C	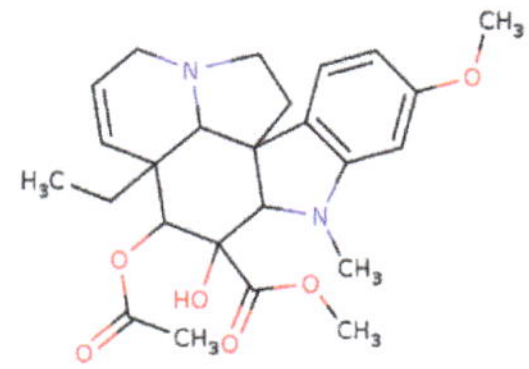
CID:525	Malic Acid	C(C(C(=O)O)O)C(=O)O	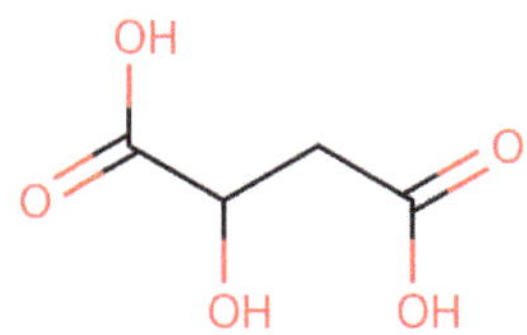
CID:1794427	Chlorogenic Acid	C1C(C(C(CC1(C(=O)O)O)OC(=O)C=CC2=CC(=C(C=C2)O)O)O)O	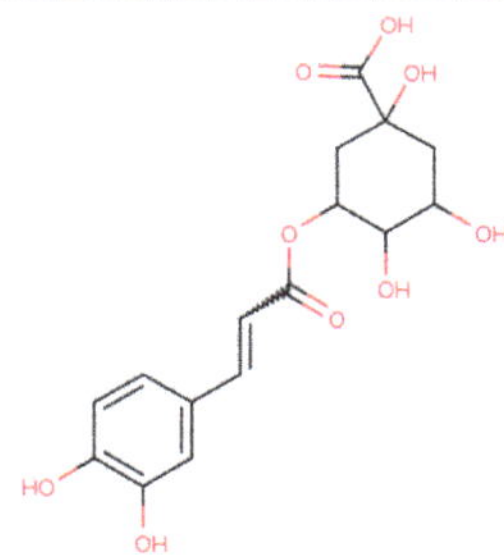
CID:444972	Fumaric Acid	C(=CC(=O)O)C(=O)O	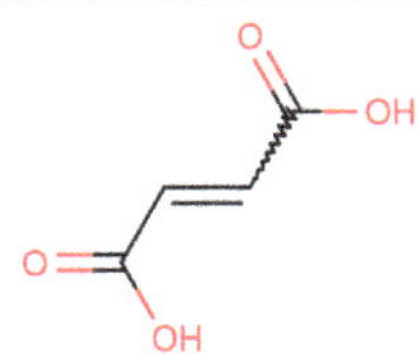
CID: 24148538	Vindolinine	CC1C23CC(C14C5(C2N(CC5)CC=C3)C6=CC=CC=C6N4)C(=O)OC	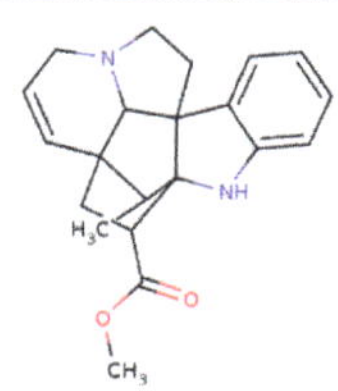
CID: 161276	Secologanin	COC(=O)C1=COC(C(C1CC=O)C=C)OC2C(C(C(C(O2)CO)O)O)O	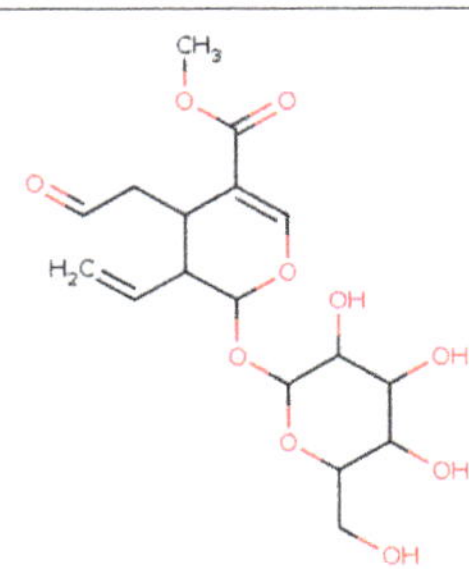

Table 2. *Cont.*

PubChem IDs	Compound Names	SMILES IDs	2D Structures
CID: 5280343	Quercetin	C1=CC(=C(C=C1C2=C(C(=O)C3=C(C=C(C=C3O2)O)O)O)O)O	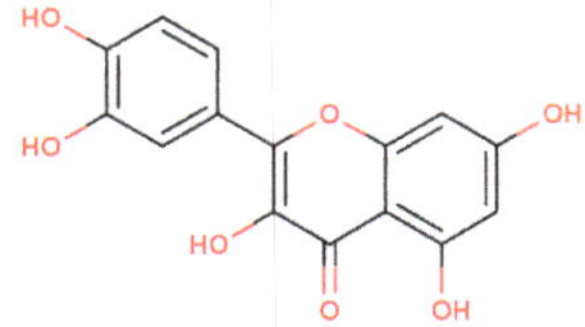

The most likely metabolites observed to be in the aqueous fraction of leaves and stems of the C. roseus plant were 2,3-Butanediol, Quinic Acid, Vindoline, Malic Acid, Chlorogenic Acid, Fumaric Acid, Vindolinine, Secologanin, and Quercetin, which were used in vertical screening. The dominant components of the aqueous extract of leaves are 2,3 butanediol, 4-0 caffeoyl, quinic acids, fumaric acids, vindolinine, glucose, glutamate, and lactate. While the most likely metabolites observed with the aqueous fraction of stem were branch chain amino lactate, alanine, pyruvate, glutamate, malic acid, glucose, chlorogenic acids, fumaric acid, secologanin, quercetin, fumaric acids, and loganic acid, The loganic acid was only observed in the aqueous fraction of the stem.

3.5. Proton Nuclear Magnetic Resonance Spectroscopy

In order to perform the 1H-NMR analysis, the samples that had been extracted were mixed with D_2O again until they reached a volume of 600 μL, which was the needed amount. Both the frozen and modified extracts were treated with 0.5 mM sodium trimethylsilyl-2,2,3,3-d4-propionate (TSP) in order to alter the chemical calibration. We prepared every single one of the samples over the course of two days, and they were then kept in storage at 4 °C. 1H-NMR A spectrometer equipped with a 5 mm broadband inverse probe was used to record spectra at MHz and 300 K. The 1H studies were conducted in one dimension using a 90° pulse angle and a little pre-saturation of the water resonance. With a capture period of s and a relaxation delay of 5 s, 512 shifts were used to collect NMR spectra. In all of these methods, a single 1H-NMR scan is all that is needed to quickly produce metabolomics data from a sample (5 s for 64–128 scans, for example). Chenomx NMR Suite 8.1 was used for processing and analysis of the spectra. To account for a line-broadening of 0.5 Hz, the spectra that had been forward-transformed were multiplied by a logarithmic weighted function. The chemical shifts of all the bands were compared to TSP, and they were all hand-corrected and adjusted for baseline. Chenomx was used to perform an analysis of the spectra that were obtained, and the specific metabolites that were found were calculated in each of the specimens. With the use of the integrated Chenomx, the Human Metabolome Database [45], and further research on plant metabolomic studies, after analysis, the metabolite-related spikes of the produced bands were assigned to the corresponding chemical shifts. The identified molecules were evaluated and validated by comparing them with the chemical shift readings obtained from additional NMR-based metabolomics investigations that were carried out in and by comparing them using the other Metabolomic databases. The identified metabolites were analyzed by Chenomx software (Chenomx NMR Suite 8.1) and with respect to the internal standard TSP. All the NMR spectral data were used to identify and characterize metabolites [46].

4. Conclusions

Given the rising death rate over the past decade and the increasing complexity of the disease, the need for innovative and safer therapeutic agents is urgent. Through this NMR analysis, 2,3 butanediol, quinic acids, vindoline, chlorogenic acids, vindolinine, secologanin, and quercetin are just some of the phytochemicals and terpenoid indole alkaloids (TIAs) that were produced in abundance in the leaves and less in the stem of *C. roseus*, a few of which as chlorogenic acid and vindolinine are likely to have their significant antibacterial activities. These chemicals are significantly extracted in polar solvents (water) and not in nonpolar solvents (hexane). The strong antibacterial properties of the aqueous extracts are seen in their ability to fight both Gram-positive and Gram-negative bacteria. The chemical constituent of this plant extracted in water could be an alternative antimicrobial molecule. Thus, the active chemical of this plant extracted in water needs to be explored more through in vivo studies.

Author Contributions: Conceptualization, Q.M.S.J. and V.A.; methodology, V.A.; software, V.A. and Q.M.S.J.; validation, V.A. and Q.M.S.J.; formal analysis, V.A.; investigation, V.A. and Q.M.S.J.; resources, V.A. and Q.M.S.J.; data curation, Q.M.S.J. and V.A.; writing—original draft preparation, V.A. and Q.M.S.J.; writing—review and editing, V.A. and Q.M.S.J.; visualization, V.A. and Q.M.S.J.; supervision, Q.M.S.J.; project administration, Q.M.S.J.; funding acquisition, Q.M.S.J. All authors have read and agreed to the published version of the manuscript.

Funding: The Deanship of Scientific Research, Qassim University, Saudi Arabia, funded the project under grant number 2023-SDG-1-HMSRC-36946.

Institutional Review Board Statement: Not applicable.

Informed Consent Statement: Not applicable.

Data Availability Statement: Data is contained within the article.

Acknowledgments: The authors gratefully acknowledge Qassim University, represented by the Deanship of Scientific Research, on the financial support for this research under the number 2023-SDG-1-HMSRC-36946 during the academic year 1445 AH/2023 AD. The authors also thank Azhar Kamal, Integral University, Lucknow, and Pradeep Kumar, Department of NMR, AIIMS, New Delhi, India, for their technical suggestions and help.

Conflicts of Interest: The authors declare no conflicts of interest.

References

1. Kahn, R.; Morozov, I.; Feldmann, H.; Richt, J.A. 6th International Conference on emerging zoonoses. *Zoonoses Public Health* **2012**, *59*, 2–31. [CrossRef] [PubMed]
2. Capita, R.; Alonso-Calleja, C. Antibiotic-resistant bacteria: A challenge for the food industry. *Crit. Rev. Food Sci. Nutr.* **2013**, *53*, 11–48. [CrossRef] [PubMed]
3. Neethirajan, S. Recent advances in wearable sensors for animal health management. *Sens. Bio-Sens. Res.* **2017**, *12*, 15–29. [CrossRef]
4. Sounkaria, S.; Sachdeva, G.; Das, A.; Verma, S.R.; Saxena, S.C.; Singh, B.P.; Rahman, S.; Chandra, P. Potentialities of nanobiotechnology in nutrient management in the livestock products. In *Nanobiotechnology for the Livestock Industry*; Elsevier: Amsterdam, The Netherlands, 2023; pp. 111–137.
5. Nisar, P.; Ali, N.; Rahman, L.; Ali, M.; Shinwari, Z.K. Antimicrobial activities of biologically synthesized metal nanoparticles: An insight into the mechanism of action. *JBIC J. Biol. Inorg. Chem.* **2019**, *24*, 929–941. [CrossRef]
6. Gold, K.; Slay, B.; Knackstedt, M.; Gaharwar, A.K. Antimicrobial activity of metal and metal-oxide based nanoparticles. *Adv. Ther.* **2018**, *1*, 1700033. [CrossRef]
7. Parham, S.; Wicaksono, D.H.; Bagherbaigi, S.; Lee, S.L.; Nur, H. Antimicrobial treatment of different metal oxide nanoparticles: A critical review. *J. Chin. Chem. Soc.* **2016**, *63*, 385–393. [CrossRef]
8. Gonelimali, F.D.; Lin, J.; Miao, W.; Xuan, J.; Charles, F.; Chen, M.; Hatab, S.R. Antimicrobial properties and mechanism of action of some plant extracts against food pathogens and spoilage microorganisms. *Front. Microbiol.* **2018**, *9*, 1639. [CrossRef] [PubMed]
9. Alhaithloul, H.A.; Soliman, M.H.; Ameta, K.L.; El-Esawi, M.A.; Elkelish, A. Changes in ecophysiology, osmolytes, and secondary metabolites of the medicinal plants of Mentha piperita and *Catharanthus roseus* subjected to drought and heat stress. *Biomolecules* **2019**, *10*, 43. [CrossRef]
10. van Dam, N.M.; van der Meijden, E. A role for metabolomics in plant ecology. In *Biology of Plant Metabolomics*; Annual Plant Reviews; Blackwell Publishing Ltd: Oxford, UK, 2011; Volume 43, pp. 87–107.
11. Taher, Z.M.; Agouillal, F.; Marof, A.Q.; Dailin, D.J.; Nurjayadi, M.; Razif, E.N.; Gomaa, S.E.; El Enshasy, H.A. Anticancer molecules from *Catharanthus roseus*. *Indones. J. Pharm.* **2019**, *30*, 147. [CrossRef]
12. Thirumaran, R.; Prendergast, G.C.; Gilman, P.B. Cytotoxic chemotherapy in clinical treatment of cancer. In *Cancer Immunotherapy*; Elsevier: Amsterdam, The Netherlands, 2007; pp. 101–116.

13. Pant, B. Application of plant cell and tissue culture for the production of phytochemicals in medicinal plants. In *Infectious Diseases and Nanomedicine II, Proceedings of the First International Conference (ICIDN–2012), Kathmandu, Nepal, 15–18 December 2012*; Springer: New Delhi, India, 2014; pp. 25–39.
14. Das, A.; Sarkar, S.; Bhattacharyya, S.; Gantait, S. Biotechnological advancements in *Catharanthus roseus* (L.) G. Don. *Appl. Microbiol. Biotechnol.* **2020**, *104*, 4811–4835. [CrossRef]
15. Farnsworth, N.R.; Akerele, O.; Bingel, A.S.; Soejarto, D.D.; Guo, Z. Medicinal plants in therapy. *Bull. World Health Organ.* **1985**, *63*, 965–981. [CrossRef] [PubMed]
16. Gajalakshmi, S.; Vijayalakshmi, S.; Devi, R.V. Pharmacological activities of *Catharanthus roseus*: A perspective review. *Int. J. Pharma Bio Sci.* **2013**, *4*, 431–439.
17. Mishra, D.; Chitara, M.K.; Chaturvedi, P. Study of phytochemicals, antioxidant activity and antimicrobial properties of *Catharanthus roseus* (L.) G. Don. *Emergent Life Sci. Res.* **2022**, *8*, 75–79. [CrossRef]
18. Karunanidhi, A.; Thomas, R.; van Belkum, A.; Neela, V. In vitro antibacterial and antibiofilm activities of chlorogenic acid against clinical isolates of Stenotrophomonas maltophilia including the trimethoprim/sulfamethoxazole resistant strain. *BioMed Res. Int.* **2013**, *2013*, 392058. [CrossRef] [PubMed]
19. Lu, H.; Tian, Z.; Cui, Y.; Liu, Z.; Ma, X. Chlorogenic acid: A comprehensive review of the dietary sources, processing effects, bioavailability, beneficial properties, mechanisms of action, and future directions. *Compr. Rev. Food Sci. Food Saf.* **2020**, *19*, 3130–3158. [CrossRef] [PubMed]
20. Muhammad, M.; Basit, A.; Wahab, A.; Li, W.-J.; Shah, S.T.; Mohamed, H.I. Response mechanism of plant stresses to secondary metabolites production. In *Fungal Secondary Metabolites*; Elsevier: Amsterdam, The Netherlands, 2024; pp. 469–492.
21. Goboza, M.; Meyer, M.; Aboua, Y.G.; Oguntibeju, O.O. In vitro antidiabetic and antioxidant effects of different extracts of catharanthus roseus and its indole alkaloid, vindoline. *Molecules* **2020**, *25*, 5546. [CrossRef] [PubMed]
22. Huang, W.; Wang, Y.; Tian, W.; Cui, X.; Tu, P.; Li, J.; Shi, S.; Liu, X. Biosynthesis investigations of terpenoid, alkaloid, and flavonoid antimicrobial agents derived from medicinal plants. *Antibiotics* **2022**, *11*, 1380. [CrossRef] [PubMed]
23. Karthikeyan, G.; Swamy, M.K.; Viknesh, M.R.; Shurya, R.; Sudhakar, N. Bioactive Phytocompounds to fight against antimicrobial resistance. In *Plant-Derived Bioactives: Production, Properties and Therapeutic Applications*; Springer: Singapore, 2020; pp. 335–381.
24. Salem, M.A.; Perez de Souza, L.; Serag, A.; Fernie, A.R.; Farag, M.A.; Ezzat, S.M.; Alseekh, S. Metabolomics in the context of plant natural products research: From sample preparation to metabolite analysis. *Metabolites* **2020**, *10*, 37. [CrossRef] [PubMed]
25. Dugé de Bernonville, T.; Foureau, E.; Parage, C.; Lanoue, A.; Clastre, M.; Londono, M.A.; Oudin, A.; Houillé, B.; Papon, N.; Besseau, S.; et al. Characterization of a second secologanin synthase isoform producing both secologanin and secoxyloganin allows enhanced de novo assembly of a *Catharanthus roseus* transcriptome. *BMC Genom.* **2015**, *16*, 619. [CrossRef]
26. Miettinen, K.; Dong, L.; Navrot, N.; Schneider, T.; Burlat, V.; Pollier, J.; Woittiez, L.; Van Der Krol, S.; Lugan, R.; Ilc, T. The seco-iridoid pathway from *Catharanthus roseus*. *Nat. Commun.* **2014**, *5*, 3606. [CrossRef]
27. Xu, F.; Zou, L.; Ong, C.N. Multiorigination of chromatographic peaks in derivatized GC/MS metabolomics: A confounder that influences metabolic pathway interpretation. *J. Proteome Res.* **2009**, *8*, 5657–5665. [CrossRef] [PubMed]
28. Guirimand, G.; Guihur, A.; Poutrain, P.; Héricourt, F.; Mahroug, S.; St-Pierre, B.; Burlat, V.; Courdavault, V. Spatial organization of the vindoline biosynthetic pathway in *Catharanthus roseus*. *J. Plant Physiol.* **2011**, *168*, 549–557. [CrossRef] [PubMed]
29. Lou, Z.; Wang, H.; Zhu, S.; Ma, C.; Wang, Z. Antibacterial activity and mechanism of action of chlorogenic acid. *J. Food Sci.* **2011**, *76*, M398–M403. [CrossRef] [PubMed]
30. Wang, S.; Yao, J.; Zhou, B.; Yang, J.; Chaudry, M.T.; Wang, M.; Xiao, F.; Li, Y.; Yin, W. Bacteriostatic Effect of Quercetin as an Antibiotic Alternative In Vivo and Its Antibacterial Mechanism In Vitro. *J. Food Prot.* **2018**, *81*, 68–78. [CrossRef] [PubMed]
31. Bentz, A.B. A Review of Quercetin: Chemistry, antioxidant properties, and bioavailability. *J. Young Investig.* **2017**, *10*, 15. Available online: https://www.jyi.org/2009-april/2017/10/15/a-review-of-quercetin-chemistry-antioxidant-properties-and-bioavailability (accessed on 24 January 2024).
32. Singh, P.; Arif, Y.; Bajguz, A.; Hayat, S. The role of quercetin in plants. *Plant Physiol. Biochem. PPB* **2021**, *166*, 10–19. [CrossRef] [PubMed]
33. Kim, J.; Cantor, A.B.; Orkin, S.H.; Wang, J. Use of in vivo biotinylation to study protein–protein and protein–DNA interactions in mouse embryonic stem cells. *Nat. Protoc.* **2009**, *4*, 506–517. [CrossRef] [PubMed]
34. Azizan, A.; Lee, A.X.; Abdul Hamid, N.A.; Maulidiani, M.; Mediani, A.; Abdul Ghafar, S.Z.; Zolkeflee, N.K.Z.; Abas, F. Potentially bioactive metabolites from pineapple waste extracts and their antioxidant and α-glucosidase inhibitory activities by 1H NMR. *Foods* **2020**, *9*, 173. [CrossRef]
35. Schripsema, J. Application of NMR in plant metabolomics: Techniques, problems and prospects. *Phytochem. Anal. Int. J. Plant Chem. Biochem. Tech.* **2010**, *21*, 14–21. [CrossRef] [PubMed]
36. Syeda, A.M.; Riazunnisa, K. Data on GC-MS analysis, in vitro anti-oxidant and anti-microbial activity of the *Catharanthus roseus* and Moringa oleifera leaf extracts. *Data Brief* **2020**, *29*, 105258. [CrossRef]
37. Kim, S.; Thiessen, P.A.; Bolton, E.E.; Chen, J.; Fu, G.; Gindulyte, A.; Han, L.; He, J.; He, S.; Shoemaker, B.A.; et al. PubChem Substance and Compound databases. *Nucleic Acids Res.* **2016**, *44*, D1202–D1213. [CrossRef]
38. Chen, J.H.; Linstead, E.; Swamidass, S.J.; Wang, D.; Baldi, P. ChemDB update—Full-text search and virtual chemical space. *Bioinformatics* **2007**, *23*, 2348–2351. [CrossRef] [PubMed]

39. Kishida, H.; Unzai, S.; Roper, D.I.; Lloyd, A.; Park, S.Y.; Tame, J.R. Crystal structure of penicillin binding protein 4 (dacB) from Escherichia coli, both in the native form and covalently linked to various antibiotics. *Biochemistry* **2006**, *45*, 783–792. [CrossRef] [PubMed]
40. Berman, H.M.; Westbrook, J.; Feng, Z.; Gilliland, G.; Bhat, T.N.; Weissig, H.; Shindyalov, I.N.; Bourne, P.E. The Protein Data Bank. *Nucleic Acids Res.* **2000**, *28*, 235–242. [CrossRef] [PubMed]
41. Dallakyan, S.; Olson, A.J. Small-molecule library screening by docking with PyRx. *Methods Mol. Biol.* **2015**, *1263*, 243–250. [CrossRef] [PubMed]
42. Morris, G.M.; Huey, R.; Lindstrom, W.; Sanner, M.F.; Belew, R.K.; Goodsell, D.S.; Olson, A.J. AutoDock4 and AutoDockTools4: Automated docking with selective receptor flexibility. *J. Comput. Chem.* **2009**, *30*, 2785–2791. [CrossRef] [PubMed]
43. Jamal, Q.M.S.; Khan, M.I.; Alharbi, A.H.; Ahmad, V.; Yadav, B.S. Identification of Natural Compounds of the Apple as Inhibitors against Cholinesterase for the Treatment of Alzheimer's Disease: An In Silico Molecular Docking Simulation and ADMET Study. *Nutrients* **2023**, *15*, 1579. [CrossRef]
44. BIOVIA Discovery Studio. Discovery Studio Visualizer. 2021, v. 21.1.0.20298. San Diego. Available online: https://discover.3ds.com/discovery-studio-visualizer-download (accessed on 8 January 2022).
45. Wishart, D.S.; Tzur, D.; Knox, C.; Eisner, R.; Guo, A.C.; Young, N.; Cheng, D.; Jewell, K.; Arndt, D.; Sawhney, S.; et al. HMDB: The Human Metabolome Database. *Nucleic Acids Res.* **2007**, *35*, D521–D526. [CrossRef]
46. Kumar, M.S.N.; Gupta, G.; Kumar, V.; Jagannathan, N.R.; Sinha, S.; Mewar, S.; Kumar, P. Differentiation between sepsis survivors and sepsis non-survivors through blood serum metabolomics: A proton nuclear magnetic resonance spectroscopy (NMR) study. *Magn. Reson. Imaging* **2022**, *89*, 49–57. [CrossRef]

pharmaceuticals

MDPI

Article

HPLC-DAD Analysis and Investigation of Biological Properties of the Leaves of *Globularia alypum* (L.), Infusion Extract

Sahar Nouir [1], Aicha Laouani [2,3], Ahmed Loghmari [4], Khaireddine Bouassida [4], Raoudha Slim [5], Rim Bouhajeb [6], Yosra Hasni [7], Khaled Saguem [2,3], Bouraoui Ouni [5] and Amira Zaïri [1,*]

1 Laboratory of Biochemistry, Faculty of Medicine of Sousse, University of Sousse, Sousse 4023, Tunisia; sanouir@yahoo.fr

2 Laboratory of Metabolic Biophysics and Applied Pharmacology (LR12/ES02), Faculty of Medicine of Sousse, University of Sousse, Sousse 4023, Tunisia; laouani_aicha@yahoo.fr (A.L.); khaledsaguem@famso.u-sousse.tn (K.S.)

3 USCR Analytical Platform UHPLC-MS & Research in Medicine and Biology, Faculty of Medicine of Sousse, University of Sousse, Sousse 4023, Tunisia

4 Urology Department, Sahloul Hospital, Sousse 4054, Tunisia; loghmariahmed@gmail.com (A.L.); bouassidakhaireddine@gmail.com (K.B.)

5 Laboratory of Bioactive Natural Substances and Biotechnology Research, Faculty of Dental Medicine of Monastir, University of Monastir, Sousse 4023, Tunisia; raoudha_slim3@yahoo.fr (R.S.); elounibouraoui@yahoo.fr (B.O.)

6 Department of Pharmacology, Faculty of Medicine of Sousse, University of Sousse, Sousse 4023, Tunisia; rimbouhajeb1993@gmail.com

7 Department of Endocrinology, Farhat Hached Hospital of Sousse, Sousse 4000, Tunisia; yosrahasnielabed@gmail.com

* Correspondence: zairi_amira@yahoo.fr

Abstract: *Globularia alypum* L. (GA) belonging to the Globulariaceae family is a Mediterranean plant which is widely used in traditional Tunisian medicine. The aim of this study was to investigate the phytochemical composition, antioxidant, anti-arthritic, antiproliferative, antibacterial and antibiofilm potential of aqueous GA leaf extracts (AGAL). Quantitative analyses of the different constituents of extracts were evaluated by high-performance liquid chromatography with photodiode-array detection (HPLC-DAD). Spectrophotometric methods and chemical tests were used for antioxidant and anti-arthritic activities. The antiproliferative study was evaluated using colorectal cancer SW620 cells, while the antibacterial assessment and analysis of the antibiofilm effects were determined by the microdilution method and the crystal violet assay, respectively. AGAL extracts presented several components, mainly Nepetin-7-Glucoside and trans-ferrulic acid. The results showed that they had an important antioxidant (IC_{50} = 0.34; 0.38 and 1.20 mg/mL) and anti-arthritic (IC_{50} = 2.94 mg/mL) properties, and these effects are displayed in a dose-dependent manner. In addition, this extract demonstrated significant antiproliferative (IC_{50} = 50 µg/mL), antibacterial (MIC = 6.25 mg/mL and MBC = 6.25 mg/mL), and antibiofilm (59.70% at 25 mg/mL) properties especially against *S. aureus*. The results achieved confirm the important role of this plant as a source of therapeutic activities.

Keywords: *Globularia alypum* L.; HPLC-DAD; antioxidant activity; anti-arthritic activity; antiproliferative effect; antibacterial and antibiofilm activities

1. Introduction

Medicinal plants can yield a wide range of bioactive substances, particularly secondary metabolites. Thus, numerous scientists have reported conducting in-depth investigations utilizing various plant extracts to evaluate the antibacterial, anti-inflammatory, analgesic, antioxidant, and many other therapeutic properties of these extracts [1]. A wild plant in the *Globulariaceae* family is *Globularia alypum* L. (GA). This shrub is perennial and can be found in the Mediterranean region. There are several uses for the plant [2]. It is one of the most popular traditional plant treatments in the Tunisian traditional pharmacopoeia and it is known by the local name Zrigua. Traditionally, its leaves have been employed as cholagogue, laxative, stomachic, purgative, and sudorific agents [3]. Additionally, ethnobotanical studies have demonstrated its effectiveness in the treatment of cardiovascular and renal illnesses [1].

Other studies showed that the active principles in leaves, stems and flowers in methanol and dichloromethane extracts of GA are supposed to antagonize the contractile response induced by different neurotransmitters [4]. More recently, GA petroleum ether extract showed anti-tuberculosis activity against *Mycobacterium tuberculosis* while a GA methanol extract has shown a potent antioxidant effect [5–7]. All these biological activities are mainly due to the abundance of secondary metabolites, such as polyphenols and iridoids [8]. It is also important to mention that several studies have stated the different activities of GA, but most of them deal with organic extracts, whereas only few studies report the bioactivities of their aqueous extracts, namely decoctions or infusions. In fact, it has been reported that the aqueous GA leaf extract (GAAE) has the potential for human male infertility treatment since the leaves contain active compounds with androgenic qualities that enhance active spermatogenesis in mice at a daily dose of 100 mg/kg for 15 days [9]. In addition, previous in vivo studies showed a laxative effect of GAAE in constipated rats, and an anti-inflammatory effect in rats with induced ulcerative colitis (UC) [10].

The hypoglycemic and hypotriglyceridemia roles are another potential of GAAE; this effect was shown in rats through repeated oral administration [4]. Additionally, it has been noted that the aqueous extracts are comparatively safe because a 10 g/kg dosage was not deadly in mice [9] and the GA LD50 value in rats was found to be above 14.5 g/kg [11]. GA aqueous extract has also been shown in other studies to have potential as an adjuvant for the management and/or prevention of oxidative stress and hypertriglyceridemia. Indeed, researchers demonstrated that offering rats fed a high-fructose diet an extra dose of GA aqueous extract protects hypertriglyceridemia while also lowering TG-VLDL levels. Furthermore, by raising SOD and GPx, GA can shield the heart from oxidative stress [12,13]. To the best of our knowledge, no data are available regarding antimicrobial or anti-arthritic activities of the aqueous extract of GA. Accordingly, the aim of the present study is to scrutinize the antioxidant, anti-arthritic, antiproliferative, and antimicrobial activities of aqueous extracts obtained by infusion of *G. alypum* leaves. Moreover, a phytochemical analysis of extracts was also carried out.

2. Results

2.1. HPLC-DAD Analysis

An HPLC-DAD analysis system was used to separate and identify the active substances contained in GA infusion. The chromatographic separation of the infusion extract is shown in Figure 1. Analysis of this chromatogram recorded at 324 nm indicated the presence of phenolic compounds. Referring to the chromatogram of the standards (Figure 2), a total of five phenolic compounds were detected and identified on the basis of their retention times. The compounds were labelled according to their order of elution. The phenolic compounds detected in the GA infusion included Cafeic Acid: peak 1, RT = 7.4 min, Trans Ferrulic Acid: peak 2, RT = 13.4 min, Verbascoside:peak 3, RT = 17.04 min, Nepetin-7-Glucoside: peak 4, RT = 19.01 and Isorhamnetin-3-O-Rutinoside: pic 5, RT = 21.13 min (Table 1). Figure 3 illustrates the superposition of the two chromatograms, the infusion chromatogram and the chromatogram of the authentic standards purchased from Sigma Aldrich. In addition to retention time, peak identification is based on the agreement between the spectra of the analyte of interest and its corresponding authentic standard.

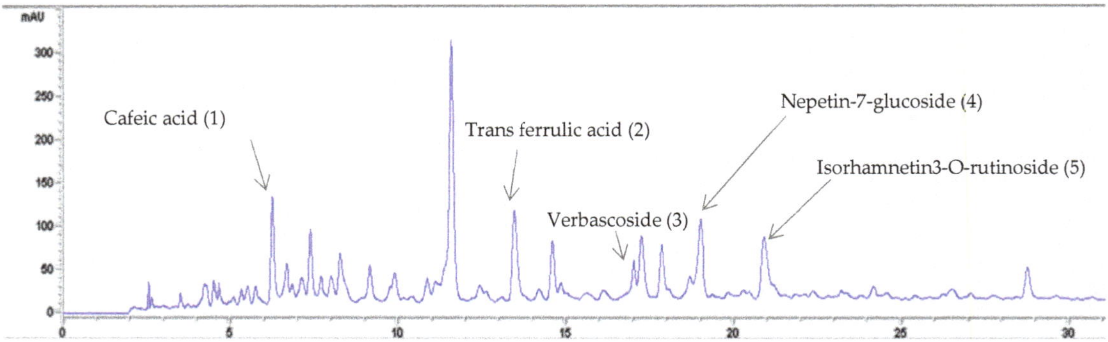

Figure 1. Chromatographic profile of *Globularia alypum* L. acquired at 324 nm.

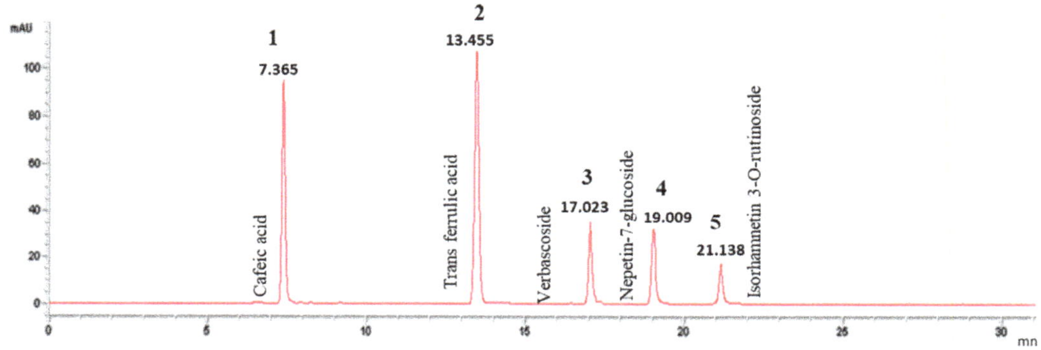

Figure 2. Chromatographic profile of standards recorded at 324 nm.

Table 1. Identification and quantification of five phenolic compounds of *Globularia alypum* L. extract acquired at 324 nm.

Peak	Retention Time (min)	Identification	Area	Quantity (µg/mL)
1	7.4	Cafeic Acid	468.3	7
2	13.4	Trans Ferrulic Acid	1011	10.33
3	17.04	Verbascoside	214.24	7
4	19.01	Nepetin-7-Glucoside	885.8	30.82
5	21.13	Isorhamnetin-3-O-Rutinoside	151.8	8.9

By recording the absorption spectra of the eluted analytes whose chromatographic peaks are illustrated in Figure 1, it is possible to distinguish three groups of analytes according to the shape and location of the spectral bands in their absorption spectra. The first group is formed by caffeic acid which represents an absorption spectrum characteristic of a phenolic acid chromophore. The second group is formed by Verbascoside and transferrulic acid; these compounds represent a characteristic absorption spectrum of a phenylpropanoid glycoside chromophore. The last group is formed by flavonoid glycosides represented by Nepetin7 glucoside and isorhamnetin 3-o rutinoside and whose absorption spectra are characteristic of a flavonoid chromophore.

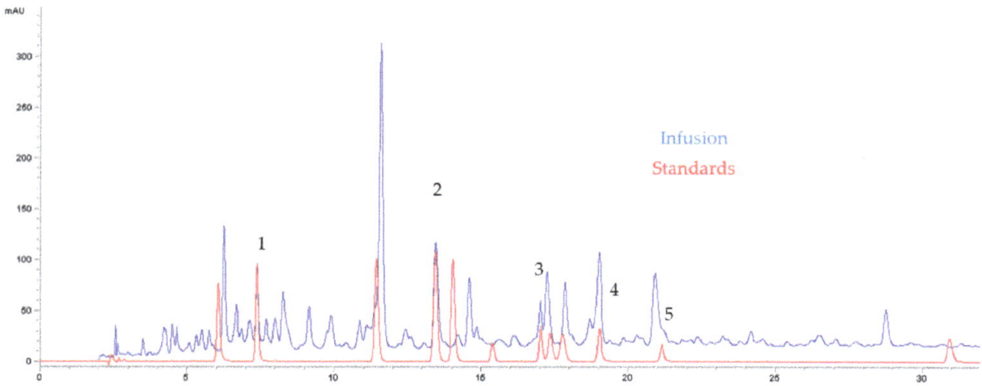

Figure 3. Chromatographic profile of *Globularia alypum* L. extract (blue) and standards (red) acquired at 324 nm.

In terms of quantity, nepetin-7-O-glucoside (30.82 μg/mL) was the most abundant component, followed by transferulic acid (10.33 μg/mL (*w/w*) (DW). Verbascoside and caffeic acid concentrations were present in smaller amounts in the plant infusion (7 μg/mL).

2.2. Antioxidant Activity

The antioxidant effect of *G. alypum.* infusion leaf extracts was performed by ABTS and β-carotene assays; the results were expressed as IC50 values. As presented in Table 2, the extract of *G. alypum* showed important antioxidant activities with significant variability between the used methods. The highest antioxidant potential with a value of IC50 = 0.24 ± 0.03 mg/mL was obtained by β-carotene assay, whereas a value of IC50 = 0.38 ± 0.02 mg/mL was obtained by ABTS. We concluded that the β-carotene activity assay was the most sensitive one in terms of IC50 by comparing the two methods used (Table 2).

Table 2. Antioxidant activity of *G. alypum* leaves. Values with different superscripts within the same column are significantly different ($p < 0.05$), and each data point is represented by the average of three repetitions ± SD of one independent experiment; IC_{50}: Half maximal Inhibitory Concentration.

IC_{50} (mg/mL)	Ascorbic Acid	Infusion
ABTS scavenging assay	0.06 ± 0.02 [a]	0.38 ± 0.02 [b]
β-carotene bleaching assay	0.59 ± 0.00 [a]	0.24 ± 0.03 [b]

2.3. Anti-Arthritic Effect

The results of in vitro anti-arthritic activity showed that aqueous extracts of *G. alypum* leaves had auspicious activity, as shown from the results on histamine releases, protein denaturation assay (Table 3).

Table 3. Evaluation of Anti-arthritic activity of *G. alypum* leaves. Results of the ANOVA test are significantly different at $p < 0.05$, and each data point is represented by the average of three repetitions ± SD of one independent experiment; IC_{50}: Half maximal Inhibitory Concentration. Values with different superscripts within the same column are significantly different ($p < 0.05$).

IC_{50} (mg/mL)	Acetyl Salicylic Acid	Infusion
Protein denaturation	0.73 ± 0.02 [a]	3.58 ± 0.02 [b]

2.4. Antiproliferative Effect

In the present study, an evaluation of the antiproliferative effect of different extracts from *G. alypum* leaves on SW620 was performed at various concentrations. After 48 h of incubation, the survival rates showed that all the extracts inhibit cell line proliferation in a concentration-dependent manner. The infusion extract presented a higher anti-proliferative effect with an IC50 = 50 µg/mL (Figure 4).

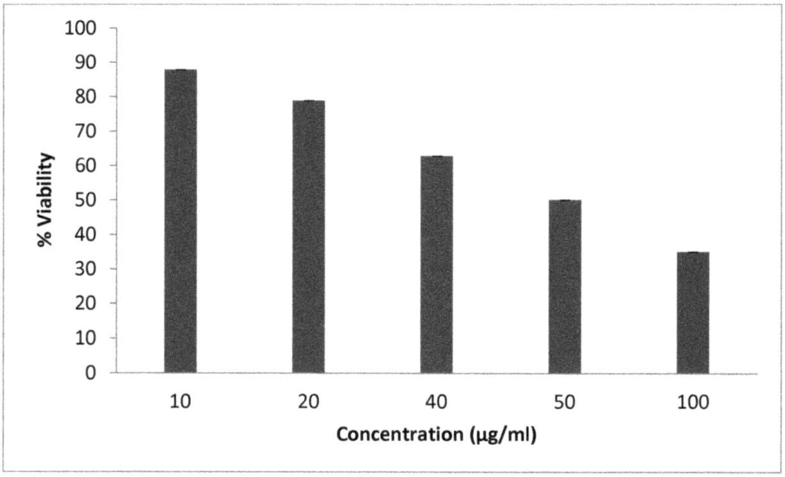

Figure 4. Antiproliferative effect of *G. alypum* leaves obtained by infusion. Viability rate (means ± standard deviations) of SW620 cells treated with the extract obtained by infusion of *G. alypum* leaves. (IC_{50} = 50 µg/mL); IC_{50}: Concentration required reducing SW620 cell viability by 50%.

2.5. Evaluation of Antibacterial Activity

Tables 4 and 5 demonstrate the aqueous *G. alypum* extracts' capacity to suppress the growth of both Gram-positive and Gram-negative planktonic cells. All the tested stains exhibited sensitivity to the extract, according to the results. *S. aureus* had the strongest effect, with a minimum inhibitory concentration (MIC) of 6.25 mg/mL and a zone of inhibition measuring 24 mm.

Table 4. Evaluation of antibacterial activity of *G. alypum* leaves at 25 mg/mL. Values are means of triplicate determination, (n = 3) ± standard deviation. N, no zone of inhibition was found.

	Zone of Inhibition (mm)	
Strains	**Tetracycline**	**Infusion**
E. coli	29.10 ± 0.00	21.00 ± 0.00
P. aeruginosa	27.20 ± 0.53	11.50 ± 1.01
S. typhimurium	25.01 ± 1.02	21.50 ± 0.31
S. aureus	21.00 ± 1.82	24.00 ± 1.31

Table 5. MIC and MBC determination of the infusion extract of *G. alypum* leaves. Minimum Inhibitory Concentration (MIC) and Minimum Bactericidal Concentration (MBC). N: not found.

Strains	**Tetracycline**		**Infusion**	
Concentrations (mg/mL)	**MIC**	**MBC**	**MIC**	**MBC**
E. coli	3.12	6.25	>25	N
P. aeruginosa	3.12	6.25	>25	N
S. typhimurium	6.25	6.25	>25	N
S. aureus	6.25	6.25	6.25	6.25

2.6. Antibiofilm Activity

In the current study, the antibiofilm effect of infusion extracts of *G. alypum* were tested at different concentrations (MIC and 1/8 MIC). The biofilm inhibition rates against *S. aureus* were 45.39% to 59.70%, and 31.69 to 45.99% against *S. thyphimirium*. Moreover, the biofilm inhibition was weaker for *E. coli* and totally absent for *P. aeuroginosa*. It is worth noting that *G. alypum*, which strongly affected *S. aureus* and *S. thyphimirium* biofilm, was the least active against *P. aeuroginosa* (Table 6).

Table 6. Percentage of biofilm inhibition after 24 h. Data are the means ± SD of three independent experiments. The values with different superscript letters show significantly ($p < 0.05$) different means.

	Percentage of Inhibition (%)			
Concentrations (mg/mL)	***E. coli*** ^{a}	***S. typhimurium*** ^{b}	***S. aureus*** ^{c}	***P. aeruginosa***
25	26.31	45.85	59.83	N
12.5	18.94	38.68	54.92	N
6.25	16.19	37.21	53.11	N
3.12	14.23	31.15	45.31	N

3. Discussion

Many substances found in nature, referred to as secondary metabolites, are derived from plants and have been used for millennia to create new therapeutics. In general, the phytochemical investigation of *Globularia alypum* revealed the presence of significant amounts of various chemical components, while the present work is aimed at analyzing the aqueous extracts of leaves of *G alypum* using the HPLC-DAD method for detecting the characteristic peak values and their functional groups. HPLC analysis revealed different characteristic peak values with various functional constituents in the extracts. The identified chemicals in Tunisian GA extracts have never been reported. The examined extracts were different from those in the results of other researchers working on Tunisian aqueous *G. alypum* species. Indeed, the phenolic fraction of *Globularia alypum* aqueous extract (GAAE) from the northwest of Tunisia is dominated by iridoids and secoiridoids with an abundance of serratoside, as demonstrated by Hajji et al. utilizing HPLC-PDA/ESI-MS analysis. They demonstrated the detection of three more flavonoids. Phellamurin comes in third, after quercetin glucoside and gallo-catechin as the primary ingredients. Verbascoside constituted the majority of GAAE's composition [10]. Furthermore, since the aqueous extracts of Bouriche et al. include distinct components, their study can be cited. In fact, the authors noted that the aqueous extracts of *G. alypum* that were collected in June 2010 from Sétif, in Eastern Algeria, showed the presence of flavonoids and phenolic acids according to the HPLC-TOF/MS analysis. The glycoside flavonoids diosmin, rutin, and scutellarin are present in significant concentrations in these extracts, with naringin and quercetin-3-β-D-glucoside having the highest concentrations. Additionally, they disclosed that of the identified phenolic acids, there was a high cinnamic acid concentration together with protocatechuic acid [14]. The variations observed in the phenolic profiles of aqueous extracts derived from diverse sources may be attributed to growth and environmental factors such as soil composition, altitude, rainfall, and climate, as well as the distinct methods employed to ascertain this composition. These elements may have a direct impact on the composition of chemical components. Given their high phenolic component content, our obtained extracts will probably show a range of biological activity [13]. For instance, Calvin et al. reveled that nepetin isolated from *Eupatorium arnottianum* (EA) was investigated in the TPA mouse ear edema and was found to be active. Nepetin reduced the TPA mouse ear edema and inhibited the NF kappaB induction as it is a major component of the EA extract [15]. Moreover, Boubaker et al. showed that isorhamnetin 3-O-rutinoside promotes apoptosis of human myelogenous erythroleukaemia cells [16]. Furthermore, as far as we know, few studies have been conducted to determine the phenolic composition of aqueous extracts of *Globularia alypum* in Tunisia. The evaluation of these extracts is very limited; only few plants have been evaluated to date, and no data have been described before to determine the polyphenol composition of decoction or infusion extracts. Almost all the available studies in the literature reported mostly on methanolic extracts or essential oils.

Nowadays, due to safety concerns for synthetic antioxidants, there is an increasing demand for natural antioxidants [16]. Herbs are great sources of antioxidants due to their natural antioxidant components, especially for food preservation. The results shown in this study revealed that aqueous extracts of *G. alypum* leaves showed important antioxidant activities and that this effect was in a dose-dependent relationship. Regarding antioxidant activity, it has been previously reported that phenolic compounds such as flavonoids, phenolic acid, and tannins contribute considerably to the antioxidant activity in medicinal plants [17]. Our extract contained the highest-level nepetin-7-O-glucoside. It has been reported that this molecule exhibits several pharmacological effects, including anti-inflammatory and antioxidant activities [15]. In addition, isorhamnetin 3-O-rutinoside is a flavonoid glycoside that exerts an antioxidant effect [16]. Our results are also in compliance with a study conducted by Jrah et al., who showed that aqueous extract of *G. alypum* showed the highest antioxidant capacity with a value of 8.9 mM TE and 4.5 mM TE by FRAP and the Reducing Power (RP) method, respectively [17]. It is interesting to note that our findings imply that our extracts have noticeably more antioxidant activity than other nearby plants. For instance, according to ABTS and β-carotene assays, *G. alypum* obtained from Oueslatia Kairouan in central Tunisia showed antioxidant activity at IC 50 = 0.89 and 0.42 mg/mL, respectively [18]. On the other hand, 0.04 and 0.15 mg/mL were sufficient to enhance the same impact. Additionally, a study conducted in January 2016 in Batna, Algeria examined the antioxidant activity of *G. alypum* collected from Ain Zaatot. Two methods were used to quantify this activity: the ferric reducing antioxidant power (FRAP) and the DPPH radical scavenging assay. The data obtained indicated that *G. alypum* exhibited significant concentrations of scavenging activity: IC50 223.04 $\pm$ 0.73 to 85.37 $\pm$ 1.48 µg/mL and EC50 0.31 $\pm$ 0.01 to 0.68 $\pm$ 0.19 mg/mL [19]. The variety seen in the antioxidant activities of G. alypum might likely be explained by the experimental setup, the methods employed, and the utilization of plants from various geographical regions. It is important to mention that aqueous extracts of *G. alypum* showed an effect on colonic antioxidant enzyme activity. A study conducted by Hajji et al. showed that GA collected from Northwest of Tunisia had a significant decrease in superoxide dismutase (SOD) and gluthation peroxidase (GPx) activities in the colon of AA-intoxicated animals compared to the controls, whereas GAAE (100, 200 and 400 mg/Kg, b.w.) or sulfasalazine (100 mg/Kg, b.w.) pretreatment over seven days significantly protected against this depletion when compared to the colitis group ($p < 0.05$) [10]. In the same context, a recent study of Hajji et al. proved that GAAE regenerates antioxidant enzymes after depletion under LOP administration enzyme levels showed depletion when treated only with LOP. However, administration of yohimbine regenerates antioxidant enzyme levels. GAAE also significantly increased SOD and GPx levels in a dose-dependent manner (400 mg/kg) [13].

The results of a second Algerian investigation demonstrated that *G. alypum* methanolic and aqueous extracts, which were obtained in June 2010 from Sétif in Eastern Algeria, could chelate ferrous ions in a concentration-dependent way. In contrast to the methanolic extract, the aqueous extract displayed more activity. In total, 52.69 μg/mL and 148.15 μg/mL, respectively, were the IC50 values. Compared to the results obtained with EDTA, the standard chelator, which produced an IC50 value of 5.97 μg/mL, this activity was less significant [14]. We draw the conclusion that the primary cause of the phenolic components of GA's antioxidant activity is their redox characteristics, which enable them to function as singlet oxygen quenchers, hydrogen donors, and reducing agents [20]. A metallic chelating potential might also exist in them [21].

According to WHO, 0.3–1% of the world population is affected by rheumatoid arthritis (RA), and among them females are three times more prone to the disease compared to males [22]. RA is a chronic, inflammatory, and systemic autoimmune disease [23]. Therapeutic agents against arthritis such as analgesics and NSAIDS reduce inflammation and joint destruction in either acute or chronic RA patients [24]. On the other hand, gastrointestinal ulcers, cardiovascular complications, myelosuppression, hepatic fibrosis, stomatitis, cirrhosis, nephrotoxicity, pulmonary toxicity, immunological reactions, and local injection-site reactions are among the long-term dangers associated with medication use. Furthermore, increased expenses and adverse effects, such as elevated chances of infections and miscarriages, necessitate ongoing surveillance [24]. As a result, fresh strategies are created to preserve the harmony between these possible hazards and recognized advantages [25]. Safer and more effective medications are currently being created from oriental sources for the treatment of RA. To lessen these negative effects and boost the positive effects, a wide range of herbal extracts and products, including polyherbal formulations, are created [24]. A review conducted by Choudhary et al. reported that about 485 plant species would have a promising anti-arthritic activity in humans. Cross-validation of information regarding the ethnic proof of historically used anti-arthritic plants was conducted using a variety of journal articles and reviews [26]. As far as we know, no such review has examined the relationship between the plant family, components utilized, and dosage form and the anti-arthritic properties of the plants. According to these data, the Papilonaceae family of plants has a higher concentration of plants with anti-arthritic action. Of these sections, leaves have been utilized most frequently in oil dose form to treat arthritis [26]. The used extracts in this study showed that aqueous extracts of *G. alypum* had an important anti-arthritic activity. In light of our knowledge, the evaluation of anti-arthritic activity of *G. alypum* is extremely limited. Only a little data relating to this activity have been reported. For instance, Friscic et al. showed that 50 μg/mL of aqueous extracts of *G. alypum* inhibited COX-1 activity and that this inhibition reached 51.3% (*G. alypum*) in the TMPD assay and 40.6% in the PGE2 assay. The authors also showed that the results obtained for *G. alypum* are comparable to those reported for the methanolic leaf (GAME) (5.33%) and the flower extract (61.05%) of the same species tested at a 33 μg/mL concentration using the TMPD assay [27]. Another study reported that the treatment of animals with GAME produced a significant decrease in the inflammatory cells; however, slight improvements in edema tissue were observed in the reference group. The authors explained that this anti-inflammatory effect of GAME may be equally related to its cinnamic acid content [28]. Additionally, they demonstrated that the outcomes for *G. alypum* are similar to those reported for the same species' methanolic leaf (GAME) (5.33%) and flower extract (61.05%) when examined using the TMPD assay at a dose of 33 μg/mL [27]. Another study found that offering GAME to rats resulted in a considerable reduction in inflammatory cells, although the reference group's edema tissue showed only modest reductions. The authors clarified that GAME's anti-inflammatory properties might be equally attributed to the amount of cinnamic acids it contains [28].

To select plant extracts with potential antitumor properties for future bio-related studies, cytotoxicity screening models provide important preliminary data [17]. To date, no reports have been found in the literature on the evaluation of the cytotoxicity of aqueous leaves extracts, as performed in this study. The present study examined, for the first time, the ability of AGAL to inhibit cancer cell proliferation, which is known to be the most promising route to treat cancer. The infusion extract presented a higher anti-proliferative effect with an IC50 = 50 μg/mL. This result can be explained by the richness of this extract of active molecules, especially ferulic acid (Figure 3). In fact, the study of Ekowati et al. performed in 2020 demonstrated that ferulic acid showed anticancer potential by suppressing angiogenesis and causing inhibition of melanoma growth in a xenograft model [29]. Comparing our result with the study of Friscic et al. [27], we distinguished that our extract has the lowest antiproliferative effect (IC_{50} = 50 and 231.43 μg/mL). In addition, no research has been performed previously to evaluate the anti-proliferative activity of aqueous extract.

Nowadays, many researchers around the world are working on plant extracts to develop new antimicrobial agents with enhanced safety and efficiency [15–19]. The prime objective of ethnopharmacology is to identify plants for medicinal importance with minimal side effects. Additionally, active compounds from the plant extracts with antibacterial activity can be transformed into possible medication. Research to develop efficient and accessible medication from active plant compounds in the interest of public health is the need of the present world. The present in vitro experimental study explored the antibacterial effect of aqueous extracts of *G. alypum* leaves against *Pseudomonas aeruginosa*, *Salmonella enterica* subsp. *enterica serovar Typhimurium*, *Escherichia coli*, and *Staphylococcus aureus*. The tested stains exhibited sensitivity to the extract, according to the results. *S. aureus* had the strongest effect, with a minimum inhibitory concentration (MIC) of 6.25 mg/mL and a zone of inhibition measuring 24 mm. The discussion is limited because, although the anti-arthritic effect of *G. alypum* aqueous extracts has been previously described, no research has been conducted to characterize its antibacterial activity. The limited information that is currently available on this activity, however, mostly reports on the antibacterial action of organic extracts [30]. For instance, we previously reported that sonication-obtained extracts of *G. alypum* demonstrated a noteworthy antibacterial effect on *S. aureus*, exhibiting a zone of inhibition of 14.5 mm that aligns with our actual study. However, these methanolic extracts demonstrated no effect against the remaining strains tested [31]. In addition to other water-soluble components that were naturally present in the plant material, Nayak et al. speculated that the anionic components, such as chlorides, thiocyanate, sulfates, and nitrate, may be responsible for the antibacterial action of aqueous extracts [32].

Since polyphenols, tannins, and flavonoids are often produced by plants and are involved in their defense against microbial infections, their presence in plant extracts may account for the antibacterial activity. Interestingly, Nepetin-7-Glucoside, a flavonoid and glycoside, is highly abundant in our extract [33]. Furthermore, trans-ferulic acid (TFA), which is abundant in the aqueous extract, possesses a variety of pharmacological qualities, such as antifungal and antibacterial activities [34].

In compliance with several other studies, the results obtained in this study showed that Gram-positive bacteria are more susceptible to plant extracts than Gram-negative bacteria. These differences may be related to the cell wall composition of bacteria. In fact, the cell wall of Gram-positive bacteria is single layered, whereas that of Gram-negative cells is multilayered [35]. Moreover, our extract also inhibited Gram-negative bacteria. This can be explained by the fact that Gram-negative bacteria have a hydrophilic membrane due to the presence of lipopolysaccharides, and thus, a small hydrophilic molecule can pass through the outer membrane as it was reported in several studies [35]. On the contrary, lipophilic compounds and macromolecules can pass through this outer membrane. Therefore, understanding of the permeation properties of the outer membrane of the microorganisms is essential to know about the antibacterial activity of a solute [35].

Extracellular polysaccharides (EPS) are a complex matrix of microorganisms that link to one another to form biofilms. These biofilms can shield cells from antibacterial agents and decrease their antibacterial effectiveness [36]. Since adhesion affects the biofilm's eventual development and maturity, it is the initial and most important stage in the formation of a biofilm [37]. Naturally occurring bacteria that produce biofilms are the main source of many illnesses in both humans and animals [38]. Bacterial biofilms can also result in major issues for the food business. These days, a lot of research has been conducted with the aim to create benign antibiofilm agents because they do not eventually induce medication resistance [39]. In the current study, an antimicrobial assay showed that our extracts displayed an antibiofilm activity especially against *S. aureus*. To the best of our knowledge, no prior information has been provided regarding the antibiofilm activity of *G. alypum*, and this is the first time that it has been documented. Furthermore, our investigation demonstrated that *G. alypum* extract exhibited clear antibiofilm efficacy against *S. aureus* biofilms at doses equal to or lower than the 1/4 MIC threshold. Many phytochemicals found in medicinal plants, including flavonoids, glycosides, tannic acid, phenolics, and chlorogenic acid, have the ability to suppress or completely eliminate biofilms by preventing the growth of bacteria that produce them, rupturing the polysaccharides in extracellular polymer (EPS), destroying the integrity of the bacteria's membrane, preventing the activity of enzymes linked to biofilm formation, rupturing the fibrils that allow bacteria adherence to one another, suppressing the expression of genes related to biofilms, or suppressing the quorum-sensing system [40–42].

G. alypum contain more than a dozen chemical constituents, including the following flavonoids: cafeic acid, trans-ferrulic acid, Verbascoside, Nepetin-7-Glucoside, Isorhamnetin-3-O-Rutinoside and other chemical constituents. We hypothesize that the combined action of *G. alypum*'s phytoconstituents, particularly the abundant flavonoids and ferrulic acid that have demonstrated both biofilm and antibacterial activity, may be responsible for both the suppression of biofilm formation and antibacterial activity. Nevertheless, a thorough explanation of the precise mechanisms at play is still required. We already demonstrated the high ferulic acid content of our extracts. One of the most prevalent phenolic acids in natural species is ferulic acid (AF), also known as 3-(4-hy-droxy-3-methoxyphenyl)-2-propenoic acid, a secondary metabolite that is a member of the phenolic chemical class [43]. After indirect studies demonstrated that ferulic acid had a high antibacterial activity against *L. monocytogenes* [44], the examination of ferulic acid's antimicrobial potential was proposed. The study of Pinheiro and his collaborators demonstrated that ferulic acid derivatives inhibit *Staphylococcus aureus* [45].

4. Materials and Methods

4.1. Plant Material

The study's use of plant material adheres to appropriate institutional, national, and international rules and regulations. *G. alypum* was collected at the full blooming stage in Tunisia's Ouardanin area in January 2019 (Table 7). Prof. Fethia Harzallah Skhiri of Tunisia's High Institute of Biotechnology in Monastir completed taxonomic identification. The plant voucher specimen was cataloged as Ga 022 in the Herbarium of the Laboratory of Bioresources: Integrative Biology and Valorization (ISBM). For 7 days, the leaves were washed and dried at room temperature. The material was dried until it reached a constant weight. To optimize phenolic extraction, the leaves were milled.

Table 7. Collection site of *Globularia. alypum* L. and its eco-geographical characteristics.

Collection Site	Geographical Location		
	Longitude (E)	Latitude (N)	Altitude (m)
Ouardanin	10°40′35″	35°42′35″	75

4.2. Preparation of the Infusion

A total of 5 g of shade-dried plant was soaked for 30 min in 100 mL of boiling distilled water. The infusion was then filtered through Whatman No. 4 paper, lyophilized and stored in an amber glass container at 4 °C until use.

4.3. HPLC-DAD Analyses

The chromatographic method adopted for analyses is based on a detection set at 324 nm. The Agilent 1100 Series HPLC system supplied with a diode array detector (DAD) is used. The chromatographic device is a computer-controlled agilent 1200. A reversed-phase Kinetex Evo C18 column placed in an oven at 30 °C is used for the separation of the different analytes in the infusion extract. The mobile phase consists of a mixture of water, acetonitrile and formic acid. Mobile phase A is formed by a combination of acetonitrile and formic acid (1%). Mobile phase B is formed by 99% water and 1% formic acid. The gradient program is conducted in the following way: 10% A, 90% B (0 min), 20% A, 80% B, (20 min), 25% A, 75% B (30 min), 35% A, 65% B, (40 min) and 10% A, 90% B10 (50 min). The rate of mobile phase elution is 1 mL/minute. Samples are filtered using a 0.20 µm filter prior to injection. The injected volume is 20 µL. Identification of the peaks of phenolic compounds is obtained by comparing their retention times as well as their UV spectra with those of available authentic standards [46,47]. All standards are purchased from Sigma-Aldrich. Peak identification is performed by congruent retention times and UV spectra compared to available authentic standards. Quantification is estimated by comparing the area of the peak of interest with that obtained in a standard chromatogram corresponding to a known concentration.

4.4. Antioxidant Activity

The method of El Arem and his collaborators based on spectrophotometric analysis was used to trap $ABTS^+$ cations [47]. To generate the ABTS radical cation, equal volumes of a solution of potassium persulfate $K_2S_2O_8$ 16 h prior to use and a stock solution of ABTS (39.2 mg) were mixed, kept at room temperature, and stored away from light. After that, ethanol was added to the solution to dilute it until the absorbance at 734 nm was between 0.7 and 0.8. For each analysis series, a volume of 975 µL of this freshly made solution was added to 25 µL of each extract, and the reading was taken at 734 nm after 20 min. A positive control was ascorbic acid. Based on the solution's discoloration, the antioxidant activity was calculated and expressed as the percentage inhibition (PI) of absorbance at 734 nm, the wavelength at which the ABTS+• radical exhibits a distinctive absorption band. Inhibition (%) = [(Abs control − Abs extract)/Abs control] × 100. All assays were performed in triplicate.

4.5. β-Carotene Bleaching Assays

The production of peroxide radicals from the oxidation of linoleic acid led to the oxidation of β-carotene, resulting in the loss of its red hue. An emulsion containing 0.5 mg β-carotene, 25 µL linoleic acid, 1 mL chloroform, 200 mg Tween 20-, and 100 mL distilled water served as the basis for this test. Subsequently, 2.5 mL of this emulsion was mixed with 0.5 mL of the extract or a control BHT (butyl hydroxytoluene) and incubated in a water bath at 50 °C for two hours. After adding the emulsion, the sample was tested many times at 20 min intervals [48], with the absorbance at T0 being recorded at 490 nm. Using the following formula, the percentage of inhibition of peroxidation was determined: IP = β-carotene after 2 h/initial β-carotene × 100. All assays were performed in triplicate.

4.6. Anti-Arthritic Effect

Using bovine serum albumin (BSA), the anti-arthritic effect of AGAL on the prevention of protein denaturation was assessed. The reaction mixture (0.5 mL) included 0.05 mL of various AGAL concentrations (0.0039–10 mg/mL) and 0.45 mL of BSA (5% aqueous solution) in addition to acetyl salicylic acid (reference drug), in that order. Using 1 N HCl, each solution was adjusted to pH 6.3. After adding 2.5 mL of phosphate buffer and incubating the samples for 30 min at 37 °C, the absorbance of the samples was determined using a spectrophotometer at 660 nm. *G. alypum* was replaced with 0.05 mL of distilled water for the test control, and BSA was absent from the product control [49]. The percentage inhibition of protein denaturation was deliberated by the following formula: Percentage inhibition = $(Abs_{Control} - Abs\ extract)/Abs_{Control}) \times 100$.

4.7. Antiproliferative Effect

Using a measurement of the SW620 cells extracted from colorectal human cells, the antiproliferative effect was assessed using the MTT assay for cellular metabolic activity. These cells were fixed at a density of 5×10^3 on a plate (MultiScreen®filtration plates, 96-well plates) in an incubator set at 37 °C with 5% CO_2. After the cells were taken out of the medium culture, they were treated with the extracts at various concentrations (100, 50, 40, 20, and 10 µg/mL) that were diluted in DMSO. This experiment was conducted three times. After 48 h of incubation, the MTT solution (1 mg/mL) treatment was started in RPMI 1640 culture media supplemented with 10% fetal bovine serum and a 10 µg/mL antibiotic: 5 µg/mL penicillin and 5 µg/mL streptomycin. The formation of purple formazan crystals from the yellow tetrazolium salt served as a marker for cells that were engaged in metabolism. After two hours of incubation at 37 °C with 5% CO_2, we evaluated the ratio (OD in the test group/OD in the control group × 100) using an ELISA reader to determine the percentage of survival of these cells. Three separate experiments were carried out.

4.8. Antibacterial Activity

The following types of bacteria were tested for AGAL's antibacterial activity using the agar disc diffusion method [50]: *Pseudomonas aeruginosa* ATCC 27853, *Salmonella enterica* subsp. *enterica serovar Typhimurium*. ATCC 14080, *Escherichia coli* ATCC 25922, and *Staphylococcus aureus* ATCC 25923. Using a sterile cotton mop, the pathogenic bacteria inoculums were adjusted to a 0.5 McFarland standard turbidity before being streaked onto Muller–Hinton (MH) agar plates. The agar mediums were covered with sterile filter discs (diameter 6 mm, Biolife, Rome, Italy), onto which 20 µL of each extract, diluted at a concentration of 25 mg/mL in sterile distilled water, was dropped. As a reference antibiotic, tetracycline (10 mg/mL; 10 µL/disc) was employed. The inhibition zone was measured to assess the antibacterial activity following a 24 h incubation period at 37 °C. Every assay was run three times. A MIC assessment was conducted [51]. The target bacteria and MH broth were added to plates containing 96 U-bottomed wells (Nunc, Roskilde, Denmark) together with serial dilutions of the extracts (0.05–25 mg/mL). Following a 24 h incubation period at 37 °C, the MBC was assessed by transferring 10 µL of the well's contents, which revealed no bacterial growth following the MIC test on MH agar. Upon examining the bacterial growth over a 24 h incubation period at 37 °C, the MBC was identified as the sample concentration with the lowest bactericidal action. Every assay was run in triplicate.

4.9. Antibiofilm Assay

The antibiofilm assay was determined using the crystal violet assay [51]. Various extract dilutions were produced at varying concentrations (0.05–25 mg/mL) in sterile distilled water. Subsequently, the mixture was added to plates containing 96 U-bottomed wells (Nunc, Roskilde, Denmark) that contained brain heart infusion (BHI) (Oxoid) with 2% glucose (*w*/*v*), containing pathogenic bacteria suspension (grown in BHI for 24 h at 37 °C; 105 CFU/mL). The negative and positive controls were BHI with 2% glucose alone and BHI with 2% glucose infected with the pathogenic strain, respectively. Following a 24 h incubation period at 37 °C, the plates underwent three PBS washes. The biofilm's cells were air-dried, fixed with methanol for 15 min, then stained with 1% crystal violet. Using a microplate reader (GIO. DE VITA E C, Roma, Italy), the absorbance at 595 nm was used to quantify the production of biofilms. Three separate experiments were conducted, and the formula used to calculate the percentage of inhibition was as follows: $(OD_{control} - OD_{Extract})/OD_{control} \times 100$ = Inhibition (%).

4.10. Statistical Analysis

The findings are shown as mean values ± standard deviation. Version 22 of SPSS was the foundation for statistical analyses. These analyses made use of the Student–Newman–Keuls test and ANOVA. For statistical significance, data were deemed different when the *p*-value was 0.05 or below.

5. Conclusions

The current investigation sheds more light on *G. alypum*'s phytochemical potential. The bioactive compounds found in the infusion extracts under investigation and their observed biological properties align with the findings of prior studies on biological activity. Additionally, these compounds offer significant health benefits not only in the treatment of oxidative stress-related diseases and reactive species production, but also in the prevention of bacterial infections.

Author Contributions: S.N.: Methodology and Draft writing; A.L. (Aicha Laouani) and K.S.: Methodology, Funding acquisition, A.L. (Ahmed Loghmari), K.B.: Resources, Software, R.S., Y.H. and B.O.: Investigation and Funding acquisition; R.B.: Methodology and A.Z.: Conceptualization, Investigation, Project Administration and Supervision. All authors have read and agreed to the published version of the manuscript.

Funding: This research received no external funding.

Institutional Review Board Statement: The study protocol was approved by the Institutional Review Board (or Ethics Committee) of the Faculty of Medicine of Sousse (protocol code CEFMS 186/2023 and date of approval: 20 June 2023).

Informed Consent Statement: Not applicable.

Data Availability Statement: Materials, data and associated protocols are promptly available to readers without undue qualifications in material transfer agreements. Concerning data information, please contact corresponding author.

Acknowledgments: We thank Faouzi Alaya Cheikh, The Norwegian University of Science and Technology, for English proof reading. We also thank Fethia Harzallah Skhiri, High Institute of Biotechnology of Monastir, for the botany identification of the plant *Globularia alypum* (L.).

Conflicts of Interest: The authors declare that they have no known competing financial interest or personal relationships that could have appeared to influence the work reported in this paper.

References

1. Jouad, H.; Haloui, M.; Rhiouani, H.; El Hilaly, J.; Eddouks, M. Ethnobotanical survey of medicinal plants used for the treatment of diabetes, cardiac and renal diseases in the North centre region of Morocco (Fez-Boulemane). *J. Ethnopharmacol.* **2001**, *77*, 175–182. [CrossRef] [PubMed]
2. Allali, H.; Benmehdi, H.; Benabadji, N. Phytotherapy of diabetes in west Algeria. *Asian. J. Chem.* **2008**, *20*, 2701–2710.
3. Skim, F.; Abderrazak, K.; Jaouhari, J.; Lazrek, H. Hypoglycaemic activity of *Globularia alypum* leaves in rats. *Fitoterapia* **1999**, *70*, 382–389. [CrossRef]
4. Bello, R.; Moreno, L.; Primo-Yufera, E.; Esplugues, J. *Globularia alypum* L. extracts reduced histamine and serotonin contraction in vitro. *Phytother. Res.* **2002**, *16*, 389–392. [CrossRef] [PubMed]
5. Ghlissi, Z.; Kallel, R.; Sila, A.; Harrabi, B.; Atheymen, R.; Zeghal, K.; Bougatef, A.; Sahnoun, Z. *Globularia alypum* methanolic extract improves burn wound healing process and inflammation in rats and possesses antibacterial and antioxidant activities. *Biomed. Pharm.* **2016**, *84*, 1488–1495. [CrossRef] [PubMed]
6. Khlifi, D.; Hamdi, M.; El Hayouni, A.; Cazaux, S.; Souchard, J.P.; Couderc, F.; Bouajila, J. Global chemical composition and antioxidant and anti-tuberculosis activities of various extracts of *Globularia alypum* L. (*Globulariaceae*) leaves. *Molecules* **2011**, *16*, 10592–10603. [CrossRef] [PubMed]
7. Taleb-Dida, N.; Krouf, D.; Bouchenak, M. *Globularia alypum* aqueous extract decreases hypertriglyceridemia and ameliorates oxidative status of the muscle, kidney, and heart in rats fed a high-fructose diet. *Nutr. Res.* **2011**, *31*, 488–495. [CrossRef] [PubMed]
8. Seca, A.M.; Pinto, D.C. Biological Potential and Medical Use of Secondary Metabolites. *Medicines* **2019**, *6*, 66. [CrossRef]
9. Fehri, B.; Aiache, J.M.; Ahmed, K.M. Active spermatogenesis induced by a reiterated administration of *Globularia alypum* L. aqueous leaf extract. *Pharmacogn. Res.* **2012**, *4*, 138–147. [CrossRef]

10. Hajji, N.; Jabri, M.A.; Tounsi, H.; Wanes, D.; Ali, I.B.E.H.; Boulila, A.; Marzouki, L.; Sebai, H. Phytochemical analysis by HPLC-PDA/ESI-MS of *Globularia alypum* aqueous extract and mechanism of its protective effect on experimental colitis induced by acetic acid in rat. *J. Funct. Foods.* **2018**, *47*, 220–228. [CrossRef]
11. Jouad, H.; Maghrani, M.; Eddouks, M. Hypoglycaemic effect of *Rubus fructicosis* L. and *Globularia alypum* L. in normal and streptozotocin-induced diabetic rats. *J. Ethnopharmacol.* **2002**, *81*, 351–356. [CrossRef] [PubMed]
12. Hajji, N.; Wannes, D.; Jabri, M.A.; Rtibi, K.; Tounsi, H.; Abdellaoui, A.; Sebai, H. Purgative/laxative actions of *Globularia alypum* aqueous extract on gastrointestinal-physiological function and against loperamide-induced constipation coupled to oxidative stress and inflammation in rats. *Neurogastroenterol. Motil.* **2020**, *32*, e13858. [CrossRef] [PubMed]
13. Hajji, N.; Russo, I.; Bianco, J.; Piazza, O.; Loino, P.; Santonicola, A.; Ciacci, C. The Role of *Globularia alypum* Explored Ex Vivo In Vitro on Human Colon Biopsies from Ulcerative Colitis Patients. *Nutrients* **2023**, *15*, 1457. [CrossRef] [PubMed]
14. Bouriche, H.; Kada, S.; Senator, A.; Demirtas, I. Phenolic Content and Biomolecule Oxidation Protective Activity of *Globularia alypum* Extracts. *Braz. Arch. Biol. Tech.* **2017**, *60*, e17160409. [CrossRef]
15. Clavin, M.; Gorzalczany, S.; Macho, A.; Munoz, E.; Ferraro, G.; Acevedo, C.; Martino, V. Anti-inflammatory activity of flavonoids from *Eupatorium arnottianum*. *J. Ethnopharmac.* **2007**, *112*, 585–589. [CrossRef] [PubMed]
16. Boubaker, J.; Bhouri, W.; Ben Sghaier, M.; Ghedira, K.; Dijoux Franca, M.G.; Chekir-Ghedira, L. Ethyl acetate extract and its major constituent, isorhamnetin 3-O-rutinoside, from *Nitraria retusa* leaves, promote apoptosis of human myelogenous erythroleukaemia cells. *Cell. Prolif.* **2011**, *44*, 453–461. [CrossRef] [PubMed]
17. Jrah Harzallah, H.; Neffati, A.; Skandrani, I.; Maaloul, E.; Chekir Ghedira, L.; Mahjoub, T. Antioxidant and antigenotoxic activities of *Globularia alypum* leaves extracts. *J. Med. Plant Res.* **2010**, *4*, 2048–2053. [CrossRef]
18. Khantouche, L.; Guesmi, F.; Motri, S.; Mejri, M.; Abderabba, M. Nutritional Composition, Analysis of Secondary Metabolites and Antioxidative Effects of the Leaves of *Globularia alypum* L. *Ind. J. Pharm. Sci.* **2018**, *80*, 274–281. [CrossRef]
19. Ouffai, K.; Azzi, R.; Abbou, F.; Lahfa, F.B. Antihemolytic and antioxidant activities of aerial parts extracts of Zygophyllum album L. and *Globularia alypum* L. from Algeria. *J. Nat. Prod. Reas.* **2022**, *1*, 41–55. [CrossRef]
20. Kamble, A.A.; Khan, N.D.; Khan, Z.H.; Mular, S.M.; Sohail, S. In vitro anti-arthritic activity of vitexnegundo and *Punica granatum*. *Res. J. Pharm. Sci.* **2017**, *6*, 5–7. [CrossRef]
21. Yan, M.; Zhu, Y.; Zhang, J.H.; Jiao, W.H.; Han, B.N.; Liu, Z.X.; Qiu, F.; Chen, W.S.; Hou-Wen Lin, H.W. Anti-Inflammatory secondary metabolites from the leaves of *Rosa laevigata*. *Bioorg. Med. Chem.* **2013**, *21*, 3290–3297. [CrossRef] [PubMed]
22. Barteková, M.; Adameová, A.; Görbe, A.; Ferenczyová, K.; Pecháňová, O.; Lazou, A.; Dhalla, N.S.; Ferdinandy, P.; Giricz, Z. Natural and synthetic antioxidants targeting cardiac oxidative stress and redox signaling in cardiometabolic diseases. *Free Radical. Biol. Med.* **2021**, *169*, 446–477. [CrossRef] [PubMed]
23. Ciampi, F.; Sordillo, L.M.; Gandy, J.C.; Caroprese, M.; Sevi, A.; Albenzio, M.; Santillo, A. Evaluation of natural plant extracts as antioxidants in a bovine in vitro model of oxidative stress. *J. Dairy. Sci.* **2020**, *103*, 8938–8947. [CrossRef] [PubMed]
24. Al-Qahtani, W.H.; Dinakarkumar, Y.; Arokiyaraj, S.; Saravanakumar, V.; Rajabathar, J.R.; Arjun, K.; Gayathri, P.K.; Appaturi, J.N. Phyto-chemical and biological activity of *Myristicafragrans*, an ayurvedic medicinal plant in Southern India and its ingredient analysis. *Saudi. J. Biol. Sci.* **2022**, *5*, 3815–3821. [CrossRef] [PubMed]
25. Tan, G.; Wang, Z.; Che, L.; Yin, S. Immunotherapeutic effects on murine pancreatic carcinoma by beta-elemene combined with dendritic cells modified with genes encoding interleukin-23. *Front. Med. China* **2007**, *1*, 41–45. [CrossRef] [PubMed]
26. Choudhary, M.; Kumar, V.; Malhotra, H.; Singh, S. Medicinal plants with potential anti- arthritic activity. *J. Intercult. Ethnopharmacol.* **2015**, *4*, 147–179. [CrossRef] [PubMed]
27. Friščić, M.; Petlevski, R.; Kosalec, I.; Madunić, J.; Matulić, M.; Bucar, F.; Hazler Pilepić, K.; Maleš, Ž. *Globularia alypum* L. and Related Species: LC-MS Profiles and Antidiabetic, Antioxidant, Anti-Inflammatory, Antibacterial and Anticancer Potential. *Pharmaceuticals* **2022**, *15*, 506. [CrossRef] [PubMed]
28. Ghlissi, Z.; Sayari, N.; Kallel, R.; Bougatef, A.; Sahnoun, Z. Antioxidant, antibacterial, anti-inflammatory and wound healing effects of Artemisia campestris aqueous extract in rat. *Biomed. Pharmacother.* **2016**, *84*, 115–122. [CrossRef]
29. Ekowati, J.; Hamid, I.S.; Diyah, N.W.; Siswandono, S. Ferulic Acid Prevents Angiogenesis Through Cyclooxygenase-2 and Vascular Endothelial Growth Factor in the Chick Embryo Chorioallantoic Membrane Model. *Turk. J. Pharm. Sci.* **2020**, *17*, 424–431. [CrossRef]
30. Da Silva, A.A.; da Silva, L.C.N.; da Fonseca, C.M.; de Araújo, J.M.; Correia, M.T.S.; Cavalcanti, M.S.; Lima, V.M. Antimicrobial Activity and Phytochemical Analysis of Organic Extracts from *Cleome spinosa* Jaqc. *Front. Microbiol.* **2016**, *28*, 963. [CrossRef]
31. Nouir, S.; Dbeibia, A.; Bouhajeb, R.; Haddad, H.; Khélifa, A.; Achour, L.; Ghardallou, M.; Zaïri, A. Phytochemical Analysis and Evaluation of the Antioxidant, Antiproliferative, Antibacterial, and Antibiofilm Effects of *Globularia alypum* (L.) Leaves. *Molecules* **2023**, *28*, 4019. [CrossRef] [PubMed]
32. Nayak, A.; Waterson, P. Global food safety as a complex adaptive system: Key concepts and future prospects. *Trends. Food. Sci. Tech.* **2019**, *91*, 409–425. [CrossRef]
33. Tim Cushnie, T.P.; Lamb, A.J. Recent advances in understanding the antibacterial properties of flavonoids. *Int. J. Antimicrob. Agents.* **2011**, *38*, 99–107. [CrossRef] [PubMed]
34. Rezaeiroshan, A.; Saeedi, M.; Samnani, K.M.; Akbari, J.; Omran, A.H.; Goli, H.; Nokhodchi, A. Vesicular Formation of Trans-Ferulic Acid: An Efficient Approach to Improve the Radical Scavenging and Antimicrobial Properties. *J. Pharmaceut. Innov.* **2022**, *17*, 652–661. [CrossRef]

35. Zaïri, A.; Nouir, S.; M'hamdi, N.; Bennani, M.; Bergaoui, I.; Mtiraoui, A.; Chaouachi, M.; Trabelsi, M. Antioxidant, Antimicrobial and the Phenolic Content of Infusion, Decoction and Methanolic Extracts of Thyme and *Rosmarinus* Species. *Cur. Phar. Biotech.* **2018**, *19*, 590–599. [CrossRef] [PubMed]
36. Lu, C.; Liu, H.; Shangguan, W.; Chen, S.; Zhong, Q. Antibiofilm activities of the cinnamon extract against *Vibrio parahaemolyticus* and *Escherichia coli*. *Arch. Microbiol.* **2021**, *203*, 125–135. [CrossRef] [PubMed]
37. Liu, Z.; Lin, Y.; Lu, Q.; Li, F.; Yu, J.; Wang, Z.; He, Y.; Song, C. In vitro and in vivo activity of EDTA and antibacterial agents against the biofilm of mucoid *Pseudomonas aeruginosa*. *Infection* **2017**, *45*, 23–31. [CrossRef]
38. Stewart, P.S.; Costerton, J.W. Antibiotic resistance of bacteria in biofilms. *Lancet* **2001**, *358*, 135–138. [CrossRef]
39. Goode, D.; Jackson, C.; Aber, K.; Shah, A.; Hensel, L. Discovery, Efficacy Testing, and Potential Target Identification of Antibiofilm Compounds. *FASEB J.* **2018**, *32*, 810–813. [CrossRef]
40. Niu, G. Colorimetric method for identifying plant essential oil components that affect biofilm formation and structure. *Appl. Environ. Microbiol.* **2004**, *70*, 6951–6956. [CrossRef]
41. Antunes, L.C.; Levandovski, R.; Dantas, G.; Caumo, G.; Hidalgo, M.P. Obesity and shift work: Chronobiological aspects. *Nutr. Res. Rev.* **2010**, *23*, 155–168. [CrossRef] [PubMed]
42. Vikram, A.; Jayaprakasha, G.K.; Jesudhasan, P.R.; Pillai, S.D.; Patil, B.S. Suppression of bacterial cell-cell signalling, biofilm formation and type III secretion system by citrus flavonoids. *J. Appl. Microbiol.* **2010**, *109*, 515–527. [CrossRef] [PubMed]
43. Chaudhary, A.; Jaswal, V.S.; Choudhary, S.; Sharma, A.; Beniwal, V.; Tuli, H.S.; Sharma, S. Ferulic Acid: A Promising Therapeutic Phytochemical and Recent Patents Advances. *Recent. Pat. Inf. Al. Drug Discov.* **2019**, *13*, 115–123. [CrossRef] [PubMed]
44. Takahashi, H.; Takahashi, T.; Miya, S.; Yokoyama, H. Growth inhibition effects of ferulic acid and glycine/sodium acetate on Listeria monocytogenes in coleslaw and egg alad. *Food Control.* **2015**, *57*, 105–109. [CrossRef]
45. Pinheiro, P.G.; Santiago, G.M.P.; da Silva, F.E.F.; de Araújo, A.C.J.; de Oliveira, C.R.T.; Freitas, P.R.; Rocha, J.E.; Neto, J.B.A.; da Silva, M.M.C.; Tintino, S.R. Ferulic acid derivatives inhibiting Staphylococcus aureus tetK and MsrA efflux pumps. *Biotechnol. Rep.* **2022**, *34*, e00717. [CrossRef] [PubMed]
46. Guyot, S.; Marnet, N.; Laraba, D.; Sanoner, P.; Drilleau, J.F. Reversed-Phase HPLC following Thiolysis for Quantitative Estimation and Characterization of the Four Main Classes of Phenolic Compounds in Different Tissue Zones of a French Cider Apple Variety (*Malus domestica* Var. Kermerrien). *J. Agric. Food Chem.* **1998**, *46*, 1698–1705. [CrossRef]
47. El Arem, A.; Saafi, E.B.; Mechri, B.; Lahouar, L.; Issaoui, M.; Hammami, M.; Achour, L. Effects of the Ripening Stage on Phenolic Profile, Phytochemical Composition and Antioxidant Activity of Date Palm Fruit. *J. Agric. Food. Chem.* **2012**, *60*, 10896–10902. [CrossRef]
48. Miraliakbari, H.; Shahidi, F. Antioxidant activity of minor components of tree nut oils. *Food. Chem.* **2008**, *111*, 421–427. [CrossRef]
49. Sree Kumari, C.; Yasmin, N.; RaffiqHussain, M.; Babuselvam, M. In Vitro Anti-inflammatory and Anti-arthritic property of *Rhizopora mucronata* leaves. *Int. J. Pharma. Sci. Reas.* **2015**, *6*, 3.
50. Dbeibia, A.; Ben Taher, F.; Altamar, K.; Haddaji, N.; Mahdi, A.; Amri, Z.; Mzoughi, R.; Jabeur, C. Control of *Staphylococcus aureus* methicillin resistant isolated from auricular infections using aqueous and methanolic extracts of Ephedra alata. *Saudi. J. Biol. Sci.* **2022**, *29*, 1021–1028. [CrossRef]
51. Chaieb, K.; Kouidhi, B.; Jrah, H.; Mahdouani, K.; Bakhrouf, A. Antibacterial activity of Thymoquinone, an active principle of Nigella sativa and its potency to prevent bacterial biofilm formation. *BMC Complement. Altern. Med.* **2011**, *11*, 29. [CrossRef] [PubMed]

pharmaceuticals

MDPI

Review

Exploring the Role of Berberine as a Molecular Disruptor in Antimicrobial Strategies

Anna Duda-Madej [1,*,†], Szymon Viscardi [2,†], Hanna Bazan [2] and Jakub Sobieraj [2]

1 Department of Microbiology, Faculty of Medicine, Wroclaw Medical University, Chałubińskiego 4, 50-368 Wrocław, Poland
2 Faculty of Medicine, Wroclaw Medical University, Ludwika Pasteura 1, 50-367 Wrocław, Poland; szymon.viscardi@student.umw.edu.pl (S.V.); hanna.bazan@student.umw.edu.pl (H.B.); jakub.sobieraj@student.umw.edu.pl (J.S.)
* Correspondence: anna.duda-madej@umw.edu.pl
† These authors contributed equally to this work.

Abstract

In recent years, one of the most important issues in public health is the rapid growth of antibiotic resistance among pathogens. Multidrug-resistant (MDR) strains (mainly *Enterobacteriaceae* and non-fermenting bacilli) cause severe infections, against which commonly used pharmaceuticals are ineffective. Therefore, there is an urgent need for new treatment options and drugs with innovative mechanisms of action. Natural compounds, especially alkaloids, are showing promising potential in this area. This review focuses on the ability of the isoquinoline alkaloid berberine (BRB) to overcome various resistance mechanisms against conventional antimicrobial agents. BRB has demonstrated significant activity in inhibiting efflux pumps of the RND (Resistance-Nodulation-Cell Division) family, such as MexAB-OprM (*P. aeruginosa*) and AdeABC (*A. baumannii*). Moreover, BRB was able to decrease quorum sensing activity in both Gram-positive and Gram-negative pathogens, resulting in reduced biofilm formation and lower bacterial virulence. Additionally, BRB has been identified as a potential inhibitor of FtsZ, a key protein responsible for bacterial cell division. Particularly noteworthy, though requiring further investigation, are reports suggesting that BRB might inhibit β-lactamase enzymes, including NDM, AmpC, and ESβL types. The pleiotropic antibacterial actions of BRB, distinct from the mechanisms of traditional antibiotics, offer hope for breaking bacterial resistance. However, more extensive studies, especially in vivo, are necessary to fully evaluate the clinical potential of BRB and determine its practical applicability in combating antibiotic-resistant infections.

Keywords: berberine; β-lactamase inhibitors; efflux pump inhibitors; FtsZ protein; isoquinoline alkaloid; multidrug resistance; quorum sensing inhibitors

1. Introduction

Antibiotic resistance among pathogenic bacteria is the "silent pandemic of the 21st century" and is a significant public health problem worldwide. It can result from (i) overuse of antibiotics [1], (ii) incorrect use of antibiotics (taking inappropriate doses or too short a duration of therapy) [2], (iii) improper disposal of antimicrobial drugs [3], and (iv) agricultural overuse [4].

According to the WHO (World Health Organization), an estimated 1.27 million deaths worldwide each year are directly caused by infections with MDR (multidrug-resistant) bacteria, and 4.95 million deaths are indirectly linked to them [5]. Statistical predictions for the near future are very alarming, as they show that, with such an increasing trend, these cases will increase 10-fold in 2050, making antibiotic resistance the number one cause of all deaths in the world, overtaking even cancer [6].

The mechanism of activity of the antibiotics known so far includes their selective action based on interference with key life processes of bacteria, different from those occurring in eukaryotic cells. Antibiotics can act via (i) inhibiting cell wall synthesis (β-lactams and glycopeptides) [7]; (ii) inhibiting protein synthesis (tetracyclines, aminoglycosides, macrolides, lincosamides, streptogramins, oxazolidinones, and chloramphenicol) [8]; (iii) inhibiting DNA/RNA synthesis (quinolones, fluoroquinolones, rifampicin, and metronidazole) [9,10]; (iv) acting as antimetabolites (sulfonamides, trimethoprim, and cotrimoxazole) [11]; and (v) cytoplasmic membrane damage (daptomycin and polymyxins) [12]. Although the field of antibiotic therapy is developing rapidly, the number of antimicrobial drugs discovered in the last half-century is negligible. There is a feeling of a constant deficit of them, especially those active against resistant strains. Indeed, it is a fact that, in recent years, compounds have been discovered promising for the future in combating infections with the etiology of resistant strains, i.e., teixobactin (discovered in 2015) [13], darobactin (discovered in 2019) [14], and lariocidin (discovered in 2025) [15]. However, despite the intense scientific efforts in the field of finding new compounds that exhibit antimicrobial activity, the rate is still far too slow to overcome the development of bacterial resistance to antibiotics.

Over the past decades, bacteria have "learned" a defense against the effective action of drugs. This involves (i) inactivation of the antibiotic [16], (ii) changing its target site of action (overproduction of molecules constituting the target site or replacing them with alternative structures) [17], (iii) reducing the permeability of cellular envelopes [18,19], and (iv) active efflux of the drug from the cell [20]. These modifications can occur as a result of genetic mutations (changes in target site proteins) [21,22] or the ability to produce enzymes hydrolyzing or modifying the antibiotic [23,24]. These comprehensive abilities acquired by bacteria have contributed to the development of resistance to most (MDR), XDR (extensively drug-resistant), and even all (PDR (pandrug-resistant)) antibiotics used in therapy and considered as "last chance" drugs [25]. Additionally, the problem is "me too drugs," i.e., the fact that most "new" antibiotics were created by modifying existing drugs [26].

Therefore, it is essential to explore novel compounds that exert their effects through mechanisms distinct from those of the currently available agents. A critical aspect of this search involves uncovering new pathways involved in bacterial cell–eukaryotic cell interactions. Furthermore, a comprehensive understanding of the intricate resistance mechanisms employed by various bacterial species is fundamental to the success in this search, as circumventing these defenses would enable the therapeutic agent to act more effectively.

Recent progress in research allowed the development of new drugs, invented in order to overcome bacterial mechanisms of antibiotic resistance. Fabimycin can serve as an example. It inhibits FabI, a rate-determining step catalyzing enzyme, which is involved in fatty acid synthesis. Its ability to accumulate inside targeted bacteria facilitates its effectiveness against resistant Gram-negative bacteria, which was proven in a mouse infection model [27,28]. Another promising compound is INF55 (5-nitro-2-phenyl-1*H*-indole), which not only blocks the pumping of antibiotics out of the bacterial cell (NorA inhibitor) but also increases the efficacy of fluoroquinolones (e.g., ciprofloxacin) [29,30]. Although it is not a stand-alone antibiotic, this compound appears to be the key that opens up a new strategy in the fight against multidrug-resistant bacteria. Acting as a resistance-modifying agent (RMA), it restores the efficacy of existing antibiotics. Notably, research has demonstrated that coupling an efflux pump inhibitor with an antibacterial agent is a highly promising approach [29]. The field of phytomedicine has gained increasing attention, with natural compounds being investigated as potential sources of new antimicrobial agents. One such development is the conjugation of berberine (BRB) with INF55, which has resulted in a hybrid molecule exhibiting potent antimicrobial activity, particularly against *Enterococcus faecalis* and methicillin-resistant *Staphylococcus aureus* (MRSA) [31–33].

In our review, we focused on summarizing reports flowing from research on the isoquinoline alkaloid BRB (Figure 1), which is widely present in plants. This compound is present in significant amounts in representatives of the *Berberidaceae,* including *Berberis aristata* or *Ranunculaceae—Coptis chinensis* [34,35]. This alkaloid has long held a prominent position among bioactive phytochemicals in traditional and natural medicine due to its broad therapeutic potential. Numerous studies have emphasized its anticancer [36], antimicrobial [37,38], and anti-inflammatory [39] properties. At the same time, BRB, due to its weak absorption from the gastrointestinal tract and high toxic dose (41.6 g/kg), is a safe compound for clinical use [40] and particularly worthy of attention. The reviews available in the literature focus primarily on the very important topic of overcoming BRB bioavailability. They extensively discuss its metabolic profile [41] and physicochemical, pharmacological, and toxicological properties [42]. They focus on the molecular action targets of this compound [43] and the impact of structural modifications to increase therapeutic effects, including improved bioavailability and absorption [44]. In addition, they discuss in detail the positive and negative sides of the formulation of BRB and its derivatives [45]. However, they do not analyze in detail the antimicrobial activity of BRB and the attractive combinations that potentiate DDIs (drug–drug interactions). After analyzing these reviews, there was a need to encapsulate the subject into a whole expanding the area of the effect of this isoquinoline alkaloid on the bacterial cell. Therefore, the main objective of this review is to provide a comprehensive overview of the antimicrobial mechanisms of action of this compound, which positions it as a promising candidate for overcoming the growing challenge of antibiotic resistance. These mechanisms include the disruption of efflux pump function, inhibition of bacterial cell division, interference with quorum sensing pathways, and suppression of β-lactamase activity. They are interesting from the point of view of antimicrobial activity and, in our opinion, worth special attention. This is because it seems that solving the problem of bioavailability and weak permeability of BRB using nanoparticles, phytosomes, or BRB derivatives is the key to overcoming multidrug resistance.

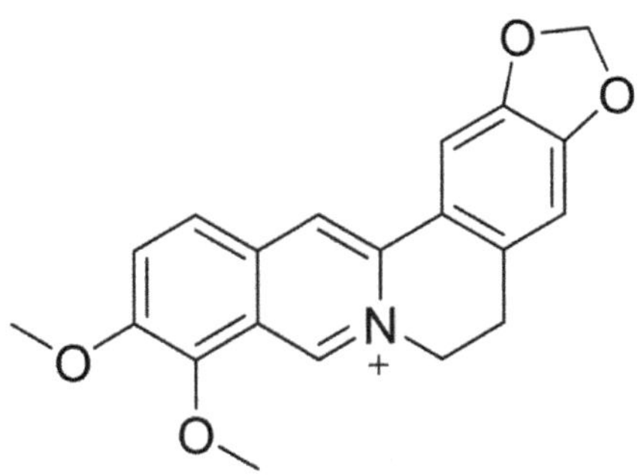

Figure 1. Molecular structure of berberine (two-dimensional).

2. Berberine Disrupting the Efficiency of Bacterial Efflux Pumps

2.1. Berberine Interference with MFS Efflux Pumps Superfamily

According to reports of numerous researchers, BRB as a cationic compound undergoes efficient efflux by MDR bacteria due to the MFS (major facilitator superfamily) efflux pump system, such as NorA [32,46,47]. The result is limited activity against these bacteria and the need for classic EPIs (efflux pump inhibitors), for example, CCCP (carbonyl cyanide 3-chlorophenylhydrazone), PaβN (Phe-Arg-β-naphthylamide), or others newly synthesized, to obtain the antibacterial effect of the alkaloid [30,32,33,48]. Ettefagh et al. also proved that the plant extract from *Hydrastis canadensis* L. can overcome the efflux of BRB conditioned by the presence of NorA in *S. aureus* [49]. In an analysis of 13 alkaloids with antibacterial potential, BRB showed the best antimicrobial profile against MRSA isolates expressing NorA and MdeA pumps (MIC = 125 μg/mL). However, the EtBr (ethidium bromide) analysis did not demonstrate the ability to interfere with the efflux pump system; no accumulation of bromide was observed [50].

However, in recent years, research indicating the ability of the alkaloid to interfere with the function of MFS effluent pumps has emerged [51,52]. Reports on this subject come from the study of Li et al., in which researchers reported on the ability of the preparation in the sub-inhibitory concentration to interfere with the function of the MdfA pump present in *Escherichia coli* [51]. For the strain overexpressing MdfA pump, an 8-fold higher MIC value for ciprofloxacin (CYP) was determined compared to the reference strain. The addition of BRB (20–50 μg/mL) resulted in the restoration of antibiotic susceptibility and the accumulation of fluoroquinolone within *E. coli* cells (decrease in MIC from 0.032 μg/mL to 0.008 and 0.004 μg/mL, respectively). At the molecular level, BRB particles have been shown to interfere with MdfA pump subunits and consequently prevented their conformational transition, which is likely to be the proper mechanism of action of the alkaloid [51]. BRB activity against efflux pump expressing MRSA isolates was also evaluated. The alkaloid showed a synergistic interaction with antibiotics: CYP, tobramycin (TOB), and oxacillin (FICI, fractional inhibitory concentration index ≤ 0.5). Moreover, the time–kill curve analysis showed that, after 24 h exposure to BRB (64 μg/mL) combined with TOB (256 μg/mL) or CYP (0.25 μg/mL), there was 99.9% inhibition of bacterial growth. In the assessment of EtBr accumulation inside *S. aureus* cells, exposure to BRB (32–64 μg/mL) resulted in a fluorescence increase, giving a comparable result to that obtained in the positive control (CCCP, 5 μM). In the docking study, alkaloid presented a significant affinity for efflux pump proteins: MepA, NorA, NorB, and SdrM (binding energy: 7.9, −7.6, −7.8, and −9.4 kcal/mol, respectively) [52].

2.2. Berberine Interference with RND Efflux Pumps Superfamily

Acinetobacter baumannii: BRB hydrochloride has been tested by Li et al. for its ability to overcome antibiotic resistance in MDR *A. baumannii* [51]. Importantly, BRB (MIC = 256 μg/mL) in combination with classical drugs led to a restoration of bacterial susceptibility to CYP, tigecycline (TGC), meropenem (MER), and sulbactam (SBT) among MDR isolates originally resistant to them (MIC reduction of antibiotics, respectively: 32-fold, 2-fold, 64-fold, and 16-fold). Importantly, the researchers showed that nearly 100% of the tested strains were characterized by the expression of the AdeABC efflux pump. In the analysis of *adeB* gene expression at BRB stimulation, an upregulation in gene expression was noted in contrast to strains not exposed to the alkaloid. This information, together with the relatively high (−7.42 kcal/mol) binding energy of BRB with AdeB, indicated that the alkaloid acts as a substrate rather than a pure pump inhibitor. Thus, BRB enhanced the effect of antibiotics by competing with them for a binding site in the efflux pump area [51]. Ahmadi et al. showed that the exposure of *A. baumannii* MDR isolates to, among others, BRB and a BRB + thioridazine combination decreased the expression level of the *adeB* gene encoding the subunit of efflux pump AdeABC [53].

Pseudomonas aeruginosa: Morita et al. evaluated the efficacy of BRB in their ability to antagonize aminoglycoside resistance in *P. aeruginosa* expressing the MexXY-OprM efflux pump [54]. Alkaloid (250 μg/mL) led to a decrease in MIC for amikacin (ACN), TOB, and gentamicin (GEN) in the two- to eight-fold range. Importantly, the tested isolates were resistant to all tested aminoglycosides, and a similar relationship in terms of MIC was not demonstrated in the case of pathogens lacking expression of the efflux pumps. BRB, in combination with GEN, has been shown to induce a synergistic relationship (FICI ≤ 0.5) against *P. aeruginosa* harboring a MexXY-OprM pump. In addition, there was a similarly spectacular decrease in MIC of the mentioned antibiotics after a combination with BRB against *Achromobacter xylosoxidans* and *Burkholderia cepacia* (for *A. xylosoxindans*, there was a MIC reduction from 512 to 16 µg/mL for TOB) [54]. Further analysis showed that the alkaloid induced in *P. aeruginosa* wild type (expression of MexAB, MexCD, MexEF, MexXY, and MexVW) a decrease in MIC for erythromycin (ERT) from 256 to 64 µg/mL (four-fold) and TET (tetracycline) from 32 to 16 g/mL (two-fold). Importantly, the knockout strain that preserved only the expression of the MexXY pump was only slightly more sensitive to ERY (eight-fold MIC reduction), which indicated the key role of BRB in blocking this particular pump [54]. The ability of the alkaloid to interfere with the function of the RND-type efflux pump was also assessed by Aghayan et al. Researchers evaluated the effect of BRB on *P. aeruginosa* isolates derived from burn wounds. Among 60 isolated pathogens, ~90% resistant isolates were significantly resistant to ceftriaxone, clindamycin, kanamycin, CYP, and rifampicin (RIF). Importantly, it was shown that the use of a combination of BRB + CYP resulted in a decrease in MIC and MBC parameters for fluoroquinolone, which, taking into account reports from the Morita et al. study, may indicate an inhibition of efflux pumps. This is reflected in the distribution of genes encoding efflux pumps of the tested isolates: ~98% was characterized by the expression of *mexA*, *-D*, and *-F*; *mexX* was found in 96.6% of isolates [55]. The summary of the BRB impact on RND-type efflux pumps is presented in Figure 2.

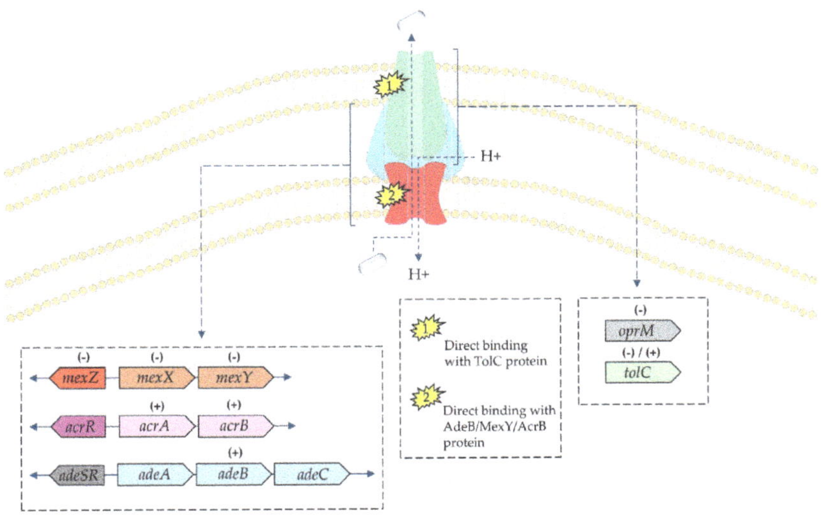

Figure 2. Berberine anti-efflux activity against Gram-negative bacteria expressing RND-type efflux pumps (*P. aeruginosa, A. baumannii,* and the *Enterobacteriaceae*). Abbreviations: *acrA,B,R*, *adeA–C,S,R*, *mexX–Z*, *oprM*, and *tolC*—genes encoding efflux pumps subunits and their negative regulators; AcrB, AdeB, MexY, and TolC—efflux pumps protein subunits; H+—proton. Upregulation was marked as (+) and downregulation as (−).

Significant reports in the field of the anti-efflux properties of alkaloid come from the Su et al. study, which assessed the effect of the BRB + imipenem (IMI) combination against the *P. aeruginosa* (PA012) isolate forming the MexXY-OprM pump. The combination of compounds induced a synergistic relationship (FICI $\leq$ 0.5) and resulted in a decrease in MIC for both compounds: four- and eight-fold, respectively. Moreover, the use of BRB and IMI in sub-inhibitory concentrations (¼ MIC for BRB) resulted in the accumulation of alkaloid within *Pseudomonas* cells. RT-qPCR analysis showed a decrease in the expression of the genes *mexX*, *mexY*, *mexZ* (~40% reduction), and *oprM* (~50% reduction) [56]. The alkaloid also demonstrated the ability to bind with the MexY protein—a component of the RND pump described above, created by *P. aeruginosa*. In silico, BRB and the aminoglycoside-TOB showed affinity for the antibiotic binding site (antibiotic site). The mentioned alkaloid was characterized by a higher affinity to protein molecules (−864 kJ/mol vs. −454 kJ/mol). The result of the study suggested the formation of a stable MexY-BRB complex protecting TOB from efflux. Moreover, in the subsequent in vitro analysis (30 isolates of *P. aeruginosa*, 100% of which harbored the *mexY* gene), a synergy between BRB (80 µg/mL) and TOB was demonstrated in 12 cases, which was manifested as a reduction in the MIC of the antibiotic $\geq$ two-fold [57]. Another study investigated the effects of BRB on efflux pumps MexXY-OprM and MexAB-OprM present in *P. aeruginosa*. The use of 200 µM BRB in combination with EtBr resulted in increased accumulation of this in *Pseudomonas* strains harboring MexXY-OprM (inhibition of the efflux ratio equal to 55%). However, the alkaloid did not show any significant effect on the isolate forming the second of mentioned efflux pumps [58]. BRB also demonstrated efficacy against the aminoglycoside-resistant *P. aeruginosa* strain harboring MexXY-OprM. Alkaloid, in a series of studies, has proven to be a candidate for an inhibitor of the protein MexY [59,60]. In the context of the pump, BRB and a number of its aromatic derivatives have been shown to be able to block the allosteric subunit of the MexY protein. A docking study demonstrated the ability of the alkaloid to bind with the described protein (−8.66 kcal/mol) present in the *P. aeruginosa* PA07 strain. Evaluation of a further five clinical isolates of *Pseudomonas* confirmed the beneficial alkaloid profile (docking study) in the dysfunction of the MexXY-OprM efflux pump [60].

Enterobacteriaceae: The ability of BRB to potentiate CYP activity against *Klebsiella pneumoniae* expressing the AcrAB-tolC pump was also evaluated. The researchers showed that the combination of an alkaloid (MIC $\geq$ 512 µg/mL) with CYP (MIC in the range of 4–512 µg/mL) induced a relationship defined in ~80% of the strains as additive. Interestingly, it was shown that, despite the ability of the alkaloid to increase the antibacterial activity of CYP, this combination of antibiotic (¼ MIC) with BRB (1024 µg/mL) induced a 14-fold increase in the expression of *acrA*, *acrB*, *tolC*, and *acrR* genes. The antimicrobial effect was likely achieved by the interaction with pump proteins or by accumulation of AcrAB in the bacterial cytoplasm, which induced cellular toxicity [61]. These reports are in conjunction with the results of the transcriptome analysis of the *Escherichia coli* K12 strain exposed to BRB. Bacteria under the influence of alkaloid increased the expression of a number of genes responsible for efflux: *acrF* (17-fold increase) and *yhdX-Z* (14–34-fold) [62]. In turn, Gokgoz et al. revealed that *E. coli* K12 exposure to BRB induced a decrease in the expression of genes encoding external membrane proteins, e.g., *ompC*, *ompF*, and *ompW*. The latter protein was described to play an important role in the development of bacterial resistance to various antibiotics [63]. The alkaloid was also effective in interfering with the resistance to COL mediated by MCR-1 (mobilized colistin resistance 1), and in disrupting the AcrAB-TolC efflux pump in *Salmonella* spp. and *E. coli* isolates. Despite the lack of significant antimicrobial activity of BRB (MIC in the range of 625–1250 µg/mL), the combination of EDTA (ethylenediaminetetraacetic acid) and alkaloid (both ¼ MIC) resulted in a decrease in MIC of COL-NS (colistin—non-susceptible) isolates (1–256-fold). The demonstrated ability to lower the MIC for COL in the range of 8–2048-fold reduction was defined as a synergistic interaction for both adjuvants. The BRB docking assay demonstrated the ability of the alkaloid to form complexes with the MCR-1 protein and RND pump subunits AcrB and TolC. Moreover, both BRB and EDTA showed the ability to reduce the expression of *mcr-1* and *tolC* genes [64].

2.3. Berberine Interference with Mycobacterium spp. Efflux Pumps

BRB also showed the potential to increase the activity of clarithromycin (CLA) against *Mycobacterium avium intracellulare* (MAC) complex isolates. The preparation, like other EPIs (CCCP, piperine, and tetrandrine), led to an improvement in mycobacteria sensitivity to CLA (in 50% of strains that were originally resistant). The alkaloid in the sub-MIC concentration (20–30 μg/mL) led to ≥four-fold reduction of MIC in 10/12 MAC isolates, and the interaction was defined as synergy. What is particularly important, the *M. avium* subsp. *hominissuis* 2373 strain obtained significant sensitivity to the antibiotic after combining with BRB, and there was a decrease in MIC from 2048 μg/mL to ≤0.25 μg/mL [65]. Puk et al. reported that the combination of BRB (16–64 μg/mL) with a number of antibiotics resulted in the development of synergistic interactions against *Mycobacterium fortuitum, chelonae,* and *peregrinum* (*Mycobacterium* other than *tuberculosis*—MOTT). Both a decrease in MICs for tuberculostatics (RIF, streptomycin, and CLA) and aminoglycoside antibiotics were observed. Taking into account the known EPI properties of the alkaloid, it can be assumed that the synergistic interaction was the effect of disturbing the function of the MOTT efflux pumps [66]. The influence of BRB and other EPIs, e.g., verapamil and CCCP, on MAC isolates expressing efflux pumps type ABC (ATP-binding cassette) was also assessed. The researchers reported that *M. avium* subsp. *hominissuis* ATCC 700898 exposure to CLA most strongly induced the overexpression of pump-encoding genes in the pathogen (ABC, MFS, and RND pumps—MmpL). Analysis with EtBr revealed that BRB (MIC = 128 μg/mL) increased the accumulation of bromide in relation to the studied bacterial isolates. What is particularly important, the combination of BRB and CLA as the only one (among the EPIs tested) resulted in an increase in macrolide activity, which was ultimately defined as synergy (FICI $\leq$ 0.5) [67].

3. Berberine Interference with Quorum Sensing

3.1. Quorum Sensing and Quorum Quenching

Quorum sensing (QS) is a mode of intercellular communication that allows the bacterial community to adapt to changing circumstances through modifications of gene expression. It can affect the metabolism of the cells in the community, as well as interactions between the cells and, therefore, i.e., the formation of a biofilm or excretion of common goods, such as extracellular enzymes. As those survival strategies are a rising concern in medicine, allowing bacteria to resist therapy, disrupting QS can be useful in combating infections. Such an approach is called quorum quenching and was proven to be effective in inhibiting the production of virulence factors and biofilm by numerous pathogens [68]. To achieve this goal, various enzymes that inactivate QS signals can be used. For example, lactonase SsoPox-I was tested in *P. aeruginosa* pneumonia in rats, in which, when inhaled, reduced PAO1 lasB virulence gene activity, pyocyanin synthesis, proteolytic activity, and biofilm formation [69]. Analogical activity is studied in the case of BRB, which activity as a QS inhibitor can, among other mechanisms, be used to combat bacterial infections.

3.2. Berberine Inhibits Quorum Sensing in Pseudomonas aeruginosa

A study by Aswathanarayan et al. investigated BRB sub-inhibitory concentrations as a potential inhibitor of biofilm formation and QS-mediated phenotypes of *P. aeruginosa,* Gram-negative, rod-shaped bacteria responsible for many cases of severe infections, especially hospital-acquired pneumonia. Two strains were used: *P. aeruginosa* PAO1, which is a wild type, and *P. aeruginosa* PAO1-JP2, a mutant unable to produce acyl-homoserine lactones

(AHLs), signaling molecules involved in quorum sensing. In the PAO1 strain, BRB at a 0.625 mg/mL concentration reduced biofilm formation by 71.70% [70]. In the case of the mutant strain, 0.078 mg/mL solution was used, and signaling molecules were added: C4-HSL (*N*-Butanoyl-L-homoserine lactone) in one trial and 3-oxo-C12-HSL (*N*-3-Oxo-Dodecanoyl-L-homoserine lactone) in the other. The reduction in biofilm formation was 65.50% and 60.74%, respectively. Compared to the control trial, it proves that BRB inhibits biofilm formation by *P. aeruginosa* through the inhibition of QS. This alkaloid was also among the bioactive metabolites of halophilic bacteria, which showed the inhibition of QS in a multidrug-resistant *P. aeruginosa* [71]. BRB was also identified using affinity chromatography as an active compound in *Phellodendron amurense* extract in a study by Yi et al., in which MIC against *P. aeruginosa* was established as 1280 µg/mL [72]. In this study, ½ MIC of BRB suppressed biofilm formation by 50.5% and reduced the production of pyocyanin, a virulence factor of *P. aeruginosa* by 45.0%. It also inhibited the production of rhamnolipid by 68.1% and significantly reduced the motility of bacteria by 60.3%. The authors suggested that those effects were due to the inhibition of QS through an interaction with the 2-heptyl-3-hydroxy-4-quinolone system (PQS), especially the PqsA protein, and conducted a molecular docking simulation, which suggested the existence of a stable binding interaction between BRB and PqsA.

Another study showed that BRB in combination with azithromycin suppressed quorum sensing more than both substances separately [73]. QS molecules secreted by *P. aeruginosa,* which decreased significantly, included violacein, lasl, lasR, rhlI, and rhlR. In the same study, the synergic activity of the alkaloid and azithromycin was tested in vivo on mice model of chronic lung infection, with *P. aeruginosa* PA03 as the etiological factor. Three days after infection, compared to the control group, and to groups where tested substances were used separately (in the same concentrations), the combined used revealed in dissected lungs of mice the alleviation of abscesses, hemorrhage, and inflammation with lower levels of proinflammatory cytokines Il-6 and IL-8 and higher levels of anti-inflammatory IL-10. In conclusion, the authors suggested that BRB is a promising synergic agent in treating *P. aeruginosa* infections, with quorum sensing inhibition being among crucial mechanisms of action.

3.3. Berberine Inhibition of Quorum Sensing and Biofilm Formation in Salmonella enterica subsp. enterica Serovar typhimurium

In the same study by Aswathanarayan et al., BRB was examined against *S. typhimurium.* In the crystal violet assay, the substance at the sub-MIC level showed significant antibiofilm activity; at 0.019 mg/mL, it reduced the biofilm biomass of *S. typhimurium* by 31.20%. In fluorescence microscopy analysis, the same concentration showed no inhibition in the initial attachment of the bacterial cells but suppressed maturing of the biofilm through the inhibition of extracellular polymeric substance production, which can be mediated by quorum signaling [74]. The adhesion and invasion potential of bacteria in the presence of BRB was also determined using human colon cell line HT29 in a monolayer. The highest concentration used in a test was 0.02 mg/mL. The effect was a reduction in adhesion by 54.68% and invasion by 55.37%. What is important, in the control group, this concentration had no negative effect on the human cells. The authors of the study also highlighted that other phytochemicals under research, punicalagin and carvacrol, reduced the invasion of *S. typhimurium* but not adhesion [39,75], which points to BRB as a more active substance. Aswathanarayan et al. also showed that the investigated alkaloid, as well as synthetic QS inhibitor furanone C30, decreased paralysis due to *S. typhimurium* infection in nematode *Caenorhabditis elegans.* BRB at 0.038 mg/mL decreased paralysis of the nematodes by 65.38%, while furanone C30 had slightly greater activity. In conclusion, BRB by disrupting QS seems to inhibit the virulence of *S. typhimurium.*

3.4. Berberine Inhibits Quorum Sensing in *Hafnia alvei*

H. alvei is a Gram-negative, facultatively anaerobic bacterium, vastly abundant in the environment and human feces but rarely causing infections. However, it is able to produce biofilms in which the QS process is crucial. Pang et al. investigated the effect of BRB on biofilm formation and quorum sensing by *H. alvei* through the analysis of gene expression using RT-qPCR and high-performance liquid chromatography (HPLC) [76]. In RT-qPCR, two genes involved in QS and AHL synthesis were investigated and their expression significantly decreased: the halI gene (even at the lowest investigated BRB concentration, 1/32 MIC) and halR gene (at 1/16 MIC and greater concentrations). HPLC revealed a decrease in the concentration of one of the AHLs, C14-HSL, from 2.189 μg/mL to 0.512 μg/mL after treatment with ½ MIC of BRB. Further docking analysis and molecular dynamics simulation showed that both the alkaloid and C14-HSL bind to the HalR protein, with BRB forming a more stable complex. In conclusion, BRB seems to inhibit the biofilm formation of *H. alvei* by inhibiting QS, and the mechanism behind it is the downregulation of *hal*I and *hal*R gene expression.

3.5. Berberine Inhibits Quorum Sensing in *Escherichia coli*

A study by Sun et al. compared the quorum quenching activity of BRB and another substance derived from Chinese traditional medicine, matrine. The effect on antimicrobial-resistant (AMR) *E. coli* biofilm formation and gene expression was examined using laser scanning confocal microscopy (LSCM) and RT-PCR. Analysis showed that BRB at ½ MIC (MIC = 2560 μg/mL for all AMR strains) significantly inhibited biofilm formation and had an impact on the morphology of the bacterial cells: they were swollen and elongated, with yellow fluorescence from BRB [77]. RT-PCR revealed the downregulating effect of the substance on the expression of the genes involved in QS: *luxS*, *pfS*, *hflX*, *ftsQ*, and *ftsE* at ½ and ¼ MIC. Additionally, the results showed greater activity of BRB than matrine.

3.6. Berberine and Quorum Sensing in Gram-Positive Bacteria

Among Gram-positive bacteria, *S. aureus* is a species with prominent clinical significance, especially strains resistant to antibiotics, such as MRSA. BRB is among the substances exhibiting potential in the treatment of MRSA. One of its proven properties is the ability to inhibit the biofilm formation of this pathogen. A study by Chu et al. examined this characteristic and suggested it is possible due to the hydrophobic interaction between BRB and the phenyl ring in phenylalanine, one of the amino acids present in phenyl soluble modulins (PSMs), particularly PSMα2, which form amyloid fibrils, constituting biofilm [78]. BRB was also among active compounds found in goldenseal (*Hydrastis canadensis*) leaf extract; however, it had lesser activity alone than the whole extract, probably due to other flavonoids' (sideroxylin, 8-desmethyl-sideroxylin, and 6-desmethyl-sideroxylin) additional effect [79]. The extract showed quorum quenching activity against MRSA isolates, which was confirmed by assay with fluorescent reporters and with a lux reporter. Researchers focused on accessory gene regulator (*agr*), a QS system responsible for the production of virulence factors in response to external conditions [80]. The study showed the inhibitory effects of *H. candensis* extract on *agr I*, *agr II*, and *agr III*; however, BRB alone at 75 μg/mL had no effect on the *agr* system.

Contradictory data came from a study by El-Hamid et al. in which the BRB effect on vancomycin-resistant *S. aureus* (VRSA) was investigated. The study suggested a complex mechanism of action of the substance, including QS inhibition [81]. Again, the *agr* system was a subject of researchers' interest. In the described study, the examined strains contained *agr I* and *agr III* alleles. Those VRSA strains exhibited high biofilm formation and virulence potential. In the study, they were exposed to free BRB and BRB-loaded mesoporous silica nanoparticles (MPS-NPs). After exposure, qRT-PCR revealed significantly lower levels of *agr* transcripts: in the case of the free substance, a 0.29-fold decrease and, in the case of MPS-NPs, a 0.11-fold decrease. The same strains were tested in vivo in mice infected with 5×10^6 CFUs subcutaneously and then treated topically with a free alkaloid and MPS-NPs. Both treatments resulted in lower rates of virulence factors and *agr* expression, as well as smaller clinical symptoms (skin lesions vs. abscesses and reduction in mice activity) and lower levels of proinflammatory cytokines. Those results are supported by a study by Gao et al., who examined BRB and amphotericin B synergic activity against biofilm formed by *S. aureus* and *Candida albicans* [82]. The authors analyzed the gene expression of *S. aureus* in the biofilm treated with 128 μg/mL BRB and 4 μg/mL amphotericin B. The mRNA expression of *agrA* underwent a 125-fold decrease. Therefore, BRB seems to act through QS inhibition, particularly the *agr* system, to reduce *S. aureus* virulence.

3.7. Summary

BRB acts as a QS inhibitor at sub-MIC concentrations. This property was proven for multiple bacterial species: *P. aeruginosa*, *S. enterica*, *S. aureus*, *E. coli*, and *H. alvei*. The molecular mechanisms involved are presented in Table 1. Possible effects of this activity include disruptions in biofilm formation and the production of virulence factors, which, in the case of human pathogens, especially antibiotic-resistant strains, can have clinical implications. Therefore, the quorum quenching properties of BRB should be investigated further, as one of the mechanisms responsible for potential application in the treatment of infections.

Table 1. Molecular effects of berberine on quorum sensing in pathogenic bacterial species.

Bacterial Species	Molecular Effect	References
P. aeruginosa	inhibition of PqsA, violacein, *lasl*, *lasR*, *rhlI* and *rhlR*	[72,73]
S. typhimurium	inhibition of EPS production	[70]
S. aureus	inhibition of *agr I*, *agr II*, *agr III* systems	[79,81]
E. coli	downregulation of *luxS*, *pfS*, *hflX*, *ftsQ* and *ftsE*	[77]
H. alvei	reduction of C14-HSL production	[76]

As it was presented, BRB may interfere with various QS pathways in numerous bacterial species, both Gram-positive and -negative. Biofilm formation is crucial for pathogen survival and resistance against the immune system and is also strictly associated with QS signaling. The mentioned process is presented in Figure 3.

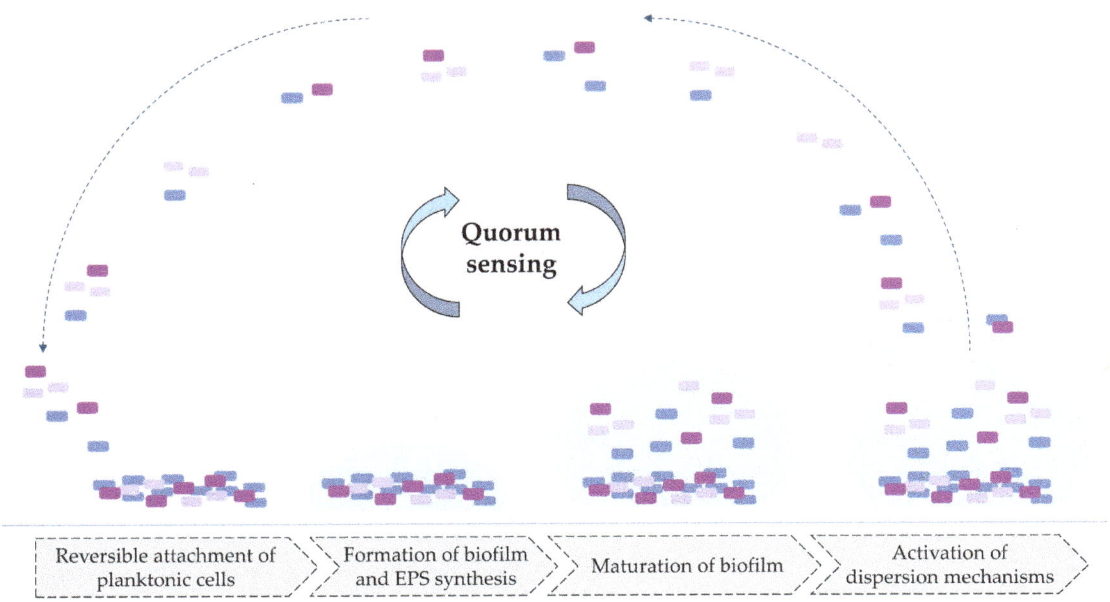

Figure 3. Molecular basis of the quorum sensing role in the process of biofilm formation (simplified scheme). Abbreviations: EPS—exopolysaccharides.

4. Berberine—Bacterial Mitosis Inhibitor

4.1. Bacterial Division

Bacteria increase their number through mitosis. This process is called division. The whole life of a bacterial cell can be split into three stages marked by the end of division, the beginning of chromosomal replication, and its end [83]. One of the most important proteins partaking in the bacterial mitosis is the FtsZ protein [84]. This tubulin homolog polymerizes into a cycle, commonly called a "Z-ring", that determines the division site and recruits other necessary proteins. It has been observed that FtsZ polymerization is highly dependent on guanosine-5′-triphosphate (GTP). Understanding of the mechanisms underlying bacterial divisions is crucial in order to come up with new antibiotics or their adjuvants.

4.2. Mechanism of Berberine and FtsZ Protein Interaction

BRB's antibacterial activity can be partly explained by its interaction with the FtsZ protein. One study proved that this alkaloid connects to the GTP-binding pocket present on FtsZ, effectively inhibiting its activity. BRB also prevents FtsZ's polymerization, as it covers its binding sides. This results in mitosis rate reduction [85]. This thesis has been supported by another study carried out in 2014, in which BRB and its derivatives' activity against various bacteria, e.g., *S. aureus*, *E. faecium*, or *E. coli*, has been compared [86]. Researchers observed a visible decrease in FtsZ protein's GTPase activity. GTPase is an enzyme that plays the role of a molecular switch that can control certain cellular processes. This may be a reason behind the observed reduction of the polymerization rate.

4.3. Berberine Activity on Gram-Positive Bacteria

One of the available studies used Gram-positive bacteria—*S. aureus* and *E. faecalis*—to verify the antimicrobial activity of BRB's derivatives in comparison to BRB [87]. Substances were applied both to antibiotic-susceptible (methicillin-susceptible *S. aureus*—MSSA and vancomycin susceptible *E. faecalis*—VSE) and antibiotic-resistant (MRSA and vancomycin-resistant *E. faecalis*—VRE) strains of those bacteria. While commonly used antibiotics, such as TET or oxacillin, demonstrated higher efficacy against MSSA and VSE compared to BRB derivatives, the latter exhibited significantly lower MIC values when tested against antibiotic-resistant strains (MRSA and VRE). The mechanism behind their efficiency has been studied in a 90° angle light scattering assay, which proved that those derivatives stimulate FtsZ polymerization. Such stimulation results in cell death due to the toxicity of the abundance of the FtsZ protein [88]. In another study, multiple derivatives of cycloberberine were synthesized in order to examine their antimicrobial properties [89]. They were tested on both methicillin-susceptible and -resistant strains of *S. aureus*, and their activity was assessed through the agar dilution method. Two compounds proved themselves to be the most effective even against MRSA, and one of them has been shown to interact with the docking side of the FtsZ protein in a computer program simulation, thus inhibiting mitosis. This corresponds to the conclusions achieved in other studies. Research conducted in 2020 tested various BRB derivatives against a few bacteria species, two of them being Gram-positive *S. aureus* and *B. subtilis* [90]. The results showed that some of those compounds are really effective against these bacteria, especially when compared to pure BRB. Like in previous research, even antibiotic-resistant strains have been proven vulnerable against tested BRB derivatives. In vitro biological assays have shown that, once again, these properties may be the result of interactions of those compounds with FtsZ, as they revealed that the BRB core of those substances links with the binding side of the protein. This mechanism results in a decreasing number of cell divisions.

4.4. *Berberine Activity on Gram-Negative Bacteria*

A study conducted in 2022 investigated the effects of berberine chloride on bacteria, including Gram-negative *Salmonella enterica* subsp. *enterica* serovar Typhi [91]. This compound was compared to other potential FtsZ inhibitors and ranked among them as the most effective. Notably, it demonstrated superior—that is, lower—MIC values against Gram-positive bacteria as compared to the Gram-negative ones. In this research, it was proven that berberine chloride prevented polymerization of the FtsZ protein and reduced its activity as a GTPase. This resulted in a decrease in mitosis. Comparable findings were reported in a study involving *Shigella flexneri*, which used berberine chloride as a reagent in both in vitro and in vivo murine models [92]. In vitro, this compound mostly presented an inhibitory effect on the FtsZ protein, thereby reducing its GTPase activity. Its antimicrobial activity against *S. flexneri* aligns with the findings of an in vivo study, which revealed a dual mechanism of action for BRB. It turned out that this substance not only slows down the mitosis rate of bacteria but, in addition, reduces inflammation and pyroptosis. It results in protection against intestinal infection caused by *S. flexneri*. The inhibitory effects of BRB's derivatives were also assessed on *E. coli*. In one of the studies, those substances were used on a recombinant FtsZ protein retrieved from *E. coli* [93]. Like in previous research, an inhibition of FtsZ polymerization was observed. Similarly to the Naz et al. study, the MIC values against Gram-positive bacteria were lower compared to the Gram-negative ones [91]. In another research, the effectiveness of simplified BRB's analogs was tested on various bacterial strains, including *E. coli* [94]. The results of this study correspond with the already named ones, as, once again, it turned out that BRB's derivatives prevent the polymerization of the FtsZ protein and reduce its GTPase activity, leading to a decrease in bacterial cell division. Their antimicrobial activity has also been assessed as higher against Gram-positive bacteria compared to Gram-negative ones.

4.5. Other Studies Concerning the Berberine Effect on Bacterial Mitosis

One of the studies has investigated the effect BRB has on *M. tuberculosis*, as it is one of the promising new antitubercular drugs [95]. In correspondence to the previous research, it turned out that BRB's analogs created stable complexes with the *M. tuberculosis* FtsZ protein, effectively inhibiting these bacterial divisions. Their efficiency appeared to be better compared to pure BRB. This research also explored pharmacokinetics through assessment of the ADMET (Absorption, Distribution, Metabolism, and Excretion) properties of these compounds, predicting their potential as orally administered drugs. BRB's antimitotic effect on bacteria was also studied on the fission yeast cells, which were genetically modified to express the FtsZ protein derived from, respectively, *S. aureus* and *Helicobacter pylori* [96]. In this research, BRB was compared to other FtsZ protein inhibitors, and its toxicity towards eukaryotic cells was also assessed. The results of the study were in accordance with the previous ones, and the inhibition of bacteria division was observed. It has been noted, though, that BRB has influenced yeast cells physiology, leading to negative side effects. Scientists have also identified a likely cause of BRB resistance in some bacteria, as certain interactions within the FtsZ protein appear to hinder it and other inhibitors from accessing the binding site. While this study confirmed once again the antimicrobial features of BRB, it also shed some light on new challenges related to it.

The mechanism of action described above of the FtsZ protein and its interaction with BRB is presented in Figure 4.

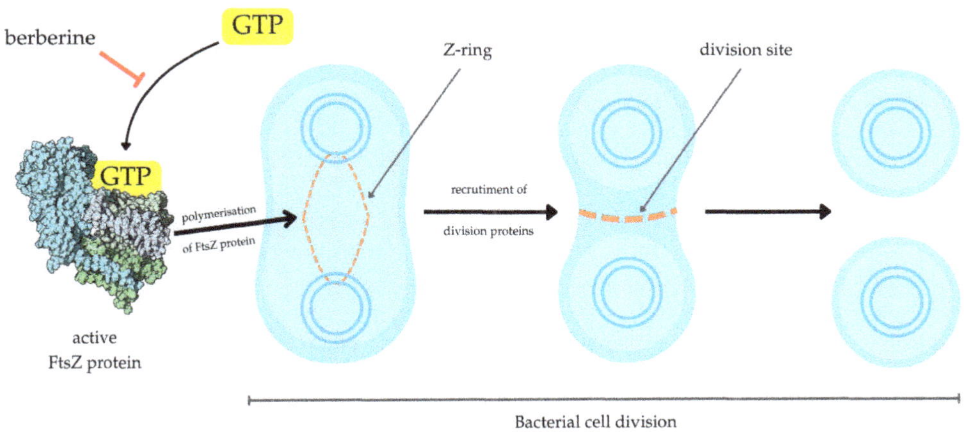

Figure 4. FtsZ protein's role in bacterial cell division and its interaction with BRB. Abbreviations: GTP—guanosine tri-phosphate.

5. Berberine—β-Lactamases Inhibitor

5.1. β-Lactamases as an Antibiotic Resistance Mechanism

One of the most commonly used groups of antibiotics are β-lactams. Those drugs are divided into four groups: penicillins, cephalosporins, monobactams, and carbapenems [97]. They all have one common structural feature, which is the β-lactam ring. β-lactams use it in order to bind with penicillin-binding proteins (PBPs), which results in the disruption of transpeptidation and thus inhibits the synthesis of bacterial cell walls. Disturbance in this process leads to bacteria cell death. One of the strategies developed by bacteria against β-lactam antibiotics is enzymatic resistance through peptides called β-lactamases [98]. They hydrolyze β-lactam rings, rendering them ineffective. Like β-lactam antibiotics, these enzymes can also be classified into several groups, the most commonly used system being the Ambler classification [99]. It is presented in Table 2 with exemplary β-lactamases.

Table 2. Ambler classification with exemplary enzymes.

<table>
<tr><th>Ambler Class</th><th>Active Site Type</th><th>Examples</th><th>References</th></tr>
<tr><td>A</td><td>Serine-β-lactamase</td><td>KPC, TEM-1</td><td>[100]</td></tr>
<tr><td>B</td><td>Metallo-β-lactamase</td><td>NDM, VIM, IMP</td><td>[99]</td></tr>
<tr><td>C</td><td rowspan="2">Serine-β-lactamase</td><td>AmpC, ADC</td><td>[101]</td></tr>
<tr><td>D</td><td>OXA-23, OXA-48</td><td>[100]</td></tr>
</table>

Abbreviations: ADC—*Acinetobacter*-derived cephalosporinase, KPC—*Klebsiella pneumoniae* carbapenemase, TEM-1—narrow spectrum β-lactamase TEM-1, OXA-23—Oxacillinase-23, OXA-48—Oxacillinase-48, NDM—New Delhi metallo-β-lactamase, VIM—Verona integron-encoded metallo-β-lactamase, IMP—Imipenemase.

5.2. Berberine as an Antibiotic Adjuvant and β-Lactamases Inhibitor

β-Lactamases pose a threat to modern medicine, as they can inactivate antibiotics used to treat infections. In order to prevent them from doing so, antibiotic adjuvants such as β-lactamase inhibitors e.g., clavulanic acid, are used [102]. Those compounds do not damage bacteria themselves but rather protect antibiotics from degradation. Promising new adjuvants also belong to BRB, which antimicrobial activity has been observed even towards highly antibiotic-resistant strains [103]. One such study evaluated BRB potential as a New Delhi metallo-β-lactamase-1 (NDM-1) inhibitor [104]. Scientists conducted molecular docking tests to assess the binding affinities of selected phyto-ligands to the active site of examined β-lactamase produced by *E. coli*. Analysis indicated that BRB effectively interacted with NDM-1, thus potentially inhibiting its activity. As there are no potent metallo-β-lactamase inhibitors for now [105], those results are quite promising. Another research conducted in 2020 analyzed BRBe's activity on β-lactamases produced by *M. tuberculosis* (BlaC) [106]. This enzyme belongs to Ambler class A [107]. Constructed models have shown that this alkaloid can bind with the catalytic side of examined β-lactamase, thus inhibiting its hydrolytic properties. Notably, BRB demonstrated a lower bond energy than the referential antibiotic (ceftazidime). This results in a more stable bond with BlaC, thereby increasing the BRB antimicrobial efficacy. BRB's activity as a potential β-Lactamase inhibitor has also been tested on β-Lactamase retrieved from *S. aureus* [108]. Docking studies against this enzyme have shown that BRBe forms bonds with key amino acid residues in the catalytic center. This may result in an inhibitory effect on this β-Lactamase. It is worth mentioning that, among the tested substances, BRB stood out due to its lowest binding energy. It contributes to the stability and efficiency of its bond with the examined *S. aureus* β-lactamase. A newer study conducted in 2024 focused on BRB interaction with class C β-lactamase (AmpC) [109]. In order to assess its inhibitory activity on AmpC, molecular docking studies have been carried out. They indicated that BRB binds with this β-lactamase with a suitable pose and low binding energy, thus stabilizing the structure. The results seem promising and validate BRB's position as a potential new β-lactamase inhibitor. In another study, BRB inhibitory properties were tested on extended-spectrum β-lactamase derived from *E. coli* [110]. This alkaloid was compared to various other compounds in a molecular docking test. While it did not emerge as the most effective one, this study nonetheless confirmed BRB's anti-β-lactamase activity, resulting in its inclusion in pharmacodynamic assessments. Notably, BRB demonstrated the largest zone of inhibition among the tested compounds, although its minimum inhibitory concentration was relatively average compared to the others.

6. Materials and Methods

In this review, we searched for articles by using the databases Scopus, PubMed, Web of Science, and Google Scholar. In total, 110 articles were cited. The articles were qualified for review by searching for the following keywords in the title and abstract of the articles:

"berberine", "efflux pump", "quorum sensing", "FtsZ", and "β-lactamase". This search excluded patent literature. The literature was selected to demonstrate the purpose of BRB on bacteria. In addition, only actives in English were included. Figure 1 shows the chemical formula of alkaloid described in the review. Figure 2 depicts a simplified scheme of the molecular action of berberine on an RND-type efflux pump. Figure 3 presents a simplified sequence of biofilm formation. Table 1 presents a summary of the BRB properties as a quorum sensing inhibitor. Table 2 stands for the Ambler classification of β-lactamases.

7. Conclusions

Given that no new class of antimicrobial agents with novel mechanisms of action has been developed over the past two decades, natural compounds—including BRB—have emerged as promising candidates for pharmaceutical research.

In this review, we summarize the current state of knowledge regarding the multiple antimicrobial mechanisms of BRB, which potentially enable it to overcome resistance among high-priority pathogens, e.g., *P. aeruginosa* and *A. baumannii*. Importantly, no effective and safe efflux-targeting antibacterial agents have yet been approved for clinical use, despite the central role of efflux in mediating multidrug resistance in critical pathogens. Thus, BRB appears to be a promising molecule in this area. BRB has demonstrated the ability to inhibit the MexAB-OprM efflux pump, a broad-substrate resistance determinant that contributes to decreased susceptibility to most therapeutic antibiotics. Furthermore, reports indicate that BRB can suppress the expression of the *AdeABC* efflux pump genes in *A. baumannii*.

Notably, BRB has also been shown to interfere with QS, thereby disrupting biofilm formation and antimicrobial resistance development in both Gram-positive and Gram-negative pathogens. By impairing QS signaling, BRB may reduce catheter-related infections, an issue of major concern in the hospital environment. QS inhibitors (QSIs) are regarded as promising antimicrobial candidates due to their ability to interfere with bacterial cell-to-cell communication and prevent infection onset. However, their clinical implementation remains distant and requires further investigation, especially under in vivo conditions.

A similar situation applies to bacterial mitosis inhibitors targeting the FtsZ protein. The unique mechanism by which BRB affects bacterial cell division is of particular interest due to the high conservation of FtsZ, suggesting that berberine-based compounds could potentially act against a broad spectrum of bacterial species.

In the context of a renewed focus on next-generation β-lactamase inhibitors, such as zidebactam, vaborbactam, taniborbactam, and relebactam, natural substances that are not structural analogs of penam have increasingly shown inhibitory activity against these enzymes. Among them, BRB appears especially promising. Due to its broad inhibitory spectrum—targeting ESβLs, AmpC, and NDM—BRB demonstrates a significant potential for the development of new β-lactamase inhibitors aimed at overcoming β-lactam resistance in multidrug-resistant bacterial strains. In particular, its activity against metallo-β-lactamases is of critical interest in light of the growing prevalence of such infections in intensive care units (ICUs) and should motivate further exploration of this compound.

In conclusion, BRB antimicrobial activity involves diverse mechanisms, including the disruption of efflux pumps, suppression of QS and mitosis, and the inhibition of β-lactamases. These properties state its potential as a future treatment option in infections caused by antibiotic-resistant bacteria. However, further research is needed to confirm the efficiency and safety in humans, assess the pharmacological properties, and invent suitable forms for medical use. BRB can also serve as a starting point for the development of even more useful derivatives or compounds with similar activity.

Author Contributions: Conceptualization, A.D.-M. and S.V.; methodology, S.V., H.B. and J.S.; software, S.V. and H.B.; validation, A.D.-M. and S.V.; investigation, A.D.-M.,S.V., H.B. and J.S.; resources,

A.D.-M.; data curation, A.D.-M., S.V.,H.B. and J.S.; writing—original draft preparation, A.D.-M., S.V., H.B. and J.S.; writing—review and editing, A.D.-M.; visualization, S.V. and J.S.; supervision, A.D.-M.; project administration, A.D.-M.; funding acquisition, A.D.-M. All authors have read and agreed to the published version of the manuscript.

Funding: This research received no external funding.

Institutional Review Board Statement: Not applicable.

Informed Consent Statement: Not applicable.

Data Availability Statement: No new data were created or analyzed in this study. Data sharing is not applicable to this article.

Conflicts of Interest: The authors declare no conflicts of interest.

Abbreviations

ACN—amikacin; ADC- *Acinetobacter*-derived cephalosporinase; ADMET—Absorption, Distribution, Metabolism, and Excretion; BRB—berberine; CCCP—carbonyl cyanide 3-chlorophenylhydrazone; CLA—clarithromycin; CYP—ciprofloxacin; C4-HSL—*N*-Butanoyl-L-homoserine lactone; EDTA—ethylenediaminetetraacetic acid; EPI -- efflux pump inhibitor; ERT—erythromycin; EtBr—ethidium bromide; FICI—fractional inhibitory concentration index; GEN—gentamicin; GTP—guanosine-5′-triphosphate; HPLC—high performance liquid chromatography; IMI—imipenem; IMP—Imipenemase; KPC—*Klebsiella pneumoniae* carbapenemase; LSCM—laser scanning confocal microscopy; MAC—*Mycobacterium avium intracellulare*; MBC—minimal bactericidal concentration; MCR-1—mobilized colistin resistance 1; MDR—multidrug-resistant; MER—meropenem; MFS—major facilitator superfamily; MIC—minimal inhibitory concentration; MOTT—*Mycobacterium* other than *tuberculosis;* MRSA—methicillin-resistant *Staphylococcus aureus;* NDM—New Delhi metallo-β-lactamase; OXA-23—Oxacillinase-23; OXA-48—Oxacillinase-48; PaβN—Phe-Arg-β-naphthylamide; PBPs—penicillin binding proteins; PDR—pandrug-resistant; PSM—phenyl soluble modulins; QS—Quorum sensing; RIF—rifampicin; RMA—resistance-modifying agent; RND—Resistance-Nodulation-Cell Division; SBT—sulbactam; TEM-1—narrow spectrum β-lactamase TEM-1; TET—tetracycline; TGC—tigecycline; TOB—tobramycin; VIM—Verona integron-encoded metallo-β-lactamase; VRE—vancomycin-resistant *E. faecalis;* VRSA—vancomycin-resistant *S. aureus;* WHO—World Health Organization; XDR—extensively drug-resistant; 3-oxo-C12-HSL—*N*-3-Oxo-Dodecanoyl-L-homoserine lactone.

References

1. Llor, C.; Bjerrum, L. Antimicrobial Resistance: Risk Associated with Antibiotic Overuse and Initiatives to Reduce the Problem. *Ther. Adv. Drug Saf.* **2014**, *5*, 229–241. [CrossRef] [PubMed]
2. Ndaki, P.M.; Mwanga, J.R.; Mushi, M.F.; Konje, E.T.; Mwita, S.M.; Mshana, S.E. Drivers of Inappropriate Use of Antibiotics among Community Members in Low- and Middle-Income Countries: A Systematic Review of Qualitative Studies. *BMC Public Health* **2025**, *25*, 705. [CrossRef] [PubMed]
3. Anwar, M.; Iqbal, Q.; Saleem, F. Improper Disposal of Unused Antibiotics: An Often Overlooked Driver of Antimicrobial Resistance. *Expert Rev. Anti-Infect. Ther.* **2020**, *18*, 697–699. [CrossRef]
4. Manyi-Loh, C.; Mamphweli, S.; Meyer, E.; Okoh, A. Antibiotic Use in Agriculture and Its Consequential Resistance in Environmental Sources: Potential Public Health Implications. *Molecules* **2018**, *23*, 795. [CrossRef]
5. World Health Organization. Antimicrobial Resistance. Available online: https://www.who.int/news-room/fact-sheets/detail/antimicrobial-resistance (accessed on 23 January 2025).
6. de Kraker, M.E.A.; Stewardson, A.J.; Harbarth, S. Will 10 Million People Die a Year Due to Antimicrobial Resistance by 2050? *PLoS Med.* **2016**, *13*, e1002184. [CrossRef]
7. Sarkar, P.; Yarlagadda, V.; Ghosh, C.; Haldar, J. A Review on Cell Wall Synthesis Inhibitors with an Emphasis on Glycopeptide Antibiotics. *Medchemcomm* **2017**, *8*, 516–533. [CrossRef]
8. Mccoy, L.S.; Xie, Y.; Tor, Y. Antibiotics That Target Protein Synthesis. *Wiley Interdiscip. Rev. RNA* **2011**, *2*, 209–232. [CrossRef]
9. Kohanski, M.A.; Dwyer, D.J.; Collins, J.J. How Antibiotics Kill Bacteria: From Targets to Networks. *Nat. Rev. Microbiol.* **2010**, *8*, 423–435. [CrossRef]

10. Santos, J.A.; Lamers, M.H. Novel Antibiotics Targeting Bacterial Replicative Dna Polymerases. *Antibiotics* **2020**, *9*, 776. [CrossRef]
11. Bhattacharjee, M.K. Antimetabolites: Antibiotics That Inhibit Nucleotide Synthesis. In *Chemistry of Antibiotics and Related Drugs*; Springer: Cham, Switzerland, 2016.
12. Ledger, E.V.K.; Sabnis, A.; Edwards, A.M. Polymyxin and Lipopeptide Antibiotics: Membrane-Targeting Drugs of Last Resort. *Microbiology* **2022**, *168*, 001136. [CrossRef]
13. Ling, L.L.; Schneider, T.; Peoples, A.J.; Spoering, A.L.; Engels, I.; Conlon, B.P.; Mueller, A.; Schäberle, T.F.; Hughes, D.E.; Epstein, S.; et al. A New Antibiotic Kills Pathogens without Detectable Resistance. *Nature* **2015**, *517*, 455–459. [CrossRef] [PubMed]
14. Imai, Y.; Meyer, K.J.; Iinishi, A.; Favre-Godal, Q.; Green, R.; Manuse, S.; Caboni, M.; Mori, M.; Niles, S.; Ghiglieri, M.; et al. A New Antibiotic Selectively Kills Gram-Negative Pathogens. *Nature* **2019**, *576*, 459–464. [CrossRef] [PubMed]
15. Jangra, M.; Travin, D.Y.; Aleksandrova, E.V.; Kaur, M.; Darwish, L.; Koteva, K.; Klepacki, D.; Wang, W.; Tiffany, M.; Sokaribo, A.; et al. A Broad-Spectrum Lasso Peptide Antibiotic Targeting the Bacterial Ribosome. *Nature* **2025**, *640*, 1022–1030. [CrossRef] [PubMed]
16. Mosaka, T.B.M.; Unuofin, J.O.; Daramola, M.O.; Tizaoui, C.; Iwarere, S.A. Inactivation of Antibiotic-Resistant Bacteria and Antibiotic-Resistance Genes in Wastewater Streams: Current Challenges and Future Perspectives. *Front. Microbiol.* **2023**, *13*, 1100102. [CrossRef]
17. Lambert, P.A. Bacterial Resistance to Antibiotics: Modified Target Sites. *Adv. Drug Deliv. Rev.* **2005**, *57*, 1471–1485. [CrossRef]
18. Ghai, I.; Ghai, S. Understanding Antibiotic Resistance via Outer Membrane Permeability. *Infect. Drug Resist.* **2018**, *11*, 523–530. [CrossRef]
19. Yang, N.J.; Hinner, M.J. Getting Across the Cell Membrane: An Overview for Small Molecules, Peptides, and Proteins. *Methods Mol. Biol.* **2015**, *1266*, 29–53. [CrossRef]
20. Gaurav, A.; Bakht, P.; Saini, M.; Pandey, S.; Pathania, R. Role of Bacterial Efflux Pumps in Antibiotic Resistance, Virulence, and Strategies to Discover Novel Efflux Pump Inhibitors. *Microbiology* **2023**, *169*, 001333. [CrossRef]
21. Faiz, S.; Irfan, M.; Farooq, S.; Khan, I.A.; Iqbal, H.; Wahab, A.-t.; Shakeel, M.; Gong, P.; Iftner, T.; Choudhary, M.I. Study of Drug Resistance-Associated Genetic Mutations, and Phylo-Genetic Analysis of HCV in the Province of Sindh, Pakistan. *Sci. Rep.* **2023**, *13*, 12213. [CrossRef]
22. Martinez, J.L.; Baquero, F. Mutation Frequencies and Antibiotic Resistance. *Antimicrob. Agents Chemother.* **2000**, *44*, 1771–1777. [CrossRef]
23. Wright, G.D. Bacterial Resistance to Antibiotics: Enzymatic Degradation and Modification. *Adv. Drug Deliv. Rev.* **2005**, *57*, 1451–1470. [CrossRef] [PubMed]
24. Egorov, A.M.; Ulyashova, M.M.; Rubtsova, M.Y. Microbial Enzyme Production. *J. Ferment. Technol.* **1988**, *66*, 365–366. [CrossRef]
25. Magiorakos, A.; Srinivasan, A.; Carey, R.B.; Carmeli, Y.; Falagas, M.E.; Giske, C.G.; Harbarth, S.; Hindler, J.F. Bacteria: An International Expert Proposal for Interim Standard Definitions for Acquired Resistance. *Microbiology* **2011**, *18*, 268–281.
26. Aronson, J.K.; Green, A.R. Me-Too Pharmaceutical Products: History, Definitions, Examples, and Relevance to Drug Shortages and Essential Medicines Lists. *Br. J. Clin. Pharmacol.* **2020**, *86*, 2114–2122. [CrossRef]
27. Parker, E.N.; Cain, B.N.; Hajian, B.; Ulrich, R.J.; Geddes, E.J.; Barkho, S.; Lee, H.Y.; Williams, J.D.; Raynor, M.; Caridha, D.; et al. An Iterative Approach Guides Discovery of the FabI Inhibitor Fabimycin, a Late-Stage Antibiotic Candidate with In Vivo Efficacy against Drug-Resistant Gram-Negative Infections. *ACS Cent. Sci.* **2022**, *8*, 1145–1158. [CrossRef]
28. Heithoff, D.M.; Mahan, S.P.; Barnes, V.L.; Leyn, S.A.; George, C.X.; Zlamal, J.E.; Limwongyut, J.; Bazan, G.C.; Fried, J.C.; Fitzgibbons, L.N.; et al. A Broad-Spectrum Synthetic Antibiotic That Does Not Evoke Bacterial Resistance. *eBioMedicine* **2023**, *89*, 104461. [CrossRef]
29. Rineh, A.; Dolla, N.K.; Ball, A.R.; Magana, M.; Bremner, J.B.; Hamblin, M.R.; Tegos, G.P.; Kelso, M.J. Attaching the NorA Efflux Pump Inhibitor INF55 to Methylene Blue Enhances Antimicrobial Photodynamic Inactivation of Methicillin-Resistant *Staphylococcus aureus* in Vitro and in Vivo. *ACS Infect. Dis.* **2017**, *3*, 756–766. [CrossRef]
30. Samosorn, S.; Bremner, J.B.; Ball, A.; Lewis, K. Synthesis of Functionalised 2-Aryl-5-Nitro-1H-Indoles and Their Activity as Bacterial NorA Efflux Pump Inhibitors. *Bioorg. Med. Chem.* **2006**, *14*, 857–865. [CrossRef]
31. Dolla, N.K.; Chen, C.; Larkins-Ford, J.; Rajamuthiah, R.; Jagadeesan, S.; Conery, A.L.; Ausubel, F.M.; Mylonakis, E.; Bremner, J.B.; Lewis, K.; et al. On the Mechanism of Berberine–INF55 (5-Nitro-2-Phenylindole) Hybrid Antibacterials. *Aust. J. Chem.* **2015**, *67*, 1471–1480. [CrossRef]
32. Ball, A.R.; Casadei, G.; Samosorn, S.; Bremner, J.B.; Ausubel, F.M.; Moy, T.I.; Lewis, K. Conjugating Berberine to a Multidrug Resistance Pump Inhibitor Creates an Effective Antimicrobial. *ACS Chem. Biol.* **2006**, *1*, 594–600. [CrossRef]
33. Samosorn, S.; Tanwirat, B.; Muhamad, N.; Casadei, G.; Tomkiewicz, D.; Lewis, K.; Suksamrarn, A.; Prammananan, T.; Gornall, K.C.; Beck, J.L.; et al. Antibacterial Activity of Berberine-NorA Pump Inhibitor Hybrids with a Methylene Ether Linking Group. *Bioorg. Med. Chem.* **2009**, *17*, 3866–3872. [CrossRef] [PubMed]

34. Neag, M.A.; Mocan, A.; Echeverría, J.; Pop, R.M.; Bocsan, C.I.; Crişan, G.; Buzoianu, A.D. Berberine: Botanical Occurrence, Traditional Uses, Extraction Methods, and Relevance in Cardiovascular, Metabolic, Hepatic, and Renal Disorders. *Front. Pharmacol.* **2018**, *9*, 557. [CrossRef] [PubMed]
35. Zhou, L.; Xu, J.; Peng, Y. Medicinal Crops. In *Encyclopedia of Agriculture and Food Systems*; Elsevier: Amsterdam, The Netherlands, 2014; pp. 223–230.
36. Duda-Madej, A.; Viscardi, S.; Szewczyk, W.; Topola, E. Natural Alkaloids in Cancer Therapy: Berberine, Sanguinarine and Chelerythrine against Colorectal and Gastric Cancer. *Int. J. Mol. Sci.* **2024**, *25*, 8375. [CrossRef] [PubMed]
37. Wu, S.; Yang, K.; Hong, Y.; Gong, Y.; Ni, J.; Yang, N.; Ding, W. A New Perspective on the Antimicrobial Mechanism of Berberine Hydrochloride Against *Staphylococcus aureus* Revealed by Untargeted Metabolomic Studies. *Front. Microbiol.* **2022**, *13*, 917414. [CrossRef]
38. Pacyga, K.; Pacyga, P.; Topola, E.; Viscardi, S.; Duda-Madej, A. Bioactive Compounds from Plant Origin as Natural Antimicrobial Agents for the Treatment of Wound Infections. *Int. J. Mol. Sci.* **2024**, *25*, 2100. [CrossRef]
39. Li, Z.; Geng, Y.-N.; Jiang, J.-D.; Kong, W.-J. Antioxidant and Anti-Inflammatory Activities of Berberine in the Treatment of Diabetes Mellitus. *Evid. Based Complement. Altern. Med.* **2014**, *2014*, 289264. [CrossRef]
40. Kheir, M.M.; Wang, Y.; Hua, L.; Hu, J.; Li, L.; Lei, F.; Du, L. Acute Toxicity of Berberine and Its Correlation with the Blood Concentration in Mice. *Food Chem. Toxicol.* **2010**, *48*, 1105–1110. [CrossRef]
41. Wang, K.; Feng, X.; Chai, L.; Cao, S.; Qiu, F. The Metabolism of Berberine and Its Contribution to the Pharmacological Effects. *Drug Metab. Rev.* **2017**, *49*, 139–157. [CrossRef]
42. Patel, P. A Bird's Eye View on a Therapeutically 'Wonder Molecule': Berberine. *Phytomedicine Plus* **2021**, *1*, 100070. [CrossRef]
43. Sun, P.; Wang, Z.; Ma, Y.; Liu, Y.; Xue, Y.; Li, Y.; Gao, X.; Wang, Y.; Chu, M. Advance in Identified Targets of Berberine. *Front. Pharmacol.* **2025**, *16*, 1500511. [CrossRef]
44. Filli, M.S.; Ibrahim, A.A.; Kesse, S.; Aquib, M.; Boakye-Yiadom, K.O.; Farooq, M.A.; Raza, F.; Zhang, Y.; Wang, B. Synthetic Berberine Derivatives as Potential New Drugs. *Braz. J. Pharm. Sci.* **2022**, *58*, e18835. [CrossRef]
45. Karimi, S.; Heidari, F.; Amraei, S. Nano Micro Biosystems Therapeutic Aspects of Berberine and Its Derivatives: Recent Advances and Challenges. *Nano Micro Biosyst.* **2023**, *2023*, 42–47.
46. Fiamegos, Y.C.; Kastritis, P.L.; Exarchou, V.; Han, H.; Bonvin, A.M.J.J.; Vervoort, J.; Lewis, K.; Hamblin, M.R.; Tegos, G.P. Antimicrobial and Efflux Pump Inhibitory Activity of Caffeoylquinic Acids from *Artemisia absinthium* against Gram-Positive Pathogenic Bacteria. *PLoS ONE* **2011**, *6*, e18127. [CrossRef]
47. Stermitz, F.R.; Lorenz, P.; Tawara, J.N.; Zenewicz, L.A.; Lewis, K. Synergy in a Medicinal Plant: Antimicrobial Action of Berberine Potentiated by 5′-Methoxyhydnocarpin, a Multidrug Pump Inhibitor. *Proc. Natl. Acad. Sci. USA* **2000**, *97*, 1433–1437. [CrossRef]
48. Musumeci, R.; Speciale, A.; Costanzo, R.; Annino, A.; Ragusa, S.; Rapisarda, A.; Pappalardo, M.S.; Iauk, L. *Berberis aetnensis* C. Presl. Extracts: Antimicrobial Properties and Interaction with Ciprofloxacin. *Int. J. Antimicrob. Agents* **2003**, *22*, 48–53. [CrossRef]
49. Ettefagh, K.; Burns, J.; Junio, H.; Kaatz, G.; Cech, N. Goldenseal (*Hydrastis canadensis* L.) Extracts Synergistically Enhance the Antibacterial Activity of Berberine via Efflux Pump Inhibition. *Planta Med.* **2011**, *77*, 835–840. [CrossRef]
50. Mohtar, M.; Johari, S.A.; Li, A.R.; Isa, M.M.; Mustafa, S.; Ali, A.M.; Basri, D.F. Inhibitory and Resistance-Modifying Potential of Plant-Based Alkaloids Against Methicillin-Resistant *Staphylococcus aureus* (MRSA). *Curr. Microbiol.* **2009**, *59*, 181–186. [CrossRef]
51. Li, Y.; Ge, X. Role of Berberine as a Potential Efflux Pump Inhibitor against MdfA from *Escherichia coli*: In Vitro and In Silico Studies. *Microbiol. Spectr.* **2023**, *11*, e03324-22. [CrossRef]
52. Seo, Y.; Kim, M.; Kim, T.-J. Enhanced Efficacy of Ciprofloxacin and Tobramycin against *Staphylococcus aureus* When Combined with Corydalis Tuber and Berberine through Efflux Pump Inhibition. *Antibiotics* **2024**, *13*, 469. [CrossRef]
53. Ahmadi, F.; Khalvati, B.; Eslami, S.; Mirzaii, M.; Roustaei, N.; Mazloomirad, F.; Khoramrooz, S.S. The Inhibitory Effect of Thioridazine on AdeB Efflux Pump Gene Expression in Multidrug-Resistant Acinetobacter Baumannii Isolates Using Real Time PCR. *Avicenna J. Med. Biotechnol.* **2022**, *14*, 132. [CrossRef]
54. Morita, Y.; Nakashima, K.; Nishino, K.; Kotani, K.; Tomida, J.; Inoue, M.; Kawamura, Y. Berberine Is a Novel Type Efflux Inhibitor Which Attenuates the MexXY-Mediated Aminoglycoside Resistance in *Pseudomonas aeruginosa*. *Front. Microbiol.* **2016**, *7*, 1223. [CrossRef]
55. Aghayan, S.S.; Kalalian Mogadam, H.; Fazli, M.; Darban-Sarokhalil, D.; Khoramrooz, S.S.; Jabalameli, F.; Yaslianifard, S.; Mirzaii, M. The Effects of Berberine and Palmatine on Efflux Pumps Inhibition with Different Gene Patterns in *Pseudomonas aeruginosa* Isolated from Burn Infections. *Avicenna J. Med. Biotechnol.* **2017**, *9*, 2–7. [PubMed]
56. Su, F.; Wang, J. Berberine Inhibits the MexXY-OprM Efflux Pump to Reverse Imipenem Resistance in a Clinical Carbapenem-resistant *Pseudomonas aeruginosa* Isolate in a Planktonic State. *Exp. Ther. Med.* **2017**, *15*, 467–472. [CrossRef] [PubMed]
57. Laudadio, E.; Cedraro, N.; Mangiaterra, G.; Citterio, B.; Mobbili, G.; Minnelli, C.; Bizzaro, D.; Biavasco, F.; Galeazzi, R. Natural Alkaloid Berberine Activity against *Pseudomonas aeruginosa* MexXY-Mediated Aminoglycoside Resistance: In Silico and in Vitro Studies. *J. Nat. Prod.* **2019**, *82*, 1935–1944. [CrossRef] [PubMed]

58. Fujiwara, M.; Yamasaki, S.; Morita, Y.; Nishino, K. Evaluation of Efflux Pump Inhibitors of MexAB- or MexXY-OprM in *Pseudomonas aeruginosa* Using Nucleic Acid Dyes. *J. Infect. Chemother.* **2022**, *28*, 595–601. [CrossRef]
59. Giorgini, G.; Mangiaterra, G.; Cedraro, N.; Laudadio, E.; Sabbatini, G.; Cantarini, M.; Minnelli, C.; Mobbili, G.; Frangipani, E.; Biavasco, F.; et al. Berberine Derivatives as *Pseudomonas aeruginosa* MexXY-OprM Inhibitors: Activity and In Silico Insights. *Molecules* **2021**, *26*, 6644. [CrossRef]
60. Giorgini, G.; Di Gregorio, A.; Mangiaterra, G.; Cedraro, N.; Minnelli, C.; Sabbatini, G.; Mobbili, G.; Simoni, S.; Vignaroli, C.; Galeazzi, R. Inhibition of Polymorphic MexXY-OprM Efflux System in *Pseudomonas aeruginosa* Clinical Isolates by Berberine Derivatives. *ChemMedChem* **2024**, *19*, e202300568. [CrossRef]
61. Zhou, X.-Y.; Ye, X.-G.; He, L.-T.; Zhang, S.-R.; Wang, R.-L.; Zhou, J.; He, Z.-S. In Vitro Characterization and Inhibition of the Interaction between Ciprofloxacin and Berberine against Multidrug-Resistant *Klebsiella pneumonia e*. *J. Antibiot.* **2016**, *69*, 741–746. [CrossRef]
62. Karaosmanoglu, K.; Sayar, N.A.; Kurnaz, I.A.; Akbulut, B.S. Assessment of Berberine as a Multi-Target Antimicrobial: A Multi-Omics Study for Drug Discovery and Repositioning. *Omics J. Integr. Biol.* **2014**, *18*, 42–53. [CrossRef]
63. Budeyri Gokgoz, N.; Avci, F.G.; Yoneten, K.K.; Alaybeyoglu, B.; Ozkirimli, E.; Sayar, N.A.; Kazan, D.; Sariyar Akbulut, B. Response of *Escherichia coli* to Prolonged Berberine Exposure. *Microb. Drug Resist.* **2017**, *23*, 531–544. [CrossRef]
64. Cui, X.; Liu, X.; Ma, X.; Li, S.; Zhang, J.; Han, R.; Yi, K.; Liu, J.; Pan, Y.; He, D.; et al. Restoring Colistin Sensitivity in Colistin-Resistant *Salmonella* and *Escherichia coli*: Combinatorial Use of Berberine and EDTA with Colistin. *mSphere* **2024**, *9*, e00182-24. [CrossRef] [PubMed]
65. Menichini, M.; Lari, N.; Rindi, L. Effect of Efflux Pump Inhibitors on the Susceptibility of *Mycobacterium avium* Complex to Clarithromycin. *J. Antibiot.* **2020**, *73*, 128–132. [CrossRef] [PubMed]
66. Puk, K.; Guz, L. Effect of Alkaloid Berberine on the Susceptibility of Nontuberculous Mycobacteria to Antibiotics. *Pol. J. Vet. Sci.* **2022**, *25*, 479–481. [CrossRef]
67. Schildkraut, J.A.; Coolen, J.P.M.; Ruesen, C.; van den Heuvel, J.J.M.W.; Aceña, L.E.; Wertheim, H.F.L.; Jansen, R.S.; Koenderink, J.B.; te Brake, L.H.M.; van Ingen, J. The Potential Role of Drug Transporters and Amikacin Modifying Enzymes in *M. avium*. *J. Glob. Antimicrob. Resist.* **2023**, *34*, 161–165. [CrossRef]
68. Schwab, M.; Bergonzi, C.; Sakkos, J.; Staley, C.; Zhang, Q.; Sadowsky, M.J.; Aksan, A.; Elias, M. Signal Disruption Leads to Changes in Bacterial Community Population. *Front. Microbiol.* **2019**, *10*, 611. [CrossRef]
69. Hraiech, S.; Hiblot, J.; Lafleur, J.; Lepidi, H.; Papazian, L.; Rolain, J.M.; Raoult, D.; Elias, M.; Silby, M.W.; Bzdrenga, J.; et al. Inhaled Lactonase Reduces *Pseudomonas aeruginosa* Quorum Sensing and Mortality in Rat Pneumonia. *PLoS ONE* **2014**, *9*, e107125. [CrossRef]
70. Aswathanarayan, J.B.; Vittal, R.R. Inhibition of Biofilm Formation and Quorum Sensing Mediated Phenotypes by Berberine in: *Pseudomonas aeruginosa* and *Salmonella typhimurium*. *RSC Adv.* **2018**, *8*, 36133–36141. [CrossRef]
71. Talaat, R.; Abu El-naga, M.N.; El-Bialy, H.A.A.; El-Fouly, M.Z.; Abouzeid, M.A. Quenching of Quorum Sensing in Multi-Drug Resistant *Pseudomonas aeruginosa*: Insights on Halo-Bacterial Metabolites and Gamma Irradiation as Channels Inhibitors. *Ann. Clin. Microbiol. Antimicrob.* **2024**, *23*, 31. [CrossRef]
72. Yi, Y.; Zhou, Y.; Lin, S.; Shi, K.; Mei, J.; Ying, G.; Wu, S. Screening and Isolation of Quorum Sensing Inhibitors of *Pseudomonas aeruginosa* from *Phellodendron amurense* Extracts Using Bio-affinity Chromatography. *J. Sep. Sci.* **2024**, *47*, 2400222. [CrossRef]
73. Li, Y.T.; Huang, J.R.; Li, L.J.; Liu, L.S. Synergistic Activity of Berberine with Azithromycin against *Pseudomonas aeruginosa* Isolated from Patients with Cystic Fibrosis of Lung in Vitro and In Vivo. *Cell. Physiol. Biochem.* **2017**, *42*, 1657–1669. [CrossRef]
74. Tan, C.H.; Koh, K.S.; Xie, C.; Tay, M.; Zhou, Y.; Williams, R.; Ng, W.J.; Rice, S.A.; Kjelleberg, S. The Role of Quorum Sensing Signalling in EPS Production and the Assembly of a Sludge Community into Aerobic Granules. *ISME J.* **2014**, *8*, 1186–1197. [CrossRef] [PubMed]
75. Inamuco, J.; Veenendaal, A.K.J.; Burt, S.A.; Post, J.A.; Tjeerdsma-van Bokhoven, J.L.M.; Haagsman, H.P.; Veldhuizen, E.J.A. Sub-Lethal Levels of Carvacrol Reduce *Salmonella* Typhimurium Motility and Invasion of Porcine Epithelial Cells. *Vet. Microbiol.* **2012**, *157*, 200–207. [CrossRef] [PubMed]
76. Pang, Y.; Wang, S.; Tao, J.; Wang, J.; Xue, Z.; Wang, R. Mechanism of Berberine Hydrochloride Interfering with Biofilm Formation of *Hafnia alvei*. *Arch. Microbiol.* **2022**, *204*, 126. [CrossRef] [PubMed]
77. Sun, T.; Li, X.D.; Hong, J.; Liu, C.; Zhang, X.L.; Zheng, J.P.; Xu, Y.J.; Ou, Z.Y.; Zheng, J.L.; Yu, D.J. Inhibitory Effect of Two Traditional Chinese Medicine Monomers, Berberine and Matrine, on the Quorum Sensing System of Antimicrobial-Resistant *Escherichia coli*. *Front. Microbiol.* **2019**, *10*, 2584. [CrossRef]
78. Chu, M.; Zhang, M.B.; Liu, Y.C.; Kang, J.R.; Chu, Z.Y.; Yin, K.L.; Ding, L.Y.; Ding, R.; Xiao, R.X.; Yin, Y.N.; et al. Role of Berberine in the Treatment of Methicillin-Resistant *Staphylococcus aureus* Infections. *Sci. Rep.* **2016**, *6*, 24748. [CrossRef]
79. Cech, N.; Junio, H.; Ackermann, L.; Kavanaugh, J.; Horswill, A. Quorum Quenching and Antimicrobial Activity of Goldenseal (*Hydrastis canadensis*) against Methicillin-Resistant *Staphylococcus aureus* (MRSA). *Planta Med.* **2012**, *78*, 1556–1561. [CrossRef]

80. Novick, R.P. Autoinduction and Signal Transduction in the Regulation of *Staphylococcal virulence*. *Mol. Microbiol.* **2003**, *48*, 1429–1449. [CrossRef]
81. Abd El-Hamid, M.I.; Ibrahim, D.; Elazab, S.T.; Gad, W.M.; Shalaby, M.; El-Neshwy, W.M.; Alshahrani, M.A.; Saif, A.; Algendy, R.M.; AlHarbi, M.; et al. Tackling Strong Biofilm and Multi-Virulent Vancomycin-Resistant *Staphylococcus aureus* via Natural Alkaloid-Based Porous Nanoparticles: Perspective towards near Future Eradication. *Front. Cell. Infect. Microbiol.* **2024**, *13*, 1287426. [CrossRef]
82. Gao, S.; Zhang, S.; Zhang, S. Enhanced in Vitro Antimicrobial Activity of Amphotericin B with Berberine against Dual-Species Biofilms of *Candida albicans* and *Staphylococcus aureus*. *J. Appl. Microbiol.* **2021**, *130*, 1154–1172. [CrossRef]
83. Wang, J.D.; Levin, P.A. Metabolism, Cell Growth and the Bacterial Cell Cycle. *Nat. Rev. Microbiol.* **2009**, *7*, 822–827. [CrossRef]
84. Barrows, J.M.; Goley, E.D. FtsZ Dynamics in Bacterial Division: What, How, and Why? *Curr. Opin. Cell Biol.* **2021**, *68*, 163–172. [CrossRef] [PubMed]
85. Domadia, P.N.; Bhunia, A.; Sivaraman, J.; Swarup, S.; Dasgupta, D. Berberine Targets Assembly of *Escherichia coli* Cell Division Protein FtsZ. *Biochemistry* **2008**, *47*, 3225–3234. [CrossRef] [PubMed]
86. Sun, N.; Chan, F.-Y.; Lu, Y.-J.; Neves, M.A.C.; Lui, H.-K.; Wang, Y.; Chow, K.-Y.; Chan, K.-F.; Yan, S.-C.; Leung, Y.-C.; et al. Rational Design of Berberine-Based FtsZ Inhibitors with Broad-Spectrum Antibacterial Activity. *PLoS ONE* **2014**, *9*, e97514. [CrossRef] [PubMed]
87. Parhi, A.; Lu, S.; Kelley, C.; Kaul, M.; Pilch, D.S.; LaVoie, E.J. Antibacterial Activity of Substituted Dibenzo[a,g]Quinolizin-7-Ium Derivatives. *Bioorg. Med. Chem. Lett.* **2012**, *22*, 6962–6966. [CrossRef]
88. Goh, S.; Boberek, J.M.; Nakashima, N.; Stach, J.; Good, L. Concurrent Growth Rate and Transcript Analyses Reveal Essential Gene Stringency in *Escherichia coli*. *PLoS ONE* **2009**, *4*, e6061. [CrossRef]
89. Fan, T.; Wang, Y.; Tang, S.; Hu, X.; Zen, Q.; Pang, J.; Yang, Y.; You, X.; Song, D. Synthesis and Antibacterial Evaluation of 13-Substituted Cycloberberine Derivatives as a Novel Class of Anti-MRSA Agents. *Eur. J. Med. Chem.* **2018**, *157*, 877–886. [CrossRef]
90. Olleik, H.; Yacoub, T.; Hoffer, L.; Gnansounou, S.M.; Benhaiem-Henry, K.; Nicoletti, C.; Mekhalfi, M.; Pique, V.; Perrier, J.; Hijazi, A.; et al. Synthesis and Evaluation of the Antibacterial Activities of 13-Substituted Berberine Derivatives. *Antibiotics* **2020**, *9*, 381. [CrossRef]
91. Naz, F.; Kumar, M.; Koley, T.; Sharma, P.; Haque, M.A.; Kapil, A.; Kumar, M.; Kaur, P.; Ethayathulla, A.S. Screening of Plant-Based Natural Compounds as an Inhibitor of FtsZ from *Salmonella Typhi* Using the Computational, Biochemical and in Vitro Cell-Based Studies. *Int. J. Biol. Macromol.* **2022**, *219*, 428–437. [CrossRef]
92. Chi, X.; Ding, J.; Zhang, Y.; Chen, Y.; Han, Y.; Lin, Y.; Jiang, J. Berberine Protects against Dysentery by Targeting Both Shigella Filamentous Temperature Sensitive Protein Z and Host Pyroptosis: Resolving in Vitro–Vivo Effect Discrepancy. *Phytomedicine* **2025**, *139*, 156517. [CrossRef]
93. Di Somma, A.; Canè, C.; Rotondo, N.P.; Cavalluzzi, M.M.; Lentini, G.; Duilio, A. A Comparative Study of the Inhibitory Action of Berberine Derivatives on the Recombinant Protein FtsZ of *E. coli*. *Int. J. Mol. Sci.* **2023**, *24*, 5674. [CrossRef]
94. Milani, G.; Cavalluzzi, M.M.; Solidoro, R.; Salvagno, L.; Quintieri, L.; Di Somma, A.; Rosato, A.; Corbo, F.; Franchini, C.; Duilio, A.; et al. Molecular Simplification of Natural Products: Synthesis, Antibacterial Activity, and Molecular Docking Studies of Berberine Open Models. *Biomedicines* **2021**, *9*, 452. [CrossRef] [PubMed]
95. Akinpelu, O.I.; Kumalo, H.M.; Mhlongo, S.I.; Mhlongo, N.N. Identifying the Analogues of Berberine as Promising Antitubercular Drugs Targeting *Mtb*-FtsZ Polymerisation through Ligand-based Virtual Screening and Molecular Dynamics Simulations. *J. Mol. Recognit.* **2022**, *35*, e2940. [CrossRef] [PubMed]
96. Sharma, A.K.; Poddar, S.M.; Chakraborty, J.; Nayak, B.S.; Kalathil, S.; Mitra, N.; Gayathri, P.; Srinivasan, R. A Mechanism of Salt Bridge–Mediated Resistance to FtsZ Inhibitor PC190723 Revealed by a Cell-Based Screen. *Mol. Biol. Cell* **2023**, *34*, ar16. [CrossRef]
97. Pandey, N.; Cascella, M. Beta-Lactam Antibiotics. In *StatPearls*; StatPearls Publishing: Treasure Island, FL, USA, 2025.
98. Smith, H.Z.; Hollingshead, C.M.; Kendall, B. Carbapenem-Resistant Enterobacterales. In *StatPearls*; StatPearls Publishing: Treasure Island, FL, USA, 2025.
99. Hammoudi Halat, D.; Ayoub Moubareck, C. The Current Burden of Carbapenemases: Review of Significant Properties and Dissemination among Gram-Negative Bacteria. *Antibiotics* **2020**, *9*, 186. [CrossRef]
100. Vrancianu, C.O.; Gheorghe, I.; Dobre, E.-G.; Barbu, I.C.; Cristian, R.E.; Popa, M.; Lee, S.H.; Limban, C.; Vlad, I.M.; Chifiriuc, M.C. Emerging Strategies to Combat β-Lactamase Producing ESKAPE Pathogens. *Int. J. Mol. Sci.* **2020**, *21*, 8527. [CrossRef]
101. Mack, A.R.; Barnes, M.D.; Taracila, M.A.; Hujer, A.M.; Hujer, K.M.; Cabot, G.; Feldgarden, M.; Haft, D.H.; Klimke, W.; van den Akker, F.; et al. A Standard Numbering Scheme for Class C β-Lactamases. *Antimicrob. Agents Chemother.* **2020**, *64*, 10–128. [CrossRef]
102. Liu, Y.; Li, R.; Xiao, X.; Wang, Z. Antibiotic Adjuvants: An Alternative Approach to Overcome Multi-Drug Resistant Gram-Negative Bacteria. *Crit. Rev. Microbiol.* **2019**, *45*, 301–314. [CrossRef]

103. Zhong, C.; Lin, S.; Li, Z.; Yang, X. Characterization of Carbapenem-Resistant *Klebsiella pneumoniae* in Bloodstream Infections: Antibiotic Resistance, Virulence, and Treatment Strategies. *Front. Cell. Infect. Microbiol.* **2025**, *15*, 1541704. [CrossRef]
104. Pallavi, T.; Raman, C.; Rajeev, G.; Shyam, G.S.; Namita, S.; Alka, N.; Rajesj, A.; Rakesh, S.K. Crystal Structure of New Delhi Metallo-Beta-Lactamase (NDM-1). *J. Adv. Bioinforma. Appl. Res.* 2011. Available online: https://www.wwpdb.org/pdb?id=pdb_00003s0z (accessed on 25 May 2025).
105. Nahar, L.; Hagiya, H.; Gotoh, K.; Asaduzzaman, M.; Otsuka, F. New Delhi Metallo-Beta-Lactamase Inhibitors: A Systematic Scoping Review. *J. Clin. Med.* **2024**, *13*, 4199. [CrossRef]
106. Sabah, D. Recherche Des Inhibiteurs Naturels de l'Enzyme Bêta-Lactamase (BlaC)À l'Origine de l'Antibiorésistance Chez Mycobacterium Tuberculosis, Agent Responsable de La Tuberculose: Approche Par Modélisation. Ph.D. Thesis, Université Ibn Khaldoun-Tiaret, Tiaret, Algeria, 2019.
107. van Alen, I.; Aguirre García, M.A.; Maaskant, J.J.; Kuijl, C.P.; Bitter, W.; Meijer, A.H.; Ubbink, M. *Mycobacterium tuberculosis* β-Lactamase Variant Reduces Sensitivity to Ampicillin/Avibactam in a Zebrafish-*Mycobacterium marinum* Model of Tuberculosis. *Sci. Rep.* **2023**, *13*, 15406. [CrossRef]
108. Sharma, H.K.; Gupta, P.; Nagpal, D.; Mukherjee, M.; Parmar, V.S.; Lather, V. Virtual Screening and Antimicrobial Evaluation for Identification of Natural Compounds as the Prospective Inhibitors of Antibacterial Drug Resistance Targets in *Staphylococcus aureus*. *Fitoterapia* **2023**, *168*, 105554. [CrossRef] [PubMed]
109. Safi, A.N.; Behrad, M.S.; Mosawi, S.H.; Bayan, A.M. Integrating Molecular Docking and Molecular Dynamics Simulation Approaches for Investigation of the Affinity and Interactions of Berberine with Class C β-Lactamase. *Afghan. J. Infect. Dis.* **2024**, *2*, 17–24. [CrossRef]
110. Ahmed, F.; Sharma, H.K.; Mukherjee, M.; Agarwal, P.; Kumar, A.; Pandita, D.; Lather, V. Exploring Synergistic Potential of Phytomolecules-Antibiotics Combination against *Escherichia coli*: An Integrated Approach Using Structure Based Drug Design. *Pharmacol. Res.—Nat. Prod.* **2025**, *6*, 100160. [CrossRef]

pharmaceuticals

MDPI

Review

Is Camphor the Future in Supporting Therapy for Skin Infections?

Anna Duda-Madej [1,*], Szymon Viscardi [2], Małgorzata Grabarczyk [3], Ewa Topola [2], Joanna Kozłowska [3], Wanda Mączka [3,*] and Katarzyna Wińska [3]

1 Department of Microbiology, Faculty of Medicine, Wroclaw Medical University, Chałubińskiego 4, 50-368 Wrocław, Poland

2 Faculty of Medicine, Wroclaw Medical University, Ludwika Pasteura 1, 50-367 Wrocław, Poland; szymon.viscardi@student.umw.edu.pl (S.V.); ewa.topola@student.umw.edu.pl (E.T.)

3 Department of Food Chemistry and Biocatalysis, Faculty of Biotechnology and Food Science, Wrocław University of Environmental and Life Sciences, C.K. Norwida 25, 50-375 Wrocław, Poland; malgorzata.grabarczyk@upwr.edu.pl (M.G.); joanna.kozlowska@upwr.edu.pl (J.K.); katarzyna.winska@upwr.edu.pl (K.W.)

* Correspondence: anna.duda-madej@umw.edu.pl (A.D.-M.); wanda.maczka@upwr.edu.pl (W.M.)

Abstract: The aim of this review is to present the potential application of camphor—a bicyclic monoterpene ketone—in the prevention of skin infections. Skin diseases represent a heterogeneous group of disorders characterized by prolonged symptoms that significantly diminish the quality of life. They affect the dermis, the epidermis, and even subcutaneous tissue. They very often have a bacterial or fungal background. Therapy for dermatological skin disorders is difficult and long-term. Therefore, it is important to find a compound, preferably of natural origin, that (i) prevents the initiation of this infection and (ii) supports the skin's repair process. Based on its documented anti-inflammatory, antibacterial, antifungal, anti-acne, anesthetic, strengthening, and warming properties, camphor can be used as a preventative measure in dermatological infectious diseases and as a component in medical and cosmetic products. This work discusses the structure and physicochemical properties of camphor, its occurrence, and methods of obtaining it from natural sources as well as through chemical synthesis. The use of camphor in industrial preparations is also presented. Additionally, after a detailed review of the literature, the metabolism of camphor, its interactions with other medicinal substances, and its antimicrobial properties against bacteria and fungi involved in skin diseases are discussed with regard to their resistance.

Keywords: camphor; antibacterial activity; antifungal activity; drug resistance; skin infections; wound healing; monoterpenoids; natural compounds

1. Introduction

Today, a growing interest in the use of natural compounds in various therapies or medical treatments can be observed. Camphor, an organic compound that belongs to the terpene group, is a great example. It is obtained from the wood of the camphor cinnamon tree that grows in Japan, China, Vietnam, Asia, Africa, Sri Lanka, Australia, Canada, and the United States. In its solid form, it is a white powder with a very intense odor that easily converts to a gas. The most commonly used form is camphor oil (*Oleum camphoratum*).

Camphor is not only a fragrant compound, as due to its properties it has also found use in the therapy of skin diseases of bacterial and fungal etiology. Camphor oil is used to support skin problems such as acne, eczema, inflammation, ulcers and wounds, psoriasis, and fungal foot infections [1–5]. Camphor provides support for this type of infection as it has been shown to have a local anesthetic effect [6]. Furthermore, it is effective against swelling and has a unique ability to remove keratinized epidermis [7,8]. As a result, it speeds up wound-healing time and facilitates faster regeneration of the damaged area.

However, it is essential to note that pure camphor, in a dose of 2 g, causes very severe poisoning. Additionally, the amount of 4 g is considered a lethal dose (calculated as >30 mg/kg of body weight in oral use) [9,10]. It should also not be applied directly to open wounds as it can easily penetrate the bloodstream and cause toxic effects on the body. Therefore, from a medical point of view, using camphor in the form of oil, preferably highly diluted, is much safer.

Camphor has also found use in cosmetology as an ingredient in ointments, lotions, and depilatories. In addition to pharmaceuticals, it is used to make gels to prevent insect bites or deliver analgesic, anti-itch, and skin cooling effects. It is also used for embalming corpses [11].

The skin is a multifunctional organ that protects tissues from the effects of environmental factors. It serves as a barrier against minor trauma that causes violation/destruction of its integrity and exposes its deeper layers to infection. crucial factors in this process are the malfunctioning of the immune system (reduced cellular and humoral immunity), coexisting diseases (e.g., diabetes),and the pathogenic properties of bacteria involved in inflammation processes [12]. In the case of a properly functioning immune response, keratinocytes prevent bacteria from taking up residence for a long time, promoting only transient colonization. In contrast, under conditions of immune imbalance, inflammation develops. Initially, it involves only the surface layer of the epidermis. However, under favorable conditions, it can also occupy the deeper layers of the skin and even progress to a generalized infection, increasing the risk of the patient's death. Skin infections can be caused by bacteria (i.e., *Staphylococcus* spp., *Streptococcus* spp., *Corynebacterium* spp., *Spirochaeta* spp., *Actinomyces* spp., and *Mycobacterium* spp.), as well as by fungi (mainly *Candida* spp. and dermatophytes) [13–19]. Nevertheless, the most commonly observed infections are staphylococcal (e.g., periungual inflammation, figwort, and boils), streptococcal (e.g., roseola) and mixed staphylococcal/streptococcal (e.g., impetigo) [20].

Skin disorders can occur either as primary infections or as secondary subinfections of pre-existing dermatosis. In primary infections, the inflammatory process is localized in the dermis (e.g., erysipelas, impetigo), in the hair follicle (folliculitis, furuncle), in the area around the nail (paronychia), or in the subcutaneous tissue (cellulitis) [21]. On the other hand, secondary infections include wound contamination due to injuries, bites, burns, pressure sores, and surgical procedures [22].

Microorganisms, both those that are constantly present and those transiently colonizing the skin and mucous membranes, are a serious source of hospitalized infections. The problem becomes even more alarming when multi-drug resistant microorganisms are involved. The presence of *Staphylococcus aureus*, particularly methicillin-resistant (MRSA), significantly increases the risk of surgical site infections, as this species is a key etiological agent of hospital-acquired infections [23]. Research by Bekka-Hadji et al. confirms the effectiveness of camphor against MRSA strains [24]. Moreover, microorganisms that naturally reside on and colonize the skin, including those that cause dermatological infections, are commonly implicated in catheter-related infections. As a results of their ability to adhere to artificial surfaces, they form a unique microenvironment called a biofilm. This directly paves the way for bloodstream infections (BSIs), which ultimately lead to sepsis [25]. This situation is particularly dangerous in the case of secondary infections (i.e., burn wounds, post-operative wounds), whose etiological agents are hospital-acquired MDR strains, mainly those of the ESKAPE group, that is, *Enterococcus faecium*, *Staphylococcus aureus*, *Klebsiella pneumoniae*, *Acinetobacter baumannii*, *Pseudomonas aeruginosa*, and *Enterobacter* spp. [26]. These pathogens represent a new paradigm related to pathogenesis, transmission, and resistance, and they are particularly dangerous from the point of view of the effectiveness of therapy for nosocomial infections. The fight against these microorganisms, and consequently the need to eradicate the biofilms formed by them, is even crucial to the effectiveness of therapy. Camphor's antimicrobial capabilities appear to be one of the available solutions [27]. A recent study is very promising and demonstrates the synergistic effects of camphor with antibiotics. It is proven that this compound not only contributes to lowering the MIC (minimal inhibitory concentration) values of antimicrobial drugs (i.e., penicillins, cephalosporins, carbapenems, monobactams, aminoglycosides, and quinolones), but also returns antibiotic sensitivity to strains that previously showed resistance to them [28,29].

One of the most dangerous contributors to bacterial superinfection is atopic dermatitis (AD). Skin infections are listed as an integral part of this condition. In people suffering from AD, the integrity of the stratum corneum is damaged and, in addition, the alkaline reaction of the skin surface results in a decrease in its antimicrobial activity. Furthermore, in these individuals a decrease in lipid content is observed in the epidermis, which hinders water binding, leading to faster moisture loss and crack formation. The skin becomes vulnerable and susceptible to microorganisms in the environment. This is particularly dangerous among children and adolescents, as recent studies conducted in 14 countries have shown an increasing trend of AD among those aged 6–14 years [30]. These data are in accordance with those presented in the Global Report on Atopic Dermatitis, which reports that AD affects up to 20% of children, 10% of young adults (20–25 years old) and 1–3% of adults [31]. The situation becomes particularly dangerous when it is additionally associated with the hospital environment, which favors the spread of multi-drug resistant strains. Retrospective studies conducted by Grossi et al. in hospitals in six European countries provide direct evidence that acute bacterial skin and skin structure infections (ABSSSI), due to their high treatment costs, constitute a significant burden on healthcare [32]. Therefore, the prevention of skin infections, including AD, is crucial not only during exacerbation, but also primarily during remission. The introduction of preparations containing compounds of natural origin, especially camphor, would: (i) strengthen the skin barrier, and accelerate its reconstruction; and also (ii) replenish lipid deficiencies and make the skin more resistant to microbial attacks. In addition, camphor exhibits soothing properties for irritations and prevents inflammatory conditions. Studies by Kang et al. have given the green light to treating this condition using leaves from *Cinnamomum camphora*. These researchers showed that the leaves have a calming effect on the production of inflammatory chemokines in vitro, resulting in relief of symptoms of dermatitis in vivo [4]. Combining the positive effects of camphor's antimicrobial properties with its therapeutic properties would be key in improving the quality of life for patients suffering from AD while simultaneously preventing potential skin superinfections of bacterial and/or fungal etiology.

In our review, we have focused on the positive impact of camphor in preventing the formation of difficult-to-heal wounds infected with strains exhibiting high resistance to antibiotics. Addressing the issues of hospital-acquired infections, we primarily focused on strains that reside in the hospital environment and exhibit the ability to acquire resistance easily while also forming biofilms. These microorganisms pose a real threat in hospitals around the world.

2. Camphor's Chemical Properties and Methods of Production

Camphor is a white solid with a characteristic odor and pungent taste, which sublimates at room temperature. It does not dissolve in water, although it dissolves well in organic solvents such as diethyl ether, ethanol, and chloroform. Chemically, camphor (1,7,7-trimethylbicyclo[2.2.1]heptan-2-one) is a cyclic terpenoid ketone with the general formula $C_{10}H_{16}O$ that occurs as two isomers: R-(+)-camphor and S-(-)-camphor (Figure 1) [33,34].

1*R*-(+)-camphor　　1*S*-(-)-camphor

Figure 1. Structure of camphor isomers.

Camphor can be obtained by chemical synthesis both as a racemic mixture and as a pure S-(-) isomer. The most common substrate used during synthesis is α-pinene. This compound is isomerized to camphene through the Wagner–Meervein rearrangement, which is a nucleophilic rearrangement involving 1,2-migration of a ring carbon atom in a bicyclic molecule. In the next step, camphene is reacted with formic or acetic acid, resulting in an isobornyl ester. This ester undergoes hydrolysis to isoborneol, which upon oxidation is converted to (±)-camphor [35].

An alternative method is to use dihydrocarvone for synthesis. Dihydrocarvone is reacted with isopropenyl acetate in the presence of p-toluenesulfonic acid as a catalyst. The ester formed in this reaction closes to (±)-camphor when subjected to the action of boron trifluoride [36].

Obtaining S-(-)-camphor requires a combination of classical chemical synthesis methods and the use of enzymes. The α-pinene chemical was used as a substrate, from which an isobornyl ester was obtained. This ester was then subjected to kinetic separation using an esterase derived from *Burkholderia gladioli* to obtain pure (+)-isoborneol, from which, after oxidation, (-)-camphor was obtained [37].

Another method is to use Oxone, which is a mixture of the three salts $2KHSO_5$, $3KHSO_4$, and $3K_2SO_4$, in which the active agent is potassium peroxymonosulfate, $KHSO_5$, as the oxidizing agent. In this case, (1*S*)-borneol is used for the reaction, which, after oxidation with Oxone, is converted to (-)-camphor [38].

3. Camphor Occurrence

Naturally occurring camphor is extracted from the wood of the camphor laurel (*Cinnamomum camphora* L.), which is native to eastern and southern Asia and now grows worldwide [34]; from the camphor tree *Dryobalanops aromatica*, which grows in Sumatra [39]; as well as from the camphor tree found in Africa *Ocotea usambarensis* [40]. As noted previously, camphor is insoluble in water; in addition, it is characterized by a high boiling point of 204 °C. These properties are used in the isolation of this monoterpenoid, because it is obtained by steam distillation followed by sublimation.

The essential oil (EO) extracted from camphor tree leaves is a mixture of volatile compounds, mainly terpenes, and is widely used in pharmaceutical, industrial, and environmental applications. Camphor tree EO extraction methods mainly include (i) steam extraction, (ii) organic solvent extraction, (iii) ionic liquid combined with microwave-assisted extraction, (iv) microwave extraction without solvents, (v) cold-pressed extraction, (vi) subcritical CO_2 extraction, (vii) ultrasound-assisted extraction, and (viii) microwave-assisted extraction, as well as the (ix) supercritical fluid extraction method. The latter method is used to split camphor tree leaves into a soluble fraction SC-CO_2 [41,42].

It is important to note that the amount of camphor in plants varies depending on the species and part of the plant. Studies have shown that *C. camphora* leaf oil is composed mainly of camphor, which accounts for as much as 93.1%, whereas in wood oil camphor is found alongside 1,8-cineol (19.8%), α-terpineol (6.2%), and safrole (3.2%), and it accounts for only 53.2% of the wood oil content [43].

Also, depending on the particular chemotype, EO extracted from the same plant species, i.e., from *C. camphora*, can contain from as much as 74% camphor (camphor chemotype) [44] down to only 5% (linalool chemotype) [45]. On the other hand, the cineole chemotype does not contain this compound [33].

Table 1 shows the camphor contents of essential oils and extracts from various plants.

Table 1. Plant resources of camphor.

Plant Cultivar	Source of EO	Percentage [%]	References
Achillea grandifolia	Inflorescences Leaves	10.0–70.5 5.5–83.2	[46]
Achillea millefolium L.	Inflorescences	13.0	[47]
Artemisia annua	Leaves and stems	11.4	[48]
Artemisia haussknechtii	Aerial parts	11.8	[49]
Artemisia khorassanica	Aerial parts	74.2	[49]
Artemisia sieberi	Aerial parts	33.6	[50]
Artemisia spicigera	Whole plant	29.6	[51]
Chrysanthemum japonense	Flowers Leaves	47.6 39.1	[52]
Cinnamomum camphora	Leaves Branch Wood	93.1 53.6 53.2	[33]
Cinnamomum camphora	Barks Leaves Fruits	51.3 40.5 28.1	[53]
Lavandula angustifolia	Leaves and inflorescences	10.7–18.8	[54]
Lavandula latifolia	Whole plant	12.2	[55]
Ocimum basilicum L.	Aerial Parts	42.1	[56]
Ocimum kilimandscharicum Guerke	Leaves	45.9	[57]
Santolina chamaecyparissus L.	Aerial part	17.7	[58]
Salvia fruticosa	Aerial part	20.3	[59]
Salvia jordanii	Aerial part	33.4	[60]
Salvia officinalis L.	Whole plant	26.6 northern Albania 43.8 southern Albania	[61]
Salvia rosmarinus	Aerial part	3.3–42.2	[60]
Stachys germanica L.	Aerial parts	52.9	[62]
Tanacetum parthenium L.	Aerial parts Stems and leaves Inflorescence Unripe seeds Ripe seeds	53.4–52.9 47.9–49.6 11.6–11.5 12.3–12.4 12.3–10.3	[63]
Thymus algeriensis	Whole plant	6.8–19.9 (vegetative stage) 8.1–15.7 (flowering stage)	[64]

4. Camphor as an Additional Ingredient in Products

Camphor is used as an ingredient in various ointments used as a broad-spectrum remedies. As pure camphor can be dangerous in overdose, in order to take advantage of its health-promoting properties it can only be used as one of the ingredients of appropriate medications.

One such ointment is Tiger Balm®, which is used as a herbal analgesic for external application. Two variants of Tiger Balm® are known, namely Red TB® and White TB®. The Red variant is recommended for use for muscle pain, whereas the White variant is recommended for use for tension headaches. Both variants contain 11% camphor in their composition. In addition, the main ingredients in both formulations for Red TB® and White TB® are, respectively, menthol (10.0% and 8.0%), clove oil (5.0% and 1.5%) and cajuput oil (7.0% and 13.0%) [65]. Another painkilling ointment is Bengay, which contains camphor, methyl salicylate, and menthol [66]. In addition, the main active ingredients of Vicks VapoRub® ointment are camphor (5%), turpentine oil (5%), L-menthol (2.75%), and eucalyptus oil (1.5%), thymol and cedarwood oil.

This ointment is used as an adjunct in the treatment of colds and other upper respiratory tract diseases in the form of rubbing the chest and back [67]. The feeling of better breathing after using this ointment is mainly due to the action of camphor and menthol, which interact with the cold receptors in the nose, causing a feeling of cold by constricting the nasal mucosa, which in turn facilitates breathing. A small amount of Vicks VapoRub® can also be dissolved in hot water and used for inhalation [67]. In 2023, Stinson et al. conducted research using rhinovirus serotype-16 (RV16)-infected A549 airway epithelial cells, in which they showed that Vicks VapoRub® modulates specific TRP (transient receptor potential) receptors and reduces the ATP release induced by RV16 [67].

There are reports in the scientific literature indicating the possibility of using Vicks VapoRub® also in the treatment of nail fungus. During in vitro tests, the ingredients of the ointment showed a broad spectrum of activity and were active against, among other microbes, *Candida, Aspergillus,* and some dermatophytes species, which encouraged further research. However, there were some errors in a 48-week clinical trial conducted by the Family Medicine Group in 2011. Unlike the phase III clinical trials for toenail fungus, this study did not exclusively enroll patients with cultured dermatophytes such as *Trichophyton rubrum* or *Trichophyton mentagrophytes* and did not limit the percentage of affected toenails to 50 or 60% [68]. At baseline, 10 of the 18 patients had more than 60% nail involvement, and some had 89% or even 100% involvement [69]. In the case of completely dystrophic nails, a 48-week treatment period may not be sufficient. However, adding a method such as nail cleaning could demonstrate the synergistic effect of this procedure and the ointment used. Additionally, in this study some patients used the ointment daily, although others used it only three to five times a week. Therefore, it cannot be ruled out that the ointment caused the formation of a more moisturized nail unit, which gives the appearance of a healthier nail, instead of actually curing the fungus [68].

In 2016, a study was conducted on the effectiveness of Vicks VapoRub® ointment in the treatment of nail fungus in people infected with HIV. In the case of these patients, it is very difficult to select an effective treatment method due to possible interactions of the therapy used with antiretroviral drugs. Of the 20 study participants, 94% of patients reported satisfaction with their toenail health and their overall treatment results at the 24-week follow-up visit [70].

Camphor has also found use as an ingredient in various types of soaps. As early as the 19th century, the so-called "medicinal soap" was used, which included camphor, and was used for the therapy of frostbite [71]. Nowadays, many types of camphor soap are available on the market. An interesting preparation is a herbal aloe-camphor soap. Its composition includes, among other things, aloe vera gel, camphor, and honey. Such soap can be used for skin prone to irritation and itching, as camphor has antibacterial and antifungal properties [72].

In addition, the properties of this monoterpenoid have been utilized in the therapy of respiratory disorders. Indeed, it is a component of multicomponent preparations, i.e., nasal and inhalation drops (e.g., Makatussin, Optipect, Sedum Balsam, and Algorhin); inhalation liquids (e.g., Cetix and Cetix Plus); syrups (e.g., Optipect and Halin); capsules (e.g., Pinimenthol); lozenges (e.g., Neo-Angin); and lotions, gels and ointments (e.g., Dracodermalin, Herbolen, Mentoklar, Rhino-tussal, Rhino-tussal S, Transpulmin, and Pulmex) [73].

5. Camphor Metabolism

Camphor is a highly lipophilic cyclic terpenoid that undergoes rapid diffusion. It can be absorbed through (i) the gastrointestinal tract (within 5 to 90 min after ingestion), (ii) the skin, and (iii) mucous membranes [74,75]. In the body, camphor is metabolized in the liver through oxidation and glucuronidation processes. Subsequently, the inactive metabolites formed as a result are excreted by the kidneys. When applied to healthy skin, its absorption volume is relatively low compared to the rate of the process [34]. Research conducted by Martin et al. revealed that the 8-h application of two patches of Satogesic™ Medicated Adhesive patch from Sato Pharmaceutical Company that contained a 1% solution of camphor led to its release into the bloodstreams of study participants below the limit of detectability. However, administration of 4 or 8 patches, corresponding to 2% and 4% solutions of this monoterpene, respectively, contributed to its penetration through the skin at levels of 26.8 ± 7.2 ng/mL vs. 41.0 ± 5.8 ng/mL (4 patches vs. 8 patches), with a mean half-life of up to 5.6 ± 1.3 h, whereas the standard half-life (3 µg/mL anethole in ethanol) does not exceed 167 min [76]. Therefore, the use of camphor on the skin should be subject to strict regulations. Poisoning from this monoterpene due to contact with the skin is commonly observed in children, especially in Asia, where there are no strict regulations regarding its use [75].

In the case of oral administration of camphor, high concentrations have been detected in the fetal brain, liver, kidneys, and blood, as well as in the amniotic fluid. Symptoms of camphor poisoning include blurred vision, nausea, vomiting, colitis, dizziness, delirium, cardiac muscle spasms, difficulty breathing, seizures, and even death [11]. The lethal dose of camphor in adults ranges from 50 to 500 mg/kg. In contrast, for children, it is 0.5–1 g, and for infants, it is 70 mg/kg [74].

Although the first studies on camphor metabolism in humans were conducted in the 1960s, it has not been fully elucidated to date [77]. Valuable insights in this field are provided by research conducted by Park et al., which indicated that camphor specifically inhibits nicotinic acetylcholine receptors (nAChR), thereby preventing the secretion of catecholamines. This action may be one of the causes of neurotoxicity, as nAChR are known to play a key role in neuromuscular junctions [78]. Moreover, camphor may modulate the activity of hepatic enzymes involved in drug metabolism. Indeed, it has been demonstrated that a drug containing this compound, when applied to the skin for cold relief, caused a transient elevation in serum liver enzymes in a 2-month-old infant [79,80]. Additionally, in the case of Swiss Albino mice treated with camphor at a dose of 300 mg/kg, an increase in hepatic enzyme activity, including CYP (cytochrome P450), cytochrome b5, aryl hydrocarbon hydroxylase, and glutathione S-transferase, was observed, leading to a significant elevation in reduced glutathione levels [34].

Identification of camphor biotransformation products in humans is only possible in cases of acute poisoning. In the urine of patients admitted to the hospital due to intoxication after ingesting 6–10 g of camphor, the main metabolites identified included camphor hydroxylated at positions 3, 5, 8, and 9, as well as further oxidation products such as 5-ketocamphor and carboxylic acids resulting from the oxidation of 8- or 9-hydroxycamphor. Interestingly, the presence of isoborneol in urine was the result of the microbiological reduction of camphor [81]. Within in vitro studies, (-)-camphor was incubated with human liver microsomes in the presence of an NADPH-generating system. Hydroxylation of this compound to 5-*exo*-hydroxycamphor was observed, which is also the main biotransformation product of camphor in dogs, rabbits, and rats [82].

Numerous studies, extending back more than 150 years, have provided valuable information regarding the transforming ability of camphor in the animal body. Indeed, the presence of the glucuronide derivative of hydroxycamphor in the urine of dogs was demonstrated, as well as 3-hydroxycamphor, 5-hydroxycamphor, and *cis* and *trans*-π-hydroxycamphor, after the administration of (+)-camphor with food [83]. On the other hand, in the case of rabbits, there was additionally a stereospecific *endo*-reduction of camphor to borneol, and a small amount of isoborneol in the liver cytosol [84,85]. The biotransformation abilities that camphor represents in the human and animal organisms are shown in Figure 2.

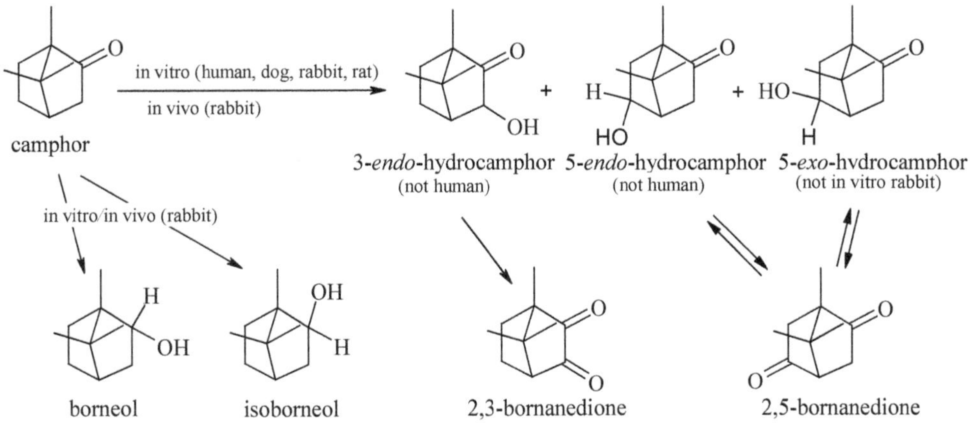

Figure 2. Camphor's biotransformation pathways in humans and animals.

In addition, in vitro studies showed that insect cells are capable of oxidizing (-)-camphor. The experiment was conducted in a human liver microsome system—an NADPH-producing system—with human recombinant enzymes (CYP1A1, CYP1A2, CYP1B1, CYP2A6, CYP2B6, CYP2C8, CYP2C9, CYP2C19, CYP2D6, CYP2E1, and CYP3A4). It was proven that only CYP2A6 was capable of catalyzing the hydroxylation of camphor [82,86].

Another significant step in camphor metabolism is the conjugation of its oxidation products with glucuronic acid in the liver, followed by excretion through the kidneys. The transferase responsible for conjugating hydroxylated derivatives of camphor is not known. However, it is understood that both borneol and isoborneol undergo extensive glucuronidation via uridine 5′-diphosphoglucuronosyltransferase UGT2B7 to form borneol-2-*O*-glucuronide and isoborneol-2-*O*-glucuronide, respectively. Subsequently, multi-drug resistance-associated proteins MRP3 and MRP4 facilitate the efflux of glucuronides into the bloodstream. They are then primarily eliminated by the kidneys, through both glomerular filtration and tubular secretion via organic anion transporters OAT3 and OAT4 [87].

It is worth noting that camphor can significantly affect the permeation of other drugs through the skin. It has been shown that this terpenoid facilitates the penetration of lipophilic drugs through the stratum corneum of the epidermis, including indomethacin, lidocaine, aspirin, antipyrine, tegafur, and 5-fluorouracil [88,89]. The mechanism of action was elucidated by studies conducted by Cui et al., which demonstrated that (+)-camphor is capable of disrupting the lipid bilayer of the rat skin, thereby increasing the partition coefficient of propranolol (PHCl) into the stratum corneum of the epidermis [90]. This ability of camphor has significant clinical implications, as propranolol, a non-selective β_1- and β_2-adrenergic receptor antagonist, is used in the treatment of hypertension, coronary artery disease, and tachyarrhythmias [91].

6. Molecular Activity of Camphor

Camphor is known as a natural bioactive compound with wide spectrum of biological activities. Those most frequently described are antibacterial, antifungal, antioxidant, anti-cancer, analgesic, and anti-inflammatory properties. The activities are usually described for EO in which camphor is a major/dominant compound. Due to its toxicity at higher concentrations, there are rarely reports on the biological activity of pure camphor.

It has been shown that the EO obtained from *Commiphora ornifolia* (Balf. fil.) Gillett was characterized by a high content of oxygenated monoterpenes (56.3%), of which camphor constituted 27.3%. It has shown significant influences on antimicrobial activity against both Gram-positive and Gram-negative bacteria. Unfortunately, investigated EOs demonstrated weak antioxidant abilities, which were calculated based on their capability to reduce 2,2-diphenyl-1-picrylhydrazyl (DPPH) [92]. Yuceturk and co-workers observed an increase in the ability to reduce the DPPH radical with a higher concentration of EO of *Thymus convolutus* Klokov. The EO consisted of 66 compounds, in which camphor was the main component (16.6%, GC/MS analysis). Authors calculated that 33.39 ± 0.25% DPPH was scavenging at a concentration of 1 mg/mL of EO. Furthermore, antiproliferative activity of EO of *T. convolutus* on human liver adenocarcinoma Hep3B cells was observed at concentrations of 250 and 125 μg/mL, although camphor was cytotoxic in high concentrations (1 mg/mL, 500, 250 and 125 μg/mL). The inhibitory effect of EO on the human colorectal adenocarcinoma HT-29 cell line at concentration of 500 μg/mL was determined. Moreover, neither EO nor camphor exhibited a significant effect on the proliferation of human umbilical vein endothelial cells (HUVEC) [93]. The antitumor activity of novel camphor-based pyrimidine derivatives was evaluated in the Zhang et al. study. It has been proven that one of the tested derivatives showed similar activity to etoposide in the inhibition of growth of the following cell lines: MDA-MB-231 (breast cancer), RPMI-8226 (multiple myeloma), and A549 (non-small cell lung cancer NSCLC). At the same time, the compounds showed lower cytotoxicity than the comparator in relation to the tested line of normal human cells (GES-1). Moreover, at the molecular level, an increase in the formation of apoptotic proteins Bax, cytochrome C, and caspase 3 was observed, although the formation of the anti-apoptotic protein Bcl-2 was significantly decreased. The proper anti-oncogenic effect was present in ROS accumulation in the cell and toxicity to mitochondria, which in turn induced the apoptosis pathway [94].

Research performed by Rawat et al. consisted of obtaining EO of *Hedychium spicatum* Sm. from Himachal Pradesh of India, in which the content of camphor was 35.6%. Studies have shown that the EO suppressed 33.57% of inflammation at 100 mg/kg b.wt. dose level, which is comparable to the standard drug ibuprofen (40.06%) [95]. Scientists from Iran tested the analgesic activity of the EO from *Artemisia sieberi* Besser, which possess 31.2% of camphor. In studies, 1 mg/kg dose of the EO significantly reduced carrageenan-induced paw edema in rats by 74.3%, which is very close to the results for the standard drug diclofenac sodium (50 mg/kg) [96]. Li and co-workers also studied the analgesic effect of camphor. Based on neuropathic pain models in mice, the scientists concluded that camphor can alleviate symptoms of hyperalgesia [6]. The molecular anti-inflammatory mechanism of EO from *Blumea balsamifera* (camphor ~9%) was also evaluated. The EO was used as a suppressor in an in vitro model of LPS (lipopolysaccharide)-related activation of macrophages of the RAW 264.7 line. The decrease in the synthesis of proinflammatory cytokines (TNF-α, IL-1β, and IL-6) and the weakening of the medio-signaling pathway mediated by NF-κB (nuclear factor kappa B) and TLR-4 (Toll-like receptor 4) were revealed. Attenuation of signaling pathways led to, among other effects, inhibition of the NLRP3 inflammasome. [97].

Due to the ability of camphor to induce the proliferation of human primary dermal fibroblasts, which are responsible for the expression of collagen IA, collagen IIIA, collagen IVA, and elastin, preparations containing camphor can be used in cosmetology as anti-wrinkle agents [98].

Molecular Effects of Camphor-Containing Essential Oils on Pathogen Cells

The Pejčić et al. study evaluated the effects of *S. officinalis* (16.6% camphor) and *Ocimum basilicum* EOs on *P. aeruginosa* biofilm-forming capacity, motility, and pyrocyanin production. MIC values of camphor-containing oil oscillated at 5–20 mg/mL against all tested isolates (including skin-wound-infection isolates). The ability of the EOs to inhibit biofilm formation was determined to be 84.1–99.6% in the concentration range of 5, 10, and 20 mg/mL. The ability to inhibit the growth of previously formed biofilms was also assessed as follows: 20 mg/mL (12.4–95.7% inhibition), 10 mg/mL (0.4–94.5% inhibition), and 5 mg/mL (11.3–94.2% inhibition). A decrease in flagellum-dependent forms of movement (swimming) of bacteria was also observed by 97% (MIC) and 81% (1/2 MIC), respectively. Similar results were observed for other forms of movement (twitching and swarming). Sage oil inhibited the production of pyrocyanin by more than 58.8% [99]. Bajalan et al. evaluated the antibacterial activity of EOs obtained from *Rosmarinus officinalis*. At the molecular level, an increase in the permeability of cell membranes of pathogens and a loss of metabolically important ions was observed [100]. In the phototoxicity test of EOs, including *Lavandula stoechas* (36.69% of camphor; white light 470, Lumen/40 watt), the ZOI increased in the case of *K. pneumoniae* (ZOI in the dark = 2.2 mm, ZOI after irradiation = 4.07 mm) [101].

Due to numerous reports on the antibacterial properties of camphor-rich essential oils against gram-negative bacteria, we have presented a summary (assessed by microdilution method (MIC) and Kirby-Bauer method) in Tables 2 and 3.

Table 2. Antibacterial activities of camphor-containing essential oils against Gram-negative bacteria (minimal dilution assay).

Bacteria	Plant Cultivar	Camphor Concentration [%]	MIC Value	Ref.
P. aeruginosa	*Salvia officinalis*	16.4%	0.125 mg/mL	[102]
	Salvia officinalis	16.6%	5 mg/mL	[99]
	Curcuma aeruginosa	29.39%	0.125 mg/mL 1 mg/mL	[103]
	Thymus hirtus ssp. *algeriensis*	19.2%	0.022 mg/mL	[104]
	Salvia pachystachys	31.0%	5 mg/mL	[105]
	Ferula communis	18.3%	0.156 mg/mL	[106]
	Rosmarinus officinalis	18.74%	2 mg/mL	[107]
	Pulicaria undulata	44.48%	6.25 mg/mL	[108]
	Rosmarinus officinalis	26.5%	2.56 mg/mL	[109]
	Oncosiphon suffruticosum	31%	6.4 mg/mL	[110]
A. baumannii	*Artemisia herba-alba* Asso	50.7%	10 mg/mL 20 mg/mL	[111]
	Rosmarinus officinalis	23.04%	12.5 mg/mL	[112]
K. pneumoniae	*Lavandula stoechas* 'avonview'	35.30%	0.39 mg/mL	[113]
	Lavandula stoechas	36.69%	0.5 mg/mL	[101]
	Withania frutescens	~24–25%	0.006125 mg/mL	[114]
E. coli	*Rosmarinus officinalis*	18.743%	1 mg/mL	[107]
	Thymus hirtus ssp. *algeriensis*	19.2%	1.8 mg/mL	[104]
	Rosmarinus officinalis	26.5%	1.28 mg/mL	[109]
	Artemisia annua	~30%	2.5 mg/mL	[115]
	Croton tetradenius	~14%	5.6 mg/mL	[116]
	Withania frutescens	~24–25%	0.006125 mg/mL	[114]
	Lavandula stoechas	36.69%	1 mg/mL	[101]
	-	pure camphor	2.75 mg/mL	[117]

Table 3. Antibacterial activities of camphor-containing essential oils against Gram-negative bacteria (Kirby-Bauer assay).

Bacteria	Plant Cultivar	Camphor Conc. [%]	ZOI Value for EO [mm]	EO Content per Disc	ZOI Value for Positive Control	Positive Control Content per Disc	Ref.
P. aeruginosa	*Curcuma aeruginosa*	29.39%	5.7	10 µL	7.6	10 µg GM	[103]
	Withania frutescens	~24–25%	16.11	10 µL	-	20 µg STR, 1.67 mg AMP	[114]
	Rosmarinus officinalis *Artemisia absinthium*	19.75% 39.1%	7.0 12.0	50 µL	ND	10 µg PCN	[118]
	Tetraclinis articulata	20.1%	20.0	6 µL	20.0 15.0	10 µg CPL 30 µg CHL	[119]
					32.0 -	30 µg GM 20/10 µg AMC	
	Pulicaria undulata	44.48%	24.0	20 µL	17.0	ND GM	[108]
					16.0	ND TET	
	Artemisia sieberi Besser	42.9% 41.6% 37.1%	10.3 8.6 10.3	5 µL	ND	ND	[120]
	-	pure camphor	10.4	ND	ND	ND	
A. baumannii	*Artemisia herba-alba* Asso	50.47%	30.6 27.3	6 µL	13.6 10.0	10 µg STR	[111]
	Rosmarinus officinalis	23.04%	34.0	ND	-	-	[112]
	Artemisia herba-alba	32.0%	15.3	10 µL	14.0 12.0	ND CIP ND AKN	[24]
	Salvia officinalis	17.1%	13.67	10 µL	ND	20 µg GM	[121]
K. pneumoniae	*Tetraclinis articulata*	20.1%	29.0	6 µL	22.0 30.0 39.0 30.0	10 µg CPL 30 µg CHL 30 µg GM 20/10 µg AMC	[119]
	Rosmarinus officinalis	24.82% 21.41%	13.12 9.06	20 µL	6.0	ND OTC	[100]
	Rosmarinus officinalis	16.99% 20.4%	8.67 9.0	5 mg	28.0	5 mg NAL	[122]
	Lavandula stoechas 'avonview'	42.47% 35.30%	10.0 8.03	30 µL	9.30	ND CHL	[123]
	Combretum hereroense	ND	18.2	10 µL	18.8	30 µg CFX	[124]
E. coli	*Rosmarinus officinalis*	16.99% 20.4%	12.67 13.67	5 mg	30.0	5 mg NAL	[122]
	Thymus hirtus ssp. *algeriensis*	19.2%	30.0	10 µL	15.0 27.0	ND STR ND CHL	[104]
	Salvia officinalis	17.1%	16.67	10 µL	ND	20 µg GM	[121]
	Pulicaria undulata	44.48%	17.0	20 µL	22.0 16.0	ND GM ND TET	[108]
	Artemisia sieberi Besser	42.9% 41.6% 37.1%	12.8 12.4 12.3	5 µL	ND	ND	[120]
	-	pure camphor	12.91	ND	ND	ND	
	Thymus algeriensis	17.45–32.56%	13.0	40 µL	27.0	25 µg AMX	[125]
	Rosmarinus officinalis	26.5%	14.2	ND	21.5	ND CIP	[109]
	Combretum hereroense	ND	15.8	10 µL	23.2	30 µg CFX	[124]

AKN—amikacin; AMC—amoxicillin/clavulanate; AMP—ampicillin; AMX—amoxicillin; CFX—cefoxitin; CHL—chloramphenicol; CIP—cyprofloxacine; CPL—colistin; GM—gentamycin; NAL—nalidixic acid; OTC—oxytetracycline; PCN—penicillin; STR—streptomycin; TET—tetracycline; ND—not defined.

The activity of the EO from *Artemisia judaica* (16.1% camphor) against pathogenic fungi was assessed in addition to its activities against *Candida albicans* ATCC 10231, *C. parapsilosis* ATCC 90018, and *C. tropicalis* ATCC 13803. The oil showed a significant inhibitory effect on germ tube formation in *C. albicans* with 80% filamentation inhibition at 0.16 μL/mL concentration. In similar tests, *C. albicans*, *C. tropicalis*, and *C. krusei* obtained MIC and MFC values that were both at the level of 1.25 μL/mL, whereas *C. parapsilosis* obtained MIC = 1.25 μL/mL and MFC = 2.5 μL/mL. At a concentration of 1/8 MIC (0.16 μL/mL), there was a decrease in filamentation of about 80%. Similarly, a significant decrease in germ tube formation was observed at the already mentioned concentration (0.16 μL/mL). A decrease in biofilm-biomass formation by more than 50% was also observed at an oil concentration of 2.5 μL/mL [126]. Cedar leaf-derived EO, as well as camphor, which is its main component, significantly inhibited the formation of *C. albicans* DAY185 *hyphae*, thus reducing the formation of biofilm. Transcriptomic analyses showed that camphor and fenchyl alcohol reduced expression levels of *ECE1*, *ECE2*, *RBT1*, and *EED1* genes specific for *hyphae* and biofilm-associated functions. In addition, camphor and fenchyl alcohol reduced the virulence of *C. albicans* in the *Caenorhabditis elegans* nematode-infection model [127]. The results of Ivanov et al.'s study showed the potential of camphor to reduce the virulence of *C. albicans*, i.e., biofilm formation and *hyphae* formation. Camphor additionally regulated the level of Cdr1- and Cdr2-efflux pumps, which belong to ATP-binding cassette transporters and play roles in the development of resistance to azole drugs. It did not affect the expression level of the *ERG1* gene, which is involved in the biosynthesis of ergosterol. The beneficial antifungal activity of camphor was achieved at an amount that was non-toxic to porcine liver cells, making it a promising antifungal compound for future studies [128].

The antifungal activity of camphor-containing oils has also been well documented. A summary of the activities of oils against *C. albicans* is presented in the form of Tables 4 and 5.

Table 4. Antifungal activities of camphor-containing essential oils against *Candida albicans* (minimal dilution assay).

Plant Cultivar	Camphor Concentration [%]	MIC Value	Ref.
Salvia lavandulifolia	29.1%	0.156 mg/mL 0.312 mg/mL	[129]
Curcuma aeruginosa	29.39%	0.25 mg/mL	[103]
-	pure camphor	0.125 mg/mL 0.35 mg/mL	[128]
Withania frutescens	24.26%	0.0004 mg/mL	[114]
Rosmarinus officinalis	26.5%	0.16 mg/mL	[109]
Cassia fistula -	~14% pure camphor	0.313 mg/mL 0.156 mg/mL	[130]
Tetraclinis articulata	20.1%	0.268 mg/mL	[119]
Brocchia cinerea	~14%	0.0168 mg/mL	[131]
Plectranthus cylindraceus Hochst. et Benth	40.93%	0.4 mg/mL	[132]
Rosmarinus officinalis	24.3% 15.52% 18.47%	0.025 mg/mL 0.00156 mg/mL 0.00078 mg/mL	[133]
Anvillea radiata	21.41%	0.01031 mg/mL 0.02275 mg/mL	[134]
Artemisia aucheri	18%	0.4 mg/mL	[135]
Salvia fruticosa	21.32%	0.079 mg/mL	[136]
Achillea grandifolia	23.4%	0.16042 mg/mL 0.525 mg/mL	[137]
Tetraclinis articulata	15.97%	0.125 mg/mL	[138]
Artemisia herba-alba var. *huguetii*	18.38%	0.00183 mg/mL	[139]

Table 5. Antifungal activities of camphor-containing essential oils against *Candida albicans* (Kirby-Bauer assay).

Plant Cultivar	Camphor Conc. [%]	ZOI Value for EO [mm]	EO Content per Disc	ZOI Value for Positive Control	Positive Control Content per Disc	Ref.
Curcuma aeruginosa	29.39%	11.6	10 μL	10.54	10 μg COM	[103]
Ocimum kilimandscharicum Guerke	52.0–57.2%	4.33–5.33 4.66–6.33	8 μL	24.33	ND KTC	[140]
Achillea odorata subsp. *pectinata*	45.01	25.33	12.5 μL	18.66	10 μg AMB	[141]
Pulicaria undulata	44.48%	23.0	20 μL	14.0	ND NYT	[108]
Withania frutescens	24.26%	47.0	10 μL	21.2	ND FLC	[114]
Suaeda vermiculata Forssk	28.74%	19.0	50 μL	16.0	10 μg CLT	[108]
Rosmarinus officinalis	33.9–41.2%	11.6–14.6	10 μL	28.0 18.0	10 μg MIC 20 μg AMB	[142]
Artemisia annua	17.0%	8.5	15–30 μL	ND	ND	[143]
Artemisia siebieri Besser	42.9% 41.6% 37.1%	16.2 14.2 16.0	5 μL	-	-	[120]
-	pure camphor	11.4	ND	-	-	
Thymus algeriensis	17.45–32.56%	13.0	80 μL	24.0	25 μg ITC	[125]
Rosmarinus officinalis	26.5%	18.2 18.6	ND	21.0 16.0	ND FLC	[109]
Tetraclinis articulata	20.1%	22.0	6 μL	10.0 18.0 19.0 10.0 0.0	100 μg AMB 50 μg ECC 50 μg MIC 50 μg CLT 1 μg 5FC	[125]
Brocchia cinerea	~14%	42.33	20 μL	21.0	ND FLC	[131]
Matricaria chamomilla	16.42%	21.07	10 μL	28.6	100 I.U. NYT	[144]
Tetraclinis articulata	15.97%	15.6	10 μL	~10 ~20	20 μg FLC 20 μg CLT	[138]
Artemisia herba-alba var. *huguetii*	18.38%	39.0	4.7 μg	24.7	ND FLC	[139]

AMB—amphotericin B; CLT—clotrimazole; COM—ciclopirox olamine; ECC—econazole; FLC—fluconazole; ITC—itraconazole; KTC—ketoconazole; MIC—miconazole; NYT—nystatin; 5FC—flucytosine; ND—not defined.

7. Mechanisms of Camphor Action on the Skin

Scientists are looking for the therapeutic effect of camphor on human skin. It is used, among others, in sunscreen creams as 4-methylbenzylidene camphor [145].

Camphor affects fibroblast proliferation by inducing phosphorylation of the PI3K/AKT and ER pathways. It prolongs the lifespan of fibroblasts in a dose-dependent manner at concentrations of 32.5, 65, 130, and 260 μM, which is responsible for the production of free radicals. The activity of elastase decreases and, consequently, the amount of elastin increases, also in a dose- and time-dependent manner. Its action inhibits skin aging by acting on beta-galactosidase, which is a marker of this process because it accumulates in the lysosomes of aging cells. The cleavage of X-Gal into blue dye was investigated with 600 and 800 μM H_2O_2, which led to an increase in the number of SA-β-gal-positive cells. At the same time, 600 and 800 μM H_2O_2 together with camphor were used in the same trial, which led to a reduction in the number of SA-β-gal-positive cells by 65% and 50%.

This indicates protection of skin fibroblasts against aging [98]. Camphor also prevents the thickening of the epidermis and subcutaneous fat tissue [146].

Camphor affects several types of receptors: heat-sensitive TRPV1, cold-sensitive TRPM8, and heat-sensitive TRPV3, and it inhibits TRPA1. TRP ion channels contain segments that are thermosensitive, called thermoTRP. Its impact on TRPV1 is linked to a desensitizing effect, resulting in analgesia. Activation of TRPV3 occurs at a temperature of 39 °C, and these receptors are found in keratinocytes, the brain, and the spinal cord [147,148].

The impact of this compound on blood circulation and temperature perception, including heat and cold, has also been investigated. Camphor increases the sensory experience when the skin temperature is between 33 to 43 °C or 33 to 18 °C. The feeling of heat or cold is perceived more strongly by people after using this compound [149]. An experiment was used in which vaseline containing 5%, 10%, and 20% camphor was placed on the skin of the subjects' forearms. It was shown that 5% camphor (with vaseline) caused a feeling of cold in the subjects with a delay of about 2 min and that lasted about 5 min, unlike vaseline itself (camphor 0%), which did not cause a feeling of cold. Higher concentrations (10% and 20%) also elicited a cold sensation lasting 9 and 7 min, respectively. Subsequently, subjects reported a sensation of warmth with delays of 3, 7, and 13 min for 5%, 10% and 20% concentrations, respectively, after the cessation of the cold sensation. Blood flow in the skin and muscles also increased with a time delay [150]. It also caused a burning sensation [151]. Camphor is a TRPV3 activator and it has been tested in the epidermal tape peel test. At temperatures of 34 and 42 °C, it did not show faster regeneration of the damaged layer. The temperature range from 36–40 °C showed accelerated regeneration in each case [152]. Applying camphor to the skin is associated with its excretion in urine [153]. Table 6 shows the molecular actions of camphor on the skin and their effects. Furthermore, Figure 3 shows a schematic mechanism of action of this compound specifically in the context of the skin.

Table 6. Molecular effects of camphor on the skin.

Molecular Actions of Camphor	Effect	Ref.
Decrease in elastase activity	Increase in the amount of elastin	[98]
Induction of phosphorylation of PI3K/AKT and ER pathways	Inhibition of fibroblast apoptosis	
Action on β-galactosidase	Inhibition of skin aging	
Activation of TRPV1	Desensitizing and analgesic effect	[147]
Activation of TRPM8	Activation of the channel, enhancement of cold sensitivity, inhibition of the response to menthol	[154]
Activation of TRPV3	Heat activation, suggestive sensitizing role	[148]
Activation and inhibition of TRPA1	Agonist–antagonist action, probable role as a cold sensor in nociceptive neurons	[151]

Methods of Treating Skin Diseases

EO containing *Cinnamomum camphora* are used as a natural remedy for soothing skin inflammation [41].

The effect of camphor on penetration into the epidermis was examined. This is important considering the possibility of better absorption of drugs when applied to the skin at the same time. It has been proven to have a weak effect on transepidermal water loss, which is a positive phenomenon. Camphor increases penetration through the skin layers [74,89]. For example, 5% camphor has been shown to improve the transdermal penetration of carvedilol in studies performed on pig skin [155]. Studies were also carried out on rats, which proved better absorption of propanolol hydrochloride when using camphor [90]. In vitro and in vivo studies (on rabbit skin) showed increased absorption of ondansetron when administered with camphor in the form of a gel. It is an antiemetic drug used, among other uses, in chemotherapy [156].

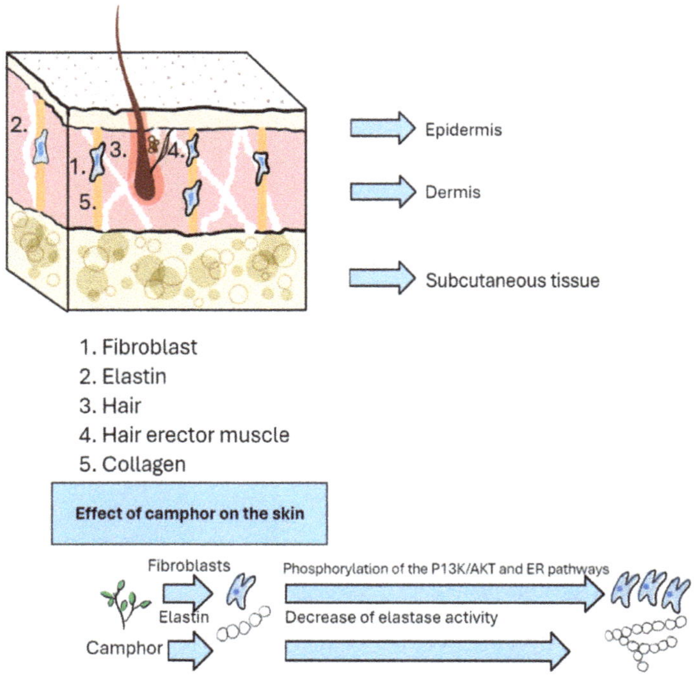

Figure 3. Simplified skin model and camphor effect.

Positive uses of camphor on the skin have an impact on the treatment of atopic dermatitis (AD). The anti-inflammatory effect of this compound has been demonstrated through the phosphorylation of transcription activator 1, Janus kinase signal transducer, and extracellular signal-regulated kinase 1/2. The synthesis of chemokines, which play a significant role in the pathogenesis of AD, was reduced [4].

Combinations of camphor and other natural compounds are also used to treat skin diseases. The use of sesame oil and honey in the treatment of second-degree burn wounds in rats is interesting. The described combination accelerated the healing process [157]. The use of the synergism of camphor with *Lavandula latifolia* was used in a checkerboard study against *S. aureus* and *L. monocytogenes*, showing better inhibitory effects against these microorganisms [55].

The combination of camphor and menthol has been used with positive effect in the treatment of itching, taking advantage of the ability of camphor to stimulate the TRPV3 receptor [158]. Camphor oil with or without glycerol dilution worked very well on facial demodeciodosis and scabies, giving complete cures in concentrations of 100%, 75% and 50% [159].

The effect of phenocamphor on mycosis of the feet, legs, and armpits caused by dermatophytes was also examined. A satisfactory effect was achieved, with a low recurrence rate [160].

Camphor, being a component of UV filters, contributes to protection against harmful radiation. To prevent the degradation of this compound (4-MBC) after dermal administration, this compound was complexed with methyl-β-cyclodextrin (RM-β-CD), which improved its effectiveness [161]. However, a case was described of a 71-year-old man who used cosmetics with a UV filter and was diagnosed with photocontact allergy to 4-methylbenzylidene camphor. The patient had been using these agents for several years [162].

An interesting combination finding is that a cream containing camphor, chondroitin sulfate, and glucosamine sulfate was used for knee osteoarthritis with better results than the placebo group. Improvement was observed after treatment with the preparation after just 4 weeks [163].

To sum up, camphor has numerous applications related to healing effects on skin diseases, and it improves the penetration of drugs into the epidermis.

However, there are reports of a negative impact on the endocrine system, as well as on the kidneys, lungs, testicles, and liver, so new solutions are being sought that will limit the penetration of the compound itself into the body. The doses used in sunscreens do not cause significant hormonal changes. Interestingly, one of the solutions being investigated is enclosing 4-MBC in microspheres [153,164,165]. The lethal dose for camphor is about 3.5 g, although the toxic dose is about 2 g [166]. However, even large amounts applied to the skin are usually not high enough to cause poisoning. One case of chronic cutaneous administration of camphor was observed, resulting in granulomatous hepatitis [10]. There are also two cases described in a hospital in the Bronx, New York, of the administration of large doses of this compound orally and one of administration to the skin, which caused epileptic seizures in children [167]. Camphor may cause dermatological side effects when applied to the skin. These include pruriginous eruptions, erythematous, and papulous oedematous [168].

8. Antimicrobial Activity of Camphor

In an era of increasing resistance of microorganisms to the antibiotics used in therapy, an important feature of the natural compounds supporting treatment is their antimicrobial activity. These properties of camphor have been confirmed against both aerobic and anaerobic bacteria, as well as against fungi. In this review, we collected information on microorganisms (bacteria and fungi) that are potential etiological agents of skin infection. We mainly selected those that are relatively easy to transmit in either the outdoor or hospital environment.

8.1. Interactions of Camphor-Containing Essential Oils with Antimicrobial Drugs

Potential pharmacological interactions between camphor and *Lavandula latifolia* EO were evaluated against *S. aureus* ATCC 25923. Based on the microdilution method, the MIC of the combination was determined at 0.16–20.0 mg/mL. The high activity of the combination of EOs and (+)-camphor (concentrations 0.31 + 1.25 mg/mL, respectively) was determined to be synergistic [55]. The EO of *Artemisia herba-alba* (32% camphor) was highly active against the MRSA S19 strain, obtaining a MIC value of 1.2 μL/mL. Moreover, synergistic properties of the combination of EOs with cefoxitin against staph were indicated [24]. The synergistic interaction was also detected in the case of *Croton tetradenius* EO with meropenem and ciprofloxacin against *S. aureus* [116]. Grimsey et al. examined the antibacterial activity of *Combretum* spp. leaf extracts (using the Kirby-Bauer method and microdilutions) against among other MRSAs. The isolate was non-susceptible to all tested β-lactams and was also characterized by a high level of resistance to GEN. It also showed only intermediate susceptibility to ciprofloxacin and chloramphenicol. *C. hereroense* extract showed, in turn, excellent activity against *S. aureus* [124]. The Cutillas et al. study evaluated the antibacterial activity of several *Salvia officinalis* EOs (camphor content in the range 10.7–19.8%) against Gram-positive bacteria. *S. aureus* was found to be susceptible to all tested oils (MIC and MBC—minimal bactericidal concentration—were in the range of 0.6–1.3 μL/mL for oils and >15 mM for camphor alone) [169]. Antibacterial and antibiofilm activities of *Salvia officinalis* and *Origanum vulgare* EOs against *S. pyogenes* ATCC 19615 and 49399 was also evaluated. Sage EO contained camphor at concentration of 16.6%. Promising results were obtained, and the MIC of the EOs was 0.5 mg/mL and was identical to the value of MBC against planktonic forms of bacteria. In addition, the oil showed at the same concentration-dependent inhibition seen for the formation of *S. pyogenes* biofilm for both strains (0.25 mg/mL) as well as leading to the eradication of an already produced pathogen biofilm (MBIC [minimum-biofilm inhibitory concentration] was established at 0.5 mg/mL) [170]. The beneficial interaction profile of essential oils rich in camphor is associated with their antibacterial properties against Gram-positive bacteria. The activity of the described substances (microdilution method and Kirby-Bauer assay) is summarized in the form of tables (Tables 7 and 8).

Table 7. Antibacterial activities of camphor-containing essential oils against Gram-positive bacteria (minimal dilution assay).

Bacteria	Plant Cultivar	Camphor Concentration [%]	MIC Value	Ref.
S. aureus	*Lavandula stoechas*	8.64%	0.01795 mg/mL	[171]
	Salvia officinalis	16.4%	0.125 mg/mL	[102]
	Ocimum tenuiflorum	31.52%	0.00225 mg/mL	[103]
	Lavandula stoechas	36.69%	0.5 mg/mL	[101]
	Rosmarinus officinalis	26.5%	0.32 mg/mL	[109]
S. pyogenes	*Satureja montana*	29.1%	0.03 mg/mL 0.63 mg/mL	[129]
	Makhlaseh	49.0–56.9%	8 mg/mL 4 mg/mL	[172]
	Salvia officinalis	16.6%	0.5 mg/mL	[170]
	Perovskia abrotanoides	21.68%	2.0 mg/mL	[173]
	Lavandula stoechas × *viridis* 'St. Brelade's'	7.13%	6.25 mg/mL	[113]
***Clostridium* spp.**	*Artemisia annua*	>60%	~1.6 mg/mL	[174]

Table 8. Antimicrobial activities of camphor-containing essential oils against *S. aureus* (Kirby-Bauer assay).

Plant Cultivar	Camphor Conc. [%]	ZOI Value for EO [mm]	EO Content per Disc	ZOI Value for Positive Control [mm]	Positive Control Content per Disc	Ref.
Ocimum kilimanscharicum Guerke	54.6% 52.0% 57.2%	7.66 6.66 5.0	8 µL/disc	18.0	ND, TET	[140]
Lavandula stoechas	8.64%	12.0 13.0 18.0	5.83 mg/disc 23.4 mg/disc 35.1 mg/disc	22.0 24.0	ND, CIP, GM	[171]
Salvia officinalis	36.92%	8.0–13.0	20 µL/disc	ND	ND	[172]
Curcuma aeruginosa	29.39%	22.0	10 µL/disc	7.28	10 µg GM	[103]
Artemisia sieberi Besser	2.8–42.9%	12.3–20.6	5 µL/disc	ND	ND	[120]
-	pure camphor	12.0	ND	ND	ND	
Thymus algeriensis	17.45–32.56%	18.0	40 µL/disc	10.0	25 µg AMX	[125]
Rosmarinus officinalis	26.5%	25.2	ND	30.0	5 µg CIP	[109]
Cinnamomum camphora	3% 6% 9%	7.0 11.0 17.0	ND	15.0	10 µg STR	[175]
Combretum hereroense	ND	21.4	10 µL/disc	7.2	5 µg/MET	[124]
				>15.0	10 µg CHL, GM 5 µg CIP	

AMX—amoxicillin; CHL—chloramphenicol; CIP—ciprofloxacine; GM—gentamycin; MET—methicillin; STR—streptomycin; TET—tetracycline; ND—not defined.

Interesting reports on the activity of the *Artemisia herba-alba* EO (32% camphor) in relation to imipenem-resistant *A. baumannii* S3310 (IRAB) include the Bekka-Hadji et al. study. Moreover, the synergistic properties of the combination of oil with ticarcillin-clavulanate, cefotaxime, imipenem, and nalidixic acid against IRAB have been demonstrated. This is an important premise in the era of increasing antibiotic resistance [24]. Another article describes the antimicrobial activity of *Salvia officinalis* EO in relation to various pathogenic bacteria, including *A. baumannii*. Camphor was the predominant component of the EO, obtaining a concentration value of 18.72%. Interestingly, the oil showed a synergistic effect in combination with cefazolin in relation to several pathogens (*S. aureus*, *K. pneumoniae*, and *A. baumannii*) [176]. In addition, the synergistic nature of the interaction of the *C. tetradenius* EO with meropenem and ciprofloxacin for *K. pneumoniae* was detected [116]. Encouraging results were also obtained in the field of antibacterial activity for that of *R. officinalis* EO against fluoroquinolone-resistant *E. coli* (*gyrA* and *parC* mutations) [122]. In the Asili et al. study, the antibacterial activity of *Artemisia annua* EO (content of ~30% camphor) was assessed in relation to MDR *E. coli* ESβL. MIC values of *A. annua* EO in relation to five clinical isolates of *E. coli* ESβL were at the level of 2.5–10 mg/mL [115]. Antibacterial activity of *C. tetradenius* EO (camphor content 13.95%) in relation to *E. coli* ATCC 25922 was described in the Siqueira et al. study. Importantly, the synergism of the EO with meropenem in the case of *E. coli* was demonstrated [116].

Due to the fact that drug resistance is a significant problem in the effectiveness and speed of treatment of skin infections, in Table 9 we summarize information on the resistance of the bacterial and fungal strains we analyzed, including the mechanism of resistance.

Table 9. Antibacterial and antifungal activity of camphor-enriched EOs and derivates, including resistance of the tested strains.

Camphor Source	MIC Value	ZOI Value	Pathogen	Resistance Mechanism	Ref.
Artemisia judaica EO (16.1% camphor)	1.25 μL/mL	-	*C. albicans*	Resistance to azoles mediated by efflux pumps Cdr1 and Cdr2	[101]
Artemisia herba-alba EO (32% camphor)	1.2 μL/mL	-	*S. aureus*	MRSA—methicillin-resistant *S. aureus*, mediated by *mecA* gene resistance to various β-lactam antibiotics	[24]
Combretum hereroense EO	0.17 mg/mL				[127]
Camphor quinoxalin-2,3(1H,4H)-dione	24 μM	-			[134]
Artemisia herba-alba EO (32% camphor)	1.2 μL/mL	-	*A. baumannii*	IRAB—imipenem-resistant *A. baumannii*	[24]
Rosmarinus officinalis EO (~23% camphor)	-	9.33–12.67 mm vs. 30.0 mm nalidixic acid	*E. coli*	Resistance to fluoroquinolones mediated by *gyrA* and *parC* genes mutations	[131]
Artemisia annua EO (~30% camphor)	2.5–10 mg/mL	-	*E. coli*	ESβL—extended spectrum β-lactamase	[132]
camphor-linked biphenyl quinoxalin-6-sulfonamide	16 μg/mL	-	*K. pneumoniae*		[134]

8.2. Antimicrobial Activity of Novel Camphor-Based Derivates

The activity of silver complexes with camphor–imine derivatives was also assessed against the *E. coli* ATCC 25922 strain. One of the compounds was characterized by strong activity against a pathogen, with an MIC value of 7.2 ± 0.1 μg/mL. The study tested derivatives also against the *S. aureus* strain Newman. One of the imine derivatives showed an excellent activity profile against *S. aureus* (MIC = 9.3 ± 1.1 μg/mL). The study also proved higher antibacterial activity on the part of camphor sulfonimine derivatives than imines.

The derivatives mentioned were also tested in relation to *P. aeruginosa* 477. The MIC for this pathogen obtained by one of the imine derivatives was 3.4 ± 0.1 μg/mL [177]. Novel camphor-based organic derivates from the Peraman et al. study showed that camphor and camphorosulfonic acid derivatives are characterized by a wide spectrum of antibacterial activities, including against MRSA. The presence of the camphor group resulted in an excellent antibacterial activity of the preparation (MIC for MRSA at the level of 24 μM). Camphor quinoxalin-2,3(1H,4H)-dione (MIC = 24 μM) and isatin-based derivates obtained a MIC values of 24 μM, 51 μM, and 82 μM, respectively, against MRSA and *P. aeruginosa* ATCC 27853. In the study, camphor-linked biphenyl quinoxalin-6-sulfonamide obtained promising results against *P. aeruginosa*, *A. baumannii*, and MDR *K. pneumoniae* ATCC 700603 (ESβL- extended spectrum β-lactamase isolate), reaching a MIC value of 16 μg/mL. Camphor and camphor-sulfonic acid derivatives were also highly active against an MDR *C. albicans* ATCC 90028 isolate. The best properties in relation to yeasts were shown by benzoin and salicylic derivatives of camphor obtaining MIC at the levels of 16 μg/mL and 8 μg/mL, respectively (positive control amphotericin B MIC = 2 μg/mL) [178].

Sancineto et al. revealed the antimicrobial activity of organoselenic compounds (including camphor diselenide) against biofilms and planktonic forms of *S. aureus* ATCC 29213 and *S. pyogenes* ATCC 20565 as important etiological factors of skin wound infections. Camphor diselenide showed moderate activity against *S. pyogenes*: MIC = 31.25 mg/L (positive control gentamycin, MIC = 2.19 mg/L). Camphor diselenide also showed an excellent biofilm inhibitory profile against *S. pyogenes* (including subinhibitory concentrations). The antimicrobial activity of camphor diselenide against biofilm and planktonic forms of *S. aureus* ATCC 29213 was also revealed. The in vitro study showed that MIC for *S. aureus* was at the level of 250 mg/L. This derivative was characterized by a strong biofilm inhibitory profile even in subinhibitory concentrations of 0.5× MIC. The antifungal properties of camphor diselenide were also revealed against *C. albicans* Sc5314. The most preferred MIC profile was that obtained by one of the derivatives (MIC = 31.25 mg/L) compared to the positive control FLC, for which MIC = 0.25 mg/L. One of the compounds at a concentration of 50 mg/L showed a decrease in biofilm formation by about 60% [27]. The Zhang et al.'s study evaluated the antibacterial properties of newly synthesized camphorylpyrimidine-amine derivatives containing bicyclic monoterpene groups. One of the derivatives (*N*-(2,4-Difluorobenzyl)-4-(4-methoxyphenyl) -8,9,9-trimethyl-5,6,7,8-tetrahydro -5,8-Methylquinazolin-2-amine) of camphor showed an interesting activity profile in relation to the tested bacteria *K. pneumoniae* (MIC = 32 μg/mL, equal to positive control of ACN). Optimism is inspired by the excellent activity of the derivative against *K. pneumoniae* and *P. aeruginosa*, which was comparable or higher than that of aminoglycosides. The preparation showed an MIC for *E. coli* at 8 μg/mL vs. 2 μg/mL for the positive control can, and 16 μg/mL for *P. aeruginosa versus* 32 μg/mL for ACN. Zhang et al. also described significant activity of one of the compounds against MRSA isolates (MIC = 8 μg/mL vs. positive control CAN's MIC = 1 μg/mL) and against pathogenic fungi *C. albicans* (MIC = 32 μg/mL vs. ketoconazole's MIC = 16 μg/mL) [94].

Carvalho et al. showed an interesting profile of antibacterial properties of silver complexes with imine and sulfoimine derivatives of camphor in relation to, among other microbes, *P. aeruginosa* 477. One of the camphor–sulphonyl–imine complexes obtained the best anti-pseudomonal properties (MIC = 36 μg/mL), which makes it an interesting option for further research in the era of increasing antibiotic resistance among *Pseudomonas aeruginosa* strains [123]. A similar report comes from the Cardoso et al. study, in which researchers assessed the effects of camphor–imine complexes with silver ions (Ag^+) against microbes such as. *P. aeruginosa* and obtained the encouraging MIC result of 19 μg/mL for one of the derivatives [179]. Another study showed the promising properties of the camphor-based 2,4-disubstituted 1,3-thiazoles in the terms of their activity against *C. albicans*. The MIC for yeasts was defined in the range of 0.12–0.98 μg/mL, which makes their activity comparable to that of tested fluconazole [180].

9. Future Perspectives of Antimicrobial Usage of Camphor Derivates

Another study determined camphor activity (concentrations 30–50%) in combination with metronidazole [Metronidazole-Loaded Camphor-Based In Situ Forming Matrix] for consideration as a therapeutic option against bacteria involved in periodontitis. The combination of 40% camphor with 5% triacetin has been shown to prolong the release of metronidazole from the substrate for up to 6 days. Activity against *S. aureus* ATCC 6538 was determined by disc diffusion assay. The test with the best parameters showed a ZOI value for *S. aureus* equal to 15.03 ± 0.6 mm, (control sample ZOI was ~23.3 mm) [181]. The Rani et al. study evaluated the antimicrobial activity of a camphor-enriched food film based on soy protein. No significant antimicrobial activity (against *E. coli*, *Listeria monocytogenes*) was demonstrated for the film as opposed to that of a 1% camphor solution alone. It has been shown that after incubation (12–16 h) of film fragments in agar, there was no significant decrease in optical density. In turn, in the case of a 1% camphor solution, this density was observed to decrease by 12.5% (*L. monocytogenes*) and 62.5% (*E. coli*). Although the study does not prove that the innovative food film had antibacterial properties, it does validate earlier reports of significant camphor activity against *E. coli* [182]. Interesting findings came from an article by Santos et al. on the use of a coating made of diamond-like carbon foil with a built-in camphor molecule. The effectiveness of a coating applied to the surface of polyurethane was assessed to combat *C. albicans'* biofilm (including yeast colonization of vascular catheters). ATCC 10231 was the strain used in the study. A significant reduction in the formation of biofilm by the fungus at the level of 91–99% has been shown, which makes the results very promising [183].

Figure 4 summarizes the average MIC values from the literature data analyzed in this review. Only those strains for which at least three antimicrobial activity values were found were considered. The very high standard deviation (SD) of the compared results is due to the fact that the analysis included studies focusing on different plants that include camphor. Nevertheless, based on the graph, it becomes clear that camphor shows an antimicrobial tendency against both Gram-positive and Gram-negative bacteria, as well as against the fungus species *C. albicans*. Therefore, its activity covers the vast majority of the panel of pathogens responsible for both primary and secondary skin infections. Thus, the preventive effect of camphor in skin disorders is very promising, not only as an additive to cosmetics, i.e., lotions, shampoos, but especially in medicine as (i) an antiseptic to be applied directly to the skin and (ii) a disinfectant applied to objects in direct contact with the skin.

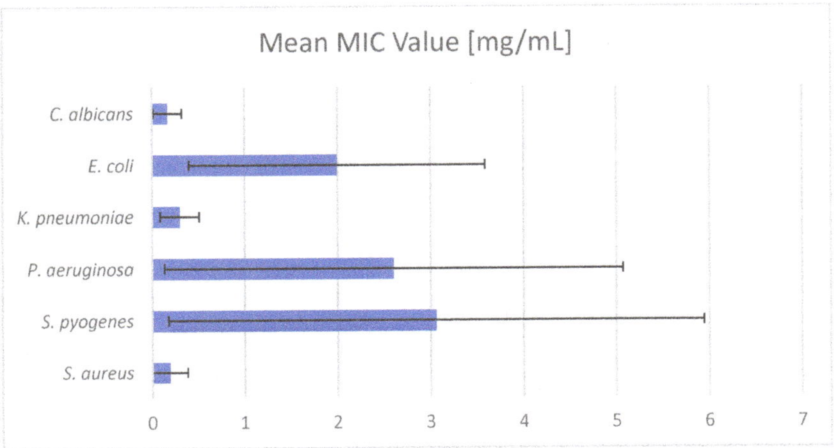

Figure 4. Camphor's averaged antimicrobial and antifungal activities (based on unified data from the literature collected from articles described and cited in Tables 4–8).

In addition, camphor, as an additive in small amounts to cosmetic products applied directly to the skin, boasts popularity. It has already found use in foot care cosmetics, such as Gehwol warming lotion and FcSynergy ointment. Its beneficial effects are also utilized in the production of body care cosmetics, such as Flos-lek gel, Ilcsi cleansing concentrate, and Gehwol herbal salt. Camphor is often an ingredient in anti-acne products, e.g., Tołpa. It is also added to shampoos, e.g., Trico Botanica, as well as antiperspirants and perfumes. Because of its wide-ranging effects (i.e., relaxing, warming, relaxing, pore-opening, pH-restoring, and purifying), camphor is a compound with many uses and it surrounds us on all sides.

10. Conclusions

In this review article, we proved that camphor is a forward-looking natural compound in medicine. It can be used with great success in the prevention of skin infections. Indeed, it shows activity against both pathogens involved in primary and secondary dermatological infections. Its addition to medical devices applied directly to the skin protects the skin from attack by microorganisms, including those showing multi-drug resistance. In addition, as an ingredient in cosmetic products, it enhances their antiseptic effect and aids in eliminating purulent eruptions. However, due to the toxicity of this compound, future research directions should focus primarily on the aspect of reducing this negative effect. These should include studies searching for associations of camphor with other compounds that would neutralize the toxic effect of camphor while simultaneously enhancing its positive activities, i.e., analgesic, antipruritic, and warming. Moreover, prospective studies around slowing the absorption and/or release of this compound are also very promising. Research supporting the possibility of using camphor in nanotechnology also deserves great attention. The use of nanoparticles carrying camphor are highly promising due to their antitoxic effects. In the future, it is worth focusing on the use of various surfaces (e.g., bandages, sponges) impregnated with nanoparticles filled with camphor. However, this idea still needs many multicenter and multidirectional experiments. There is a need for in vivo studies that would give us the green light regarding the safety of future therapies. Such research could provide guidance on using these nanoparticles not only for preventing skin disorders but mainly as a therapeutic agent in cases of skin barrier disruption. In addition, future research should be based primarily on finding new ways for this compound to interact with, for example, antibiotics on bacterial and fungal cells involved in skin diseases. Therefore, further research using camphor as a wound-healing aid are important. The results of such experiments are even desirable from the point of view of eradicating resistant strains colonizing wounds.

Author Contributions: Conceptualization, A.D.-M.; software, E.T.; investigation, A.D.-M., S.V., E.T., J.K., M.G., W.M. and K.W.; resources A.D.-M., S.V., E.T., J.K., M.G., W.M. and K.W.; data curation, A.D.-M., S.V., E.T., J.K., M.G., W.M. and K.W.; writing—original draft preparation, A.D.-M., S.V., E.T., J.K., M.G., W.M. and K.W.; writing—review and editing, A.D.-M. and S.V.; visualization, A.D.-M. and S.V.; supervision, A.D.-M. All authors have read and agreed to the published version of the manuscript.

Funding: This research received no external funding.

Institutional Review Board Statement: Not applicable.

Informed Consent Statement: Not applicable.

Data Availability Statement: Not applicable.

Conflicts of Interest: The authors declare no conflicts of interest.

References

1. Nurzyńska-Wierdak, R.; Pietrasik, D.; Walasek-Janusz, M. Essential Oils in the Treatment of Various Types of Acne—A Review. *Plants* **2023**, *12*, 90. [CrossRef]
2. Chandrasekaran, S.; Murthykumar, K.; Nirmalkumar, H.; Chandrasekar, H. Role of camphor in oral health care. *Int. J. Pharm. Sci. Health Care* **2014**, *2*, 1–5.
3. Bubley, J.A.; Alharthi, M.; Arbiser, J.L. Successful Treatment of Palmoplantar Psoriasis with Chemical Peeling and Gentian Violet. *JAAD Case Rep.* **2021**, *17*, 28–30. [CrossRef]
4. Kang, N.J.; Han, S.C.; Yoon, S.H.; Sim, J.Y.; Maeng, Y.H.; Kang, H.K.; Yoo, E.S. *Cinnamomum camphora* Leaves Alleviate Allergic Skin Inflammatory Responses In Vitro and In Vivo. *Toxicol. Res.* **2019**, *35*, 279–285. [CrossRef]
5. Abdollahi, D.; Jafariazar, Z.; Afshar, M. Effect of Monoterpenes on Ex Vivo Transungual Delivery of Itraconazole for the Management of Onychomycosis. *J. Cosmet. Dermatol.* **2020**, *19*, 2745–2751. [CrossRef]
6. Li, Z.; Gan, Y.; Kang, T.; Ke, B.; Zhao, Y.; Huang, T.; Chen, Y.; Liu, J. Camphor Attenuates Hyperalgesia in Neuropathic Pain Models in Mice. *J. Pain Res.* **2023**, *16*, 785–795. [CrossRef]
7. Silva-Filho, S.E.; de Silva-Comar, F.M.S.; Wiirzler, L.A.M.; do Pinho, R.J.; Grespan, R.; Bersani-Amado, C.A.; Cuman, R.K.N. Effect of Camphor on the Behavior of Leukocytes In Vitro and In Vivo in Acute Inflammatory Response. *Trop. J. Pharm. Res.* **2014**, *13*, 2031–2037. [CrossRef]
8. Gabbanini, S.; Lucchi, E.; Carli, M.; Berlini, E.; Minghetti, A.; Valgimigli, L. In Vitro Evaluation of the Permeation through Reconstructed Human Epidermis of Essentials Oils from Cosmetic Formulations. *J. Pharm. Biomed. Anal.* **2009**, *50*, 370–376. [CrossRef]
9. Narayan, S.; Singh, N. Camphor Poisoning—An Unusual Cause of Seizure. *Med. J. Armed Forces India* **2012**, *68*, 252–253. [CrossRef]
10. Manoguerra, A.; Erdman, A.; Wax, P.; Nelson, L.; Martin Caravati, E.; Cobaugh, D.; Chyka, P.; Olson, K.; Booze, L.; Woolf, A.; et al. Camphor Poisoning: An Evidence-Based Practice Guideline for out-of-Hospital Management. *Clin. Toxicol.* **2006**, *44*, 357–370. [CrossRef]
11. Babaei, M.; Hesari, A.K.; Soltani, S. Evaluation of the Camphor Effects on Histological Parameters of Skin in Adult Mice and the Protective Role of Vitamin E. *J. Basic Res. Med. Sci.* **2021**, *8*, 53–62.
12. Nguyen, A.V.; Soulika, A.M. The Dynamics of the Skin's Immune System. *Int. J. Mol. Sci.* **2019**, *20*, 1811. [CrossRef]
13. Del Giudice, P. Skin Infections Caused by Staphylococcus Aureus. *Acta Derm. Venereol.* **2020**, *100*, 208–215. [CrossRef]
14. Amy Stanway MB ChB Streptococcal Skin Infection. Available online: https://dermnetnz.org/Topics/Streptococcal-Skin-Infections (accessed on 23 January 2024).
15. Klitgaard, K.; Nielsen, M.W.; Ingerslev, H.C.; Boye, M.; Jensen, T.K. Discovery of Bovine Digital Dermatitis-Associated Treponema Spp. in the Dairy Herd Environment by a Targeted Deep-Sequencing Approach. *Appl. Environ. Microbiol.* **2014**, *80*, 4427–4432. [CrossRef]
16. Könönen, E.; Wade, W.G. Actinomyces and Related Organisms in Human Infections. *Clin. Microbiol. Rev.* **2015**, *28*, 419–442. [CrossRef]
17. Gardini, G.; Gregori, N.; Matteelli, A.; Castelli, F. Mycobacterial Skin Infection. *Curr. Opin. Infect. Dis.* **2022**, *35*, 79–87. [CrossRef]
18. Espinosa-Hernández, V.M.; Morales-Pineda, V.; Martínez-Herrera, E. Skin Infections Caused by Emerging Candida Species. *Curr. Fungal Infect. Rep.* **2020**, *14*, 99–105. [CrossRef]
19. Blaise, G.; Nikkels, A.; Hermanns-Lê, T.; Nikkels-Tassoudji, N.; Piérard, G.E. Corynebacterium-associated Skin Infections. *Int. J. Dermatol.* **2008**, *47*, 884–890. [CrossRef]
20. Ghahramani, G. Superficial Staphylococcal and Streptococcal Infections. In *Inpatient Dermatology*; Springer: Cham, Switzerland, 2018; pp. 99–103. [CrossRef]
21. Allen, C.H.; Patel, B.; Endom, E.E. Primary Bacterial Infections of the Skin and Soft Tissues Changes in Epidemiology and Management. *Clin. Pediatr. Emerg. Med.* **2004**, *5*, 246–255. [CrossRef]
22. Bikowski, J. Secondarily Infected Wounds and Dermatoses: A Diagnosis and Treatment Guide. *J. Emerg. Med.* **1999**, *17*, 197–206. [CrossRef]
23. Siddiqui, A.H.; Koirala, J. Methicillin-Resistant *Staphylococcus aureus*. In *StatPearls [Internet]*; StatPearls Publishing: Treasure Island, FL, USA, 2023. [PubMed]
24. Bekka-Hadji, F.; Bombarda, I.; Djoudi, F.; Bakour, S.; Touati, A. Chemical Composition and Synergistic Potential of *Mentha pulegium* L. and Artemisia Herba Alba Asso. Essential Oils and Antibiotic against Multi-Drug Resistant Bacteria. *Molecules* **2022**, *27*, 1095. [CrossRef]
25. Gahlot, R.; Nigam, C.; Vikas Kumar, G.; Yadav, H.; Anupurba, S. Catheter-Related Blood Stream Infections. *Int. J. Crit. Illn. Inj. Sci.* **2014**, *4*, 162–167. [CrossRef]
26. Ayobami, O.; Brinkwirth, S.; Eckmanns, T.; Markwart, R. Antibiotic Resistance in Hospital-Acquired ESKAPE-E Infections in Low- and Lower-Middle-Income Countries: A Systematic Review and Meta-Analysis. *Emerg. Microbes Infect.* **2022**, *11*, 443–451. [CrossRef]
27. Sancineto, L.; Piccioni, M.; De Marco, S.; Pagiotti, R.; Nascimento, V.; Braga, A.L.; Santi, C.; Pietrella, D. Diphenyl Diselenide Derivatives Inhibit Microbial Biofilm Formation Involved in Wound Infection. *BMC Microbiol.* **2016**, *16*, 220. [CrossRef]

28. Apinundecha, C.; Teethaisong, Y.; Suknasang, S.; Ayamuang, I.O.; Eumkeb, G. Synergistic Interaction between *Boesenbergia rotunda* (L.) Mansf. Essential Oil and Cloxacillin on Methicillin-Resistant Staphylococcus Aureus (MRSA) Inhibition. *Evid.-Based Complement. Altern. Med.* **2023**, *2023*, 3453273. [CrossRef]
29. Roman, H.; Niculescu, A.G.; Lazăr, V.; Mitache, M.M. Antibacterial Efficiency of Tanacetum Vulgare Essential Oil against ESKAPE Pathogens and Synergisms with Antibiotics. *Antibiotics* **2023**, *12*, 1635. [CrossRef]
30. Langan, S.M.; Mulick, A.R.; Rutter, C.E.; Silverwood, R.J.; Asher, I.; García-Marcos, L.; Ellwood, E.; Bissell, K.; Chiang, C.Y.; El Sony, A.; et al. Trends in Eczema Prevalence in Children and Adolescents: A Global Asthma Network Phase I Study. *Clin. Exp. Allergy* **2023**, *53*, 337–352. [CrossRef]
31. Flohr, C.; French', L.; Bissonnette, R.; Taieb, A.; Deleuran, M.; Austin, J. *Global Report on Atopic Dermatitis 2022*; International League of Dermatological Societies (ILDS): London, UK, 2022.
32. Grossi, A.P.; Ruggieri, A.; Del Vecchio, A.; Comandini, A.; Corio, L.; Calisti, F.; Di Loreto, G.; Almirante, B. Skin Infections in Europe: A Retrospective Study of Incidence, Patient Characteristics and Practice Patterns. *Int. J. Antimicrob. Agents* **2022**, *60*, 106637. [CrossRef]
33. Malabadi, R.B.; Kolkar, K.P.; Meti, N.T.; Chalannavar, R.K. Camphor Tree, *Cinnamomum camphora* (L.); Ethnobotany and Pharmacological Updates. *Biomedicine* **2021**, *41*, 181–184. [CrossRef]
34. Zuccarini, P.; Soldani, G. Camphor: Benefits and Risks of a Widely Used Natural Product. *Acta Biol. Szeged.* **2009**, *53*, 77–82. [CrossRef]
35. Ponomarev, D.A.; Mettee, H. Camphor and Its Industrial Synthesis. *Chem. Educ. J.* **2017**, *18*, 2–5.
36. Mahdy, A.-H.S.; Zayed, S.E.; Abo-Bakr, A.M.; Hassan, E.A. Camphor: Synthesis, Reactions and Uses as a Potential Moiety in the Development of Complexes and Organocatalysts. *Tetrahedron* **2022**, *121*, 132913. [CrossRef]
37. Calderini, E.; Drienovská, I.; Myrtollari, K.; Pressnig, M.; Sieber, V.; Schwab, H.; Hofer, M.; Kourist, R. Simple Plug-In Synthetic Step for the Synthesis of (−)-Camphor from Renewable Starting Materials. *ChemBioChem* **2021**, *22*, 2951–2956. [CrossRef]
38. Lang, P.T.; Harned, A.M.; Wissinger, J.E. Oxidation of Borneol to Camphor Using Oxone and Catalytic Sodium Chloride: A Green Experiment for the Undergraduate Organic Chemistry Laboratory. *J. Chem. Educ.* **2011**, *88*, 652–656. [CrossRef]
39. Aswandi, A.; Kholibrina, C.R. New Insights into Sumatran Camphor (*Dryobalanops aromatica* Gaertn) Management and Conservation in Western Coast Sumatra, Indonesia. *IOP Conf. Ser. Earth Environ. Sci.* **2021**, *739*, 012061. [CrossRef]
40. Renvall, P.; Niemela, T. Ocotea Usambarensis and Its Fungal Decayers in Natural Stands. *Bull. Jard. Bot. Natl. Belgique/Bull. Natl. Plantentuin Belgiё* **1993**, *62*, 403–414. [CrossRef]
41. Lee, S.-H.; Kim, D.-S.; Park, S.-H.; Park, H. Phytochemistry and Applications of *Cinnamomum camphora* Essential Oils. *Molecules* **2022**, *27*, 2695. [CrossRef]
42. Zhang, H.; Huang, T.; Liao, X.; Zhou, Y.; Chen, S.; Chen, J.; Xiong, W. Extraction of Camphor Tree Essential Oil by Steam Distillation and Supercritical CO_2 Extraction. *Molecules* **2022**, *27*, 5385. [CrossRef]
43. Poudel, D.K.; Rokaya, A.; Ojha, P.K.; Timsina, S.; Satyal, R.; Dosoky, N.S.; Satyal, P.; Setzer, W.N. The Chemical Profiling of Essential Oils from Different Tissues of *Cinnamomum camphora* L. and Their Antimicrobial Activities. *Molecules* **2021**, *26*, 5132. [CrossRef]
44. Pragadheesh, V.S.; Saroj, A.; Yadav, A.; Chanotiya, C.S.; Alam, M.; Samad, A. Chemical Characterization and Antifungal Activity of *Cinnamomum camphora* Essential Oil. *Ind. Crops Prod.* **2013**, *49*, 628–633. [CrossRef]
45. Chen, J.; Tang, C.; Zhang, R.; Ye, S.; Zhao, Z.; Huang, Y.; Xu, X.; Lan, W.; Yang, D. Metabolomics Analysis to Evaluate the Antibacterial Activity of the Essential Oil from the Leaves of *Cinnamomum camphora* (Linn.) Presl. *J. Ethnopharmacol.* **2020**, *253*, 112652. [CrossRef]
46. Tsiftsoglou, O.S.; Atskakani, M.-E.; Krigas, N.; Stefanakis, M.K.; Gounaris, C.; Hadjipavlou-Litina, D.; Lazari, D. Exploring the Medicinal Potential of Achillea Grandifolia in Greek Wild-Growing Populations: Characterization of Volatile Compounds, Anti-Inflammatory and Antioxidant Activities of Leaves and Inflorescences. *Plants* **2023**, *12*, 613. [CrossRef]
47. Schepetkin, I.A.; Özek, G.; Özek, T.; Kirpotina, L.N.; Klein, R.A.; Khlebnikov, A.I.; Quinn, M.T. Composition and Biological Activity of the Essential Oils from Wild Horsemint, Yarrow, and Yampah from Subalpine Meadows in Southwestern Montana: Immunomodulatory Activity of Dillapiole. *Plants* **2023**, *12*, 2643. [CrossRef]
48. Oftadeh, M.; Sendi, J.J.; Ebadollahi, A. Toxicity and Deleterious Effects of Artemisia Annua Essential Oil Extracts on Mulberry Pyralid (*Glyphodes pyloalis*). *Pestic. Biochem. Physiol.* **2020**, *170*, 104702. [CrossRef]
49. Shahrivari, S.; Alizadeh, S.; Ghassemi-Golezani, K.; Aryakia, E. A Comprehensive Study on Essential Oil Compositions, Antioxidant, Anticholinesterase and Antityrosinase Activities of Three Iranian Artemisia Species. *Sci. Rep.* **2022**, *12*, 7234. [CrossRef]
50. Ghasemi, G.; Alirezalu, A.; Ishkeh, S.R.; Ghosta, Y. Phytochemical Properties of Essential Oil from *Artemisia Sieberi* Besser (Iranian Accession) and Its Antioxidant and Antifungal Activities. *Nat. Prod. Res.* **2021**, *35*, 4154–4158. [CrossRef]
51. Ghorbani, S.; Kosari-Nasab, M.; Mahjouri, S.; Talebpour, A.H.; Movafeghi, A.; Maggi, F. Enhancement of In Vitro Production of Volatile Organic Compounds by Shoot Differentiation in *Artemisia spicigera*. *Plants* **2021**, *10*, 208. [CrossRef]
52. Usami, A.; Ono, T.; Marumoto, S.; Miyazawa, M. Comparison of Volatile Compounds with Characteristic Odor in Flowers and Leaves of Nojigiku (*Chrysanthemum japonense*). *J. Oleo Sci.* **2013**, *62*, 631–636. [CrossRef]
53. Guo, S.; Geng, Z.; Zhang, W.; Liang, J.; Wang, C.; Deng, Z.; Du, S. The Chemical Composition of Essential Oils from *Cinnamomum camphora* and Their Insecticidal Activity against the Stored Product Pests. *Int. J. Mol. Sci.* **2016**, *17*, 1836. [CrossRef]

54. Najafian, S.; Afshar, M.; Radi, M. Annual Phytochemical Variations and Antioxidant Activity within the Aerial Parts of *Lavandula Angustifolia*, an Evergreen Medicinal Plant. *Chem. Biodivers.* **2022**, *19*, e202200536. [CrossRef]
55. Karaca, N.; Şener, G.; Demirci, B.; Demirci, F. Synergistic Antibacterial Combination of *Lavandula latifolia* Medik. Essential Oil with Camphor. *Z. Naturforsch. C* **2021**, *76*, 169–173. [CrossRef]
56. Purkayastha, J.; Nath, S.C. Composition of the Camphor-Rich Essential Oil of *Ocimum Basilicum* L. Native to Northeast India. *J. Essent. Oil Res.* **2006**, *18*, 332–334. [CrossRef]
57. Joshi, R.K. Chemical Composition of the Essential Oil of Camphor Basil (*Ocimum kilimandscharicum* Guerke). *Glob. J. Med. Plant Res.* **2013**, *1*, 207–209.
58. Sufer, Ö.; Ceylan, A.; Onbasili, D.; Çelik Yuvali, G.; Bozok, F. Chemical Compounds and Biological Activity of Turkish *Santolina chamaecyparissus* L. Essential Oil by Microwave Assisted Distillation. *Kastamonu Üniv. Orman Fakültesi Derg.* **2021**, *21*, 165–175. [CrossRef]
59. Bozyel, M.E.; Canli, K.; Benek, A.; Simsek, O.; Akata, I.; Altuner, E.M. Biochemical Composition, a Nd in Vitro Antimicrobial and Antioxidant Activities of Salva Fruticosa, an Ethnomedicinal Plant. *Appl. Ecol. Environ. Res.* **2023**, *21*, 3243–3256. [CrossRef]
60. Pieracci, Y.; Ciccarelli, D.; Giovanelli, S.; Pistelli, L.; Flamini, G.; Cervelli, C.; Mancianti, F.; Nardoni, S.; Bertelloni, F.; Ebani, V.V. Antimicrobial Activity and Composition of Five *Rosmarinus* (Now *salvia* spp. and Varieties) Essential Oils. *Antibiotics* **2021**, *10*, 1090. [CrossRef]
61. Tosun, A.; Khan, S.; Kim, Y.; Calín-Sánchez, A.; Hysenaj, X.; Carbonell-Barrachina, A. Essential Oil Composition and Anti-Inflammatory Activity of *Salvia officinalis* L (Lamiaceae) in Murin Macrophages. *Trop. J. Pharm. Res.* **2014**, *13*, 937. [CrossRef]
62. Ivanova, S.; Pashova, S.; Dyankov, S.; Georgieva, Y.; Ivanov, K.; Benbassat, N.; Koleva, N.; Bozhkova, M.; Karcheva-Bahchevanska, D. Chemical Composition and Future Perspectives of Essential Oil Obtained from a Wild Population of *Stachys germanica* L. Distributed in the Balkan Mountains in Bulgaria. *Int. J. Anal. Chem.* **2023**, *2023*, 4275213. [CrossRef]
63. Izadi, Z.; Esna-Ashari, M.; Piri, K.; Davoodi, P. Chemical Composition and Antimicrobial Activity of Feverfew (*Tanacetum parthenium*) Essential Oil. *Int. J. Agric. Biol.* **2010**, *12*, 759–763.
64. Zouari, N.; Ayadi, I.; Fakhfakh, N.; Rebai, A.; Zouari, S. Variation of Chemical Composition of Essential Oils in Wild Populations of *Thymus algeriensis* Boiss. et Reut., a North African Endemic Species. *Lipids Health Dis.* **2012**, *11*, 28. [CrossRef]
65. Antonelli, M.; Donelli, D.; Valussi, M. Efficacy, Safety and Tolerability of Tiger Balm® Ointments: A Systematic Review and a Meta-Analysis of Prevalence. *J. Pharm. Pharmacogn. Res.* **2020**, *8*, 1–17. [CrossRef]
66. Goodnough, C.L.; Wu, Y.; Gross, E.R. Topical Analgesic BENGAY® Reduces Myocardial Infarct Size in Rodents. *Br. J. Anaesth.* **2021**, *127*, e163–e166. [CrossRef]
67. Stinson, R.J.; Morice, A.H.; Ahmad, B.; Sadofsky, L.R. Ingredients of Vicks VapoRub Inhibit Rhinovirus-Induced ATP Release. *Drugs Context* **2023**, *12*, 1–18. [CrossRef]
68. Vlahovic, T.C.; Dawes, C.L. Myths in Treating Onychomycosis. In *Onychomycosis: An Illustrated Guide to Diagnosis and Treatment*; Springer: Cham, Switzerland, 2017; pp. 215–222. [CrossRef]
69. Derby, R.; Rohal, P.; Jackson, C.; Beutler, A.; Olsen, C. Novel Treatment of Onychomycosis Using Over-the-Counter Mentholated Ointment: A Clinical Case Series. *J. Am. Board Fam. Med.* **2011**, *24*, 69–74. [CrossRef]
70. Snell, M.; Klebert, M.; Önen, N.F.; Hubert, S. A Novel Treatment for Onychomycosis in People Living With HIV Infection: Vicks VapoRub™ Is Effective and Safe. *J. Assoc. Nurses AIDS Care* **2016**, *27*, 109–113. [CrossRef]
71. Coiffard, L.; Couteau, C. Soap and Syndets: Differences and Analogies, Sources of Great Confusion. *Eur. Rev. Med. Pharmacol. Sci.* **2020**, *24*, 11432–11439. [CrossRef]
72. Patil, J.N.; Patil, K.C.; Patil, P.K.; Chaudhari, H.S. Formulation and evaluation of camphor aloe soap. *World J. Pharm. Res.* **2023**, *12*, 1257–1273. [CrossRef]
73. Kędzia, A.; Kędzia, A.W. Activity of camphor oil to anaerobic bacteria. *Postępy Fitoter.* **2009**, *3*, 147–151.
74. Santos, C.D.; Cabot, J.C. Persistent Effects after Camphor Ingestion: A Case Report and Literature Review. *J. Emerg. Med.* **2015**, *48*, 298–304. [CrossRef]
75. Wojtunik-kulesza, K.A. Toxicity of Selected Monoterpenes and Essential Oils Rich in These Compounds. *Molecules* **2022**, *27*, 1716. [CrossRef]
76. Martin, D.; Valdez, J.; Boren, J.; Mayersohn, M. Dermal Absorption of Camphor, Menthol, and Methyl Salicylate in Humans. *J. Clin. Pharmacol.* **2004**, *44*, 1151–1157. [CrossRef]
77. Robertson, J.S.; Hussain, M. Metabolism of Camphors and Related Compounds. *Biochem. J.* **1969**, *113*, 57–65. [CrossRef]
78. Park, T.J.; Seo, H.K.; Kang, B.J.; Kim, K.T. Noncompetitive Inhibition by Camphor of Nicotinic Acetylcholine Receptors. *Biochem. Pharmacol.* **2001**, *61*, 787–793. [CrossRef]
79. Zárybnický, T.; Boušová, I.; Ambrož, M.; Skálová, L. Hepatotoxicity of Monoterpenes and Sesquiterpenes. *Arch. Toxicol.* **2018**, *92*, 1–13. [CrossRef]
80. Uc, A.; Bishop, W.P.; Sanders, K.D. Camphor Hepatotoxicity. *South Med. J.* **2000**, *93*, 596–598. [CrossRef]
81. Köppel, C.; Tenczer, J.; Schirop, T.; Ibe, K. Camphor Poisoning—Abuse of Camphor as a Stimulant. *Arch. Toxicol.* **1982**, *51*, 101–106. [CrossRef]
82. Zehetner, P.; Höferl, M.; Buchbauer, G. Essential Oil Components and Cytochrome P450 Enzymes: A Review. *Flavour Fragr. J.* **2019**, *34*, 223–240. [CrossRef]
83. Santhanakrishnan, T.S. Tetrahedron Report Number 172. *Tetrahedron* **1984**, *40*, 3597–3609. [CrossRef]

84. Leibman, K.C.; Ortiz, E. Mammalian Metabolism of Terpenoids. I. Reduction and Hydroxylation of Camphor and Related Compounds. *Drug Metab. Dispos.* **1973**, *1*, 543–551.
85. Baser, K.H.C.; Buchbauer, G. *Handbook of Essential Oils Science, Technology, and Applications*; CRC Press: Boca Raton, FL, USA, 2020; ISBN 9780815370965.
86. Gyoubu, K.; Miyazawa, M. In Vitro Metabolism of (−)-Camphor Using Human Liver Microsomes and CYP2A6. *Biol. Pharm. Bull.* **2007**, *30*, 230–233. [CrossRef]
87. He, R.; Li, H.; Chu, Z.; Wang, F.; Du, F.; Xu, F. Circulating Metabolites of *Borneolum syntheticum* (Bingpian) Inhibit Foam-Cell Formation in Macrophages Induced by Oxidized Low-Density Lipoprotein. *bioRxiv* **2023**. [CrossRef]
88. Chen, J.; Jiang, Q.D.; Chai, Y.P.; Zhang, H.; Peng, P.; Yang, X.X. Natural Terpenes as Penetration Enhancers for Transdermal Drug Delivery. *Molecules* **2016**, *21*, 1709. [CrossRef]
89. Xie, F.; Chai, J.K.; Hu, Q.; Yu, Y.H.; Ma, L.; Liu, L.Y.; Zhang, X.L.; Li, B.L.; Zhang, D.H. Transdermal Permeation of Drugs with Differing Lipophilicity: Effect of Penetration Enhancer Camphor. *Int. J. Pharm.* **2016**, *507*, 90–101. [CrossRef]
90. Cui, Y.; Li, L.; Zhang, L.; Li, J.; Gu, J.; Gong, H.; Guo, P.; Tong, W. Enhancement and Mechanism of Transdermal Absorption of Terpene-Induced Propranolol Hydrochloride. *Arch. Pharm. Res.* **2011**, *34*, 1477–1485. [CrossRef]
91. Steenen, S.A.; Van Wijk, A.J.; Van Der Heijden, G.J.M.G.; Van Westrhenen, R.; De Lange, J.; De Jongh, A. Propranolol for the Treatment of Anxiety Disorders: Systematic Review and Meta-Analysis. *J. Psychopharmacol.* **2016**, *30*, 128–139. [CrossRef]
92. Mothana, R.A.; Al-Rehaily, A.J.; Schultze, W. Chemical Analysis and Biological Activity of the Essential Oils of Two Endemic Soqotri Commiphora Species. *Molecules* **2010**, *15*, 689–698. [CrossRef]
93. Celen Yuceturk, S.; Aydogan Turkoglu, S.; Kockar, F.; Kucukbay, F.Z.; Azaz, A.D. Essential Oil Chemical Composition, Antimicrobial, Anticancer, and Antioxidant Effects of Thymus Convolutus Klokov in Turkey. *Z. Naturforsch. Sect. C J. Biosci.* **2021**, *76*, 193–203. [CrossRef]
94. Zhang, Y.; Wang, Y.; Zhao, Y.; Gu, W.; Zhu, Y.; Wang, S. Novel Camphor-Based Pyrimidine Derivatives Induced Cancer Cell Death through a ROS-Mediated Mitochondrial Apoptosis Pathway. *RSC Adv.* **2019**, *9*, 29711–29720. [CrossRef]
95. Rawat, A.; Rawat, M.; Prakash, O.; Kumar, R.; Punetha, H.; Rawat, D.S. Comparative Study on Eucalyptol and Camphor Rich Essential Oils from Rhizomes of *Hedychium spicatum* Sm. and Their Pharmacological, Antioxidant and Antifungal Activities. *An. Acad. Bras. Cienc.* **2022**, *94*, e20210932. [CrossRef]
96. Pishgahzadeh, E.; Shafaroodi, H.; Asgarpanah, J. Analgesic and Antiinflammatory Activities of the Essential Oil from Artemisia Sieberi Besser. *Braz. J. Pharm. Sci.* **2019**, *55*, e17011. [CrossRef]
97. Liao, J.; Xie, X.; Wang, W.; Gao, Y.; Cai, Y.; Peng, J.; Li, T.; Yi, Q.; He, C.; Wang, L. Anti-Inflammatory Activity of Essential Oil from Leaves of *Blumea balsamifera* (L.) DC through Inhibiting TLR4/NF-KB Signaling Pathways and NLRP3 Inflammasome Activation in LPS-Induced RAW264.7 Macrophage Cells. *J. Essent. Oil Bear. Plants* **2021**, *24*, 160–176. [CrossRef]
98. Tran, T.A.; Ho, M.T.; Song, Y.W.; Cho, M.; Cho, S.K. Camphor Induces Proliferative and Anti-Senescence Activities in Human Primary Dermal Fibroblasts and Inhibits UV-Induced Wrinkle Formation in Mouse Skin. *Phyther. Res.* **2015**, *29*, 1917–1925. [CrossRef]
99. Pejčić, M.; Stojanović-Radić, Z.; Genčić, M.; Dimitrijević, M.; Radulović, N. Anti-Virulence Potential of Basil and Sage Essential Oils: Inhibition of Biofilm Formation, Motility and Pyocyanin Production of Pseudomonas Aeruginosa Isolates. *Food Chem. Toxicol.* **2020**, *141*, 111431. [CrossRef]
100. Bajalan, I.; Rouzbahani, R.; Pirbalouti, A.G.; Maggi, F. Antioxidant and Antibacterial Activities of the Essential Oils Obtained from Seven Iranian Populations of Rosmarinus Officinalis. *Ind. Crops Prod.* **2017**, *107*, 305–311. [CrossRef]
101. Erdogan Eliuz, E.A.; Ayas, D.; Goksen, G. In Vitro Phototoxicity and Antimicrobial Activity of Volatile Oil Obtained from Some Aromatic Plants. *J. Essent. Oil Bear. Plants* **2017**, *20*, 758–768. [CrossRef]
102. Farahpour, M.R.; Pirkhezr, E.; Ashrafian, A.; Sonboli, A. Accelerated Healing by Topical Administration of *Salvia officinalis* Essential Oil on Pseudomonas Aeruginosa and Staphylococcus Aureus Infected Wound Model. *Biomed. Pharmacother.* **2020**, *128*, 110120. [CrossRef]
103. Yamani, H.A.; Pang, E.C.; Mantri, N.; Deighton, M.A. Antimicrobial Activity of Tulsi (*Ocimum tenuiflorum*) Essential Oil and Their Major Constituents against Three Species of Bacteria. *Front. Microbiol.* **2016**, *7*, 195885. [CrossRef]
104. Fatma, G.; Mouna, B.F.; Mondher, M.; Ahmed, L. In-Vitro Assessment of Antioxidant and Antimicrobial Activities of Methanol Extracts and Essential Oil of Thymus Hirtus Sp. Algeriensis. *Lipids Health Dis.* **2014**, *13*, 114. [CrossRef]
105. Shakeri, A.; Sharifi, M.J.; Fazly Bazzaz, B.S.; Emami, A.; Soheili, V.; Sahebkar, A.; Asili, J. Bioautography Detection of Antimicrobial Compounds from the Essential Oil of Salvia Pachystachys. *Curr. Bioact. Compd.* **2018**, *14*, 80–85. [CrossRef]
106. Nguir, A.; Mabrouk, H.; Douki, W.; Ben Ismail, M.; Ben Jannet, H.; Flamini, G.; Hamza, M.A. Chemical Composition and Bioactivities of the Essential Oil from Different Organs of *Ferula communis* L. Growing in Tunisia. *Med. Chem. Res.* **2016**, *25*, 515–525. [CrossRef]
107. Bouyahya, A.; Et-Touys, A.; Bakri, Y.; Talbaui, A.; Fellah, H.; Abrini, J.; Dakka, N. Chemical Composition of Mentha Pulegium and Rosmarinus Officinalis Essential Oils and Their Antileishmanial, Antibacterial and Antioxidant Activities. *Microb. Pathog.* **2017**, *111*, 41–49. [CrossRef]
108. Mohammed, H.A.; Al-Omar, M.S.; Aly, M.S.A.; Hegazy, M.M. Essential Oil Constituents and Biological Activities of the Halophytic Plants, *Suaeda Vermiculata* Forssk and *Salsola Cyclophylla* Bakera Growing in Saudi Arabia. *J. Essent. Oil Bear. Plants* **2019**, *22*, 82–93. [CrossRef]

109. Stappen, I.; Ali, A.; Tabanca, N.; Khan, I.; Wanner, J.; Gochev, V.; Singh, V.; Lal, B.; Jaitak, V.; Kaul, V.; et al. Antimicrobial and Repellent Activity of the Essential Oils of Two Lamiaceae Cultivated in Western Himalaya. *Curr. Bioact. Compd.* **2015**, *11*, 23–30. [CrossRef]
110. Adewinogo, S.O.; Sharma, R.; Africa, C.W.J.; Marnewick, J.L.; Hussein, A.A. Chemical Composition and Cosmeceutical Potential of the Essential Oil of *Oncosiphon suffruticosum* (L.) Källersjö. *Plants* **2021**, *10*, 1315. [CrossRef]
111. Bertella, A.; Benlahcen, K.; Abouamama, S.; Pinto, D.C.G.A.; Maamar, K.; Kihal, M.; Silva, A.M.S. Artemisia Herba-Alba Asso. Essential Oil Antibacterial Activity and Acute Toxicity. *Ind. Crops Prod.* **2018**, *116*, 137–143. [CrossRef]
112. Tawfeeq, A.A.; Mahdi, M.F.; Abaas, I.S.; Alwan, A.H. Isolation, quantification, and identification of rosmarinic acid, gas chromatography-mass spectrometry analysis of essential oil, cytotoxic effect, and antimicrobial investigation of rosmarinus officinalis leaves. *Asian J. Pharm. Clin. Res.* **2018**, *11*, 126. [CrossRef]
113. Insawang, S.; Pripdeevech, P.; Tanapichatsakul, C.; Khruengsai, S.; Monggoot, S.; Nakham, T.; Artrod, A.; D'Souza, P.E.; Panuwet, P. Essential Oil Compositions and Antibacterial and Antioxidant Activities of Five *Lavandula stoechas* Cultivars Grown in Thailand. *Chem. Biodivers.* **2019**, *16*, e1900371. [CrossRef]
114. El Moussaoui, A.; Bourhia, M.; Jawhari, F.Z.; Salamatullah, A.M.; Ullah, R.; Bari, A.; Majid Mahmood, H.; Sohaib, M.; Serhii, B.; Rozhenko, A.; et al. Chemical Profiling, Antioxidant, and Antimicrobial Activity against Drug-Resistant Microbes of Essential Oil from *Withania frutescens* L. *Appl. Sci.* **2021**, *11*, 5168. [CrossRef]
115. Asili, J.; Emami, S.A.; Eynolghozat, R.; Noghab, Z.S.; Bazzaz, B.S.F.; Sahebkar, A. Chemical Composition and In Vitro Efficacy of Essential Oil of Seven *Artemisia* Species Against ESBL Producing Multidrug-Resistant *Escherichia coli*. *J. Essent. Oil Bear. Plants* **2015**, *18*, 124–145. [CrossRef]
116. Siqueira, I.B.; Teixeira Barbosa, A.A.; Jain, S.; Miranda Fernandes, R.P.; Tavares Silva, A.R.S.; Ferreira Barbosa, F.H.; Schimieguel, D.M.; Blank, A.F.; Sacramento, A.G.; de Castro Nizio, D.A.; et al. In Vitro Antibacterial Activity of Essential Oils of *Croton tetradenius* Baill. From the Brazilian Caatinga Biome and Its Synergistic Effect With Ciprofloxacin and Meropenem. *J. Essent. Oil Bear. Plants* **2021**, *24*, 12–21. [CrossRef]
117. Pandey, M.; Pandey, A.; Shukla, S.K.; Kumar, R.; Pathak, A.; Mishra, R.K.; Dikshit, A. A Comparative Analysis of In Vitro Growth Inhibition of Waterborne Bacteria with Bioactive Plant *Lippia nodiflora* L. and Camphor. *Desalin. Water Treat.* **2016**, *57*, 26250–26256. [CrossRef]
118. Mhiri, R.; Kchaou, M.; Belhadj, S.; El Feki, A.; Allouche, N. Characterization of Aromatic Compounds and Biological Activities of Essential Oils from Tunisian Aromatic Plants. *J. Food Meas. Charact.* **2018**, *12*, 839–847. [CrossRef]
119. Bahri, F.; Romane, A.; Höferl, M.; Wanner, J.; Schmidt, E.; Jirovetz, L. Chemical Composition and Antimicrobial Activity of Essential Oil of Algerian *Tetraclinis articulata* (Vahl) Masters. *J. Essent. Oil Res.* **2016**, *28*, 42–48. [CrossRef]
120. Mahboubi, M.; Valian, M.; Kazempour, N. Chemical Composition, Antioxidant and Antimicrobial Activity of *Artemisia Sieberi* Oils from Different Parts of Iran and France. *J. Essent. Oil Res.* **2015**, *27*, 140–147. [CrossRef]
121. Ovidi, E.; Laghezza Masci, V.; Zambelli, M.; Tiezzi, A.; Vitalini, S.; Garzoli, S. Laurus Nobilis, Salvia Sclarea and *Salvia officinalis* Essential Oils and Hydrolates: Evaluation of Liquid and Vapor Phase Chemical Composition and Biological Activities. *Plants* **2021**, *10*, 707. [CrossRef]
122. Farhat, A.; Benmoussa, H.; Bachoual, R.; Nasfi, Z.; Elfalleh, W.; Romdhane, M.; Bouajila, J. Efficiency of the Optimized Microwave Assisted Extractions on the Yield, Chemical Composition and Biological Activities of Tunisian *Rosmarinus officinalis* L. Essential Oil. *Food Bioprod. Process.* **2017**, *105*, 224–233. [CrossRef]
123. Carvalho, M.F.N.N.; Leite, S.; Costa, J.P.; Galvão, A.M.; Leitão, J.H. Ag(I) Camphor Complexes: Antimicrobial Activity by Design. *J. Inorg. Biochem.* **2019**, *199*, 110791. [CrossRef]
124. Grimsey, L.; Van Vuuren, S.F.; Wright, M.H.; Cock, I.E. Selected South African *Combretum* Spp. Extracts Inhibit Methicillin-Resistant Staphylococcus Aureus and ESBL Strains of Escherichia Coli and Klebsiella Pneumoniae. *S. Afr. J. Bot.* **2024**, *165*, 49–58. [CrossRef]
125. Ouakouak, H.; Benarfa, A.; Messaoudi, M.; Begaa, S.; Sawicka, B.; Benchikha, N.; Simal-Gandara, J. Biological Properties of Essential Oils from Thymus Algeriensis Boiss. *Plants* **2021**, *10*, 786. [CrossRef]
126. Abu-Darwish, M.S.; Cabral, C.; Gonçalves, M.J.; Cavaleiro, C.; Cruz, M.T.; Zulfiqar, A.; Khan, I.A.; Efferth, T.; Salgueiro, L. Chemical Composition and Biological Activities of Artemisia Judaica Essential Oil from Southern Desert of Jordan. *J. Ethnopharmacol.* **2016**, *191*, 161–168. [CrossRef]
127. Manoharan, R.K.; Lee, J.-H.; Lee, J. Antibiofilm and Antihyphal Activities of Cedar Leaf Essential Oil, Camphor, and Fenchone Derivatives against Candida Albicans. *Front. Microbiol.* **2017**, *8*, 278535. [CrossRef]
128. Ivanov, M.; Kannan, A.; Stojković, D.S.; Glamočlija, J.; Calhelha, R.C.; Ferreira, I.C.F.R.; Sanglard, D.; Soković, M. Camphor and Eucalyptol—Anticandidal Spectrum, Antivirulence Effect, Efflux Pumps Interference and Cytotoxicity. *Int. J. Mol. Sci.* **2021**, *22*, 483. [CrossRef]
129. Nikolić, M.; Jovanović, K.K.; Marković, T.; Marković, D.; Gligorijević, N.; Radulović, S.; Soković, M. Chemical Composition, Antimicrobial, and Cytotoxic Properties of Five Lamiaceae Essential Oils. *Ind. Crops Prod.* **2014**, *61*, 225–232. [CrossRef]
130. Satyal, P.; Dosoky, N.S.; Poudel, A.; Setzer, W.N. Essential Oil Constituents and Their Biological Activities from the Leaves of Cassia Fistula Growing in Nepal. *Open Access J. Med. Aromat. Plants* **2012**, *3*, 1–4.

131. Agour, A.; Mssillou, I.; Mechchate, H.; Es-safi, I.; Allali, A.; El Barnossi, A.; Al Kamaly, O.; Alshawwa, S.Z.; El Moussaoui, A.; Bari, A.; et al. *Brocchia cinerea* (Delile) Vis. Essential Oil Antimicrobial Activity and Crop Protection against Cowpea Weevil *Callosobruchus maculatus* (Fab.). *Plants* **2022**, *11*, 583. [CrossRef]
132. Asres, K.; Tadesse, S.; Mazumder, A.; Bucar, F. Essential Oil of *Plectranthus Cylindraceus* Hochst. Ex. Benth from Ethiopia: Chemical Composition and Antimicrobial Activity. *J. Essent. Oil Bear. Plants* **2013**, *16*, 136–143. [CrossRef]
133. Al-Maharik, N.; Jaradat, N.; Hawash, M.; Al-Lahham, S.; Qadi, M.; Shoman, I.; Jaber, S.; Rahem, R.A.; Hussein, F.; Issa, L. Chemical Composition, Antioxidant, Antimicrobial and Anti-Proliferative Activities of Essential Oils of Rosmarinus Officinalis from Five Different Sites in Palestine. *Separations* **2022**, *9*, 339. [CrossRef]
134. Beniaich, G.; Hafsa, O.; Maliki, I.; Bin Jardan, Y.A.; El Moussaoui, A.; Chebaibi, M.; Agour, A.; Zouirech, O.; Nafidi, H.-A.; Khallouki, F.; et al. GC-MS Characterization, In Vitro Antioxidant, Antimicrobial, and In Silico NADPH Oxidase Inhibition Studies of Anvillea Radiata Essential Oils. *Horticulturae* **2022**, *8*, 886. [CrossRef]
135. Mohamadi Sani, A.; Khiabani, A.; Yaghooti, F. Chemical Composition and Antimicrobial Activity of the Essential Oil of *Artemisia aucheri* Aerial Parts. *J. Essent. Oil Bear. Plants* **2016**, *19*, 875–884. [CrossRef]
136. Bahadirli, N.P. Comparison of Chemical Composition and Antimicrobial Activity of *Salvia Fruticosa* Mill. and *S. Aramiensis* Rech. Fill. (Lamiaceae). *J. Essent. Oil Bear. Plants* **2022**, *25*, 716–727. [CrossRef]
137. Drobac, M.; Kukic-Markovic, J.; Milenkovic, M.; Niketic, M.; Petrovic, S. The Chemical Composition, Antimicrobial and Antiradical Properties of the Essential Oil of Achillea Grandifolia Aerial Parts from Serbia. *Bot. Serbica* **2021**, *45*, 233–240. [CrossRef]
138. El Hachlafi, N.; Fikri-Benbrahim, K.; Al-Mijalli, S.H.; Elbouzidi, A.; Jeddi, M.; Abdallah, E.M.; Assaggaf, H.; Bouyahya, A.; Alnasser, S.M.; Attar, A.; et al. *Tetraclinis articulata* (Vahl) Mast. Essential Oil as a Promising Source of Bioactive Compounds with Antimicrobial, Antioxidant, Anti-Inflammatory and Dermatoprotective Properties: In Vitro and in Silico Evidence. *Heliyon* **2024**, *10*, e23084. [CrossRef]
139. Sanae, A.A.; Ferdinand, K.E.; Bruno, E.; Hamzaoui Najia, E.; Amal, B.; Malika, M.S.; Touriya, Z. The Antifungal Effect of the Main Monoterpenes of the Essential Oil of *Artemisia herba alba* Var. Huguetii (Caball.) Maire of the Region of Ouarzazate-Morocco When Tested against Strains of Candida. *Res. J. Chem. Environ.* **2020**, *24*, 111–117.
140. Chaturvedi, T.; Kumar, A.; Kumar, A.; Verma, R.S.; Padalia, R.C.; Sundaresan, V.; Chauhan, A.; Saikia, D.; Singh, V.R.; Venkatesha, K. Chemical Composition, Genetic Diversity, Antibacterial, Antifungal and Antioxidant Activities of Camphor-Basil (*Ocimum kilimandscharicum* Guerke). *Ind. Crops Prod.* **2018**, *118*, 246–258. [CrossRef]
141. Benali, T.; Habbadi, K.; Khabbach, A.; Marmouzi, I.; Zengin, G.; Bouyahya, A.; Chamkhi, I.; Chtibi, H.; Aanniz, T.; Achbani, E.H.; et al. GC–MS Analysis, Antioxidant and Antimicrobial Activities of Achillea Odorata Subsp. Pectinata and Ruta Montana Essential Oils and Their Potential Use as Food Preservatives. *Foods* **2020**, *9*, 668. [CrossRef]
142. Hendel, N.; Napoli, E.; Sarri, M.; Saija, A.; Cristani, M.; Nostro, A.; Ginestra, G.; Ruberto, G. Essential Oil from Aerial Parts of Wild Algerian Rosemary: Screening of Chemical Composition, Antimicrobial and Antioxidant Activities. *J. Essent. Oil Bear. Plants* **2019**, *22*, 1–17. [CrossRef]
143. Santomauro, F.; Donato, R.; Sacco, C.; Pini, G.; Flamini, G.; Bilia, A. Vapour and Liquid-Phase Artemisia Annua Essential Oil Activities against Several Clinical Strains of Candida. *Planta Med.* **2016**, *82*, 1016–1020. [CrossRef]
144. Qasem, A.; Assaggaf, H.; Montesano, D.; Khalil, Z.; Al-Mijalli, S.H.; El Baaboua, A.; El Omari, N.; El Menyiy, N.; Bakrim, S.; Sheikh, R.A.; et al. Determination of Chemical Compounds and Investigation of Biological Properties of Matricaria Chamomilla Essential Oils, Honey, and Their Mixture. *Molecules* **2022**, *27*, 5850. [CrossRef]
145. Schneider, S.L.; Lim, H.W. Review of Environmental Effects of Oxybenzone and Other Sunscreen Active Ingredients. *J. Am. Acad. Dermatol.* **2019**, *80*, 266–271. [CrossRef]
146. Berganayeva, G.; Kudaibergenova, B.; Litvinenko, Y.; Nazarova, I.; Sydykbayeva, S.; Vassilina, G.; Izdik, N.; Dyusebaeva, M. Medicinal Plants of the Flora of Kazakhstan Used in the Treatment of Skin Diseases. *Molecules* **2023**, *28*, 4192. [CrossRef]
147. Xu, H.; Blair, N.T.; Clapham, D.E. Camphor Activates and Strongly Desensitizes the Transient Receptor Potential Vanilloid Subtype 1 Channel in a Vanilloid-Independent Mechanism. *J. Neurosci.* **2005**, *25*, 8924–8937. [CrossRef]
148. Vogt-Eisele, A.K.; Weber, K.; Sherkheli, M.A.; Vielhaber, G.; Panten, J.; Gisselmann, G.; Hatt, H. Monoterpenoid Agonists of TRPV3. *Br. J. Pharmacol.* **2007**, *151*, 530–540. [CrossRef]
149. Green, B.G. Sensory Characteristics of Camphor. *J. Investig. Dermatol.* **1990**, *94*, 662–666. [CrossRef]
150. Kotaka, T.; Kimura, S.; Kashiwayanagi, M.; Iwamoto, J. Camphor Induces Cold and Warm Sensations with Increases in Skin and Muscle Blood Flow in Human. *Biol. Pharm. Bull.* **2014**, *37*, 1913–1918. [CrossRef]
151. Alpizar, Y.A.; Gees, M.; Sanchez, A.; Apetrei, A.; Voets, T.; Nilius, B.; Talavera, K. Bimodal Effects of Cinnamaldehyde and Camphor on Mouse TRPA1. *Pflug. Arch. Eur. J. Physiol.* **2013**, *465*, 853–864. [CrossRef]
152. Denda, M.; Sokabe, T.; Fukumi-Tominaga, T.; Tominaga, M. Effects of Skin Surface Temperature on Epidermal Permeability Barrier Homeostasis. *J. Investig. Dermatol.* **2007**, *127*, 654–659. [CrossRef]
153. Janjua, N.R.; Mogensen, B.; Andersson, A.M.; Petersen, J.H.; Henriksen, M.; Skakkebæk, N.E.; Wulf, H.C. Systemic Absorption of the Sunscreens Benzophenone-3, Octyl-Methoxycinnamate, and 3-(4-Methyl-Benzylidene) Camphor after Whole-Body Topical Application and Reproductive Hormone Levels in Humans. *J. Investig. Dermatol.* **2004**, *123*, 57–61. [CrossRef]
154. Selescu, T.; Ciobanu, A.C.; Dobre, C.; Reid, G.; Babes, A. Camphor Activates and Sensitizes Transient Receptor Potential Melastatin 8 (TRPM8) to Cooling and Icilin. *Chem. Senses* **2013**, *38*, 563–575. [CrossRef]

155. Gannu, R.; Vishnu, Y.V.; Kishan, V.; Rao, Y.M. In Vitro Permeation of Carvedilol through Porcine Skin: Effect of Vehicles and Penetration Enhancers. *PDA J. Pharm. Sci. Technol.* **2008**, *62*, 256–263.
156. Patel, D.R.; Joshi, A.; Patel, H.H.; Stagni, G. Development and In-Vivo Evaluation of Ondansetron Gels for Transdermal Delivery. *Drug Dev. Ind. Pharm.* **2015**, *41*, 1030–1036. [CrossRef]
157. Vaghardoost, R.; Mousavi Majd, S.G.; Tebyanian, H.; Babavalian, H.; Malaei, L.; Niazi, M.; Javdani, A. The Healing Effect of Sesame Oil, Camphor and Honey on Second Degree Burn Wounds in Rat. *World J. Plast. Surg.* **2018**, *7*, 67–71.
158. Haught, J.M.; Jukic, D.M.; English, J.C. Hydroxyethyl Starch-Induced Pruritus Relieved by a Combination of Menthol and Camphor. *J. Am. Acad. Dermatol.* **2008**, *59*, 151–153. [CrossRef]
159. Gavale, A.G.; Wagh, P.R. Herbal Drugs Use in a Skin Disorders Review Article. *World J. Pharm. Res.* **2023**, *12*, 2655–2676. [CrossRef]
160. Phillips, B. The phenol-camphor treatment of dermatophytosis. *Br. J. Dermatol.* **1944**, *56*, 219–227. [CrossRef]
161. Scalia, S.; Tursilli, R.; Iannuccelli, V. Complexation of the Sunscreen Agent, 4-Methylbenzylidene Camphor with Cyclodextrins: Effect on Photostability and Human Stratum Corneum Penetration. *J. Pharm. Biomed. Anal.* **2007**, *44*, 29–34. [CrossRef]
162. Schmidt, T.; Ring, J.; Abeck, D. Photoallergic Contact Dermatitis Due to Combined UVB (4-Methylbenzylidene camphor/octyl methoxycinnamate) and UVA (Benzophenone-3/butyl methoxydibenzoylmethane) Absorber Sensitization. *Dermatology* **1998**, *196*, 354–357. [CrossRef]
163. Cohen, M.; Wolfe, R.; Mai, T.; Lewis, D. A Randomized, Double Blind, Placebo Controlled Trial of a Topical Cream Containing Glucosamine Sulfate, Chondroitin Sulfate, and Camphor for Osteoarthritis of the Knee. *J. Rheumatol.* **2003**, *30*, 523–528.
164. Monti, D.; Chetoni, P.; Burgalassi, S.; Tampucci, S.; Centini, M.; Anselmi, C. 4-Methylbenzylidene Camphor Microspheres: Reconstituted Epidermis (Skinethic®) Permeation and Distribution. *Int. J. Cosmet. Sci.* **2015**, *37*, 298–305. [CrossRef]
165. Somade, O.T. Camphor Toxicity: A Review of Recent Findings. *Proc. Natl. Acad. Sci. India Sect. B Biol. Sci.* **2023**, *93*, 775–790. [CrossRef]
166. Chen, W.; Vermaak, I.; Viljoen, A. Camphor—A Fumigant during the Black Death and a Coveted Fragrant Wood in Ancient Egypt and Babylon—A Review. *Molecules* **2013**, *18*, 5434–5454. [CrossRef]
167. Khine, H.; Weiss, D.; Graber, N.; Hoffman, R.S.; Esteban-Cruciani, N.; Avner, J.R. A Cluster of Children with Seizures Caused by Camphor Poisoning. *Pediatrics* **2009**, *123*, 1269–1272. [CrossRef]
168. Ernst, E. Adverse Effects of Herbal Drugs in Dermatology. *Br. J. Dermatol.* **2000**, *143*, 923–929. [CrossRef]
169. Cutillas, A.; Carrasco, A.; Martinez-Gutierrez, R.; Tomas, V.; Tudela, J. *Salvia officinalis* L. Essential Oils from Spain: Determination of Composition, Antioxidant Capacity, Antienzymatic, and Antimicrobial Bioactivities. *Chem. Biodivers.* **2017**, *14*. [CrossRef]
170. Wijesundara, N.M.; Rupasinghe, H.P.V. Essential Oils from Origanum Vulgare and *Salvia officinalis* Exhibit Antibacterial and Anti-Biofilm Activities against Streptococcus Pyogenes. *Microb. Pathog.* **2018**, *117*, 118–127. [CrossRef]
171. Canlı, K.; Yetgin, A.; Benek, A.; Bozyel, M.E.; Murat Altuner, E. In Vitro Antimicrobial Activity Screening of Ethanol Extract of *Lavandula stoechas* and Investigation of Its Biochemical Composition. *Adv. Pharmacol. Sci.* **2019**, *2019*, 3201458. [CrossRef]
172. Aouf, A.; Bouaouina, S.; Abdelgawad, M.A.; Abourehab, M.A.S.; Farouk, A. In Silico Study for Algerian Essential Oils as Antimicrobial Agents against Multidrug-Resistant Bacteria Isolated from Pus Samples. *Antibiotics* **2022**, *11*, 1317. [CrossRef]
173. Ghavam, M. In Vitro Biological Potential of the Essential Oil of Some Aromatic Species Used in Iranian Traditional Medicine. *Inflammopharmacology* **2022**, *30*, 855–874. [CrossRef]
174. Ivarsen, E.; Fretté, X.C.; Christensen, K.B.; Christensen, L.P.; Engberg, R.M.; Grevsen, K.; Kjaer, A. Bioassay-Guided Chromatographic Isolation and Identification of Antibacterial Compounds from *Artemisia annua* L. That Inhibit Clostridium Perfringens Growth. *J. AOAC Int.* **2014**, *97*, 1282–1290. [CrossRef]
175. Al-Askar, A.A.; Rashad, Y.M.; Abdulkhair, W.M. Evaluation of the Antimicrobial Potential of Selected Medicinal Plant Extracts against Some Plant and Human Pathogens. *J. Pure Appl. Microbiol.* **2014**, *8*, 159–168.
176. Oukil, N.; Hamri, S.; Bedjou, F. Antimicrobial Effects of Combinations between Essential Oils, Antibiotics, and Major Components of Essential Oils. *Phytothérapie* **2023**, *21*, 10–18. [CrossRef]
177. Costa, J.; Sousa, S.; Galvão, A.; Mata, J.; Leitão, J.; Carvalho, M. Key Parameters on the Antibacterial Activity of Silver Camphor Complexes. *Antibiotics* **2021**, *10*, 135. [CrossRef]
178. Peraman, R.; Tiwari, A.K.; Geetha Vani, M.; Hemanth, J.; Geetha Sree, Y.; Karthik, K.; Ashby, C.R.; Padmanabha Reddy, Y.; Pemmidi, R.V. New Camphor Hybrids: Lipophilic Enhancement Improves Antimicrobial Efficacy against Drug-Resistant Pathogenic Microbes and Intestinal Worms. *Med. Chem. Res.* **2018**, *27*, 1728–1739. [CrossRef]
179. Cardoso, J.M.S.; Galvão, A.M.; Guerreiro, S.I.; Leitão, J.H.; Suarez, A.C.; Carvalho, M.F.N.N. Antibacterial Activity of Silver Camphorimine Coordination Polymers. *Dalton Trans.* **2016**, *45*, 7114–7123. [CrossRef]
180. Laczkowski, K.; Misiura, K.; Biernasiuk, A.; Malm, A.; Siwek, A.; Plech, T.; Ciok-Pater, E.; Skowron, K.; Gospodarek, E. Synthesis, In Vitro Biological Screening and Molecular Docking Studies of Novel Camphor-Based Thiazoles. *Med. Chem.* **2014**, *10*, 600–608. [CrossRef]
181. Jitrangsri, K.; Lertsuphotvanit, N.; Kabthong, N.; Phaechamud, T. Metronidazole-Loaded Camphor-Based In Situ Forming Matrix for Periodontitis Treatment. *AAPS PharmSciTech* **2023**, *24*, 185. [CrossRef]

182. Rani, P.; Kumari, C.; Kumar, K.D.; Kumar, R. Effect of Camphor Incorporation on the Material and Antibacterial Properties of Soy Protein Isolate Films. *J. Res. Updates Polym. Sci.* **2023**, *12*, 162–170. [CrossRef]
183. Santos, T.B.; Vieira, A.A.; Paula, L.O.; Santos, E.D.; Radi, P.A.; Khouri, S.; Maciel, H.S.; Pessoa, R.S.; Vieira, L. Flexible Camphor Diamond-like Carbon Coating on Polyurethane to Prevent Candida Albicans Biofilm Growth. *J. Mech. Behav. Biomed. Mater.* **2017**, *68*, 239–246. [CrossRef]

MDPI AG
Grosspeteranlage 5
4052 Basel
Switzerland
Tel.: +41 61 683 77 34

Pharmaceuticals Editorial Office
E-mail: pharmaceuticals@mdpi.com
www.mdpi.com/journal/pharmaceuticals

www.ingramcontent.com/pod-product-compliance
Lightning Source LLC
Chambersburg PA
CBHW040833250926
51850CB00007BA/1301
* 9 7 8 3 7 2 5 8 6 0 8 3 8 *